mostly plant-based

100 DELICIOUS **PLANT-FORWARD** RECIPES
USING **10 INGREDIENTS** OR LESS

MIA SYN, MS, RDN

VICTORY BELT PUBLISHING INC.
Las Vegas

First published in 2023 by Victory Belt Publishing Inc.

ISBN-13: 978-1-628604-84-9

The information included in this book is for educational purposes only. It is not intended or implied to be a substitute for professional medical advice. The reader should always consult their healthcare provider to determine the appropriateness of the information for their own situation or if they have any questions regarding a medical condition or treatment plan. Reading the information in this book does not constitute a physician-patient relationship.

Cover design by Kat Lannom and Justin-Aaron Velasco

Interior design and illustrations by Yordan Terziev and Boryana Yordanova

Printed in Canada

TC 0122

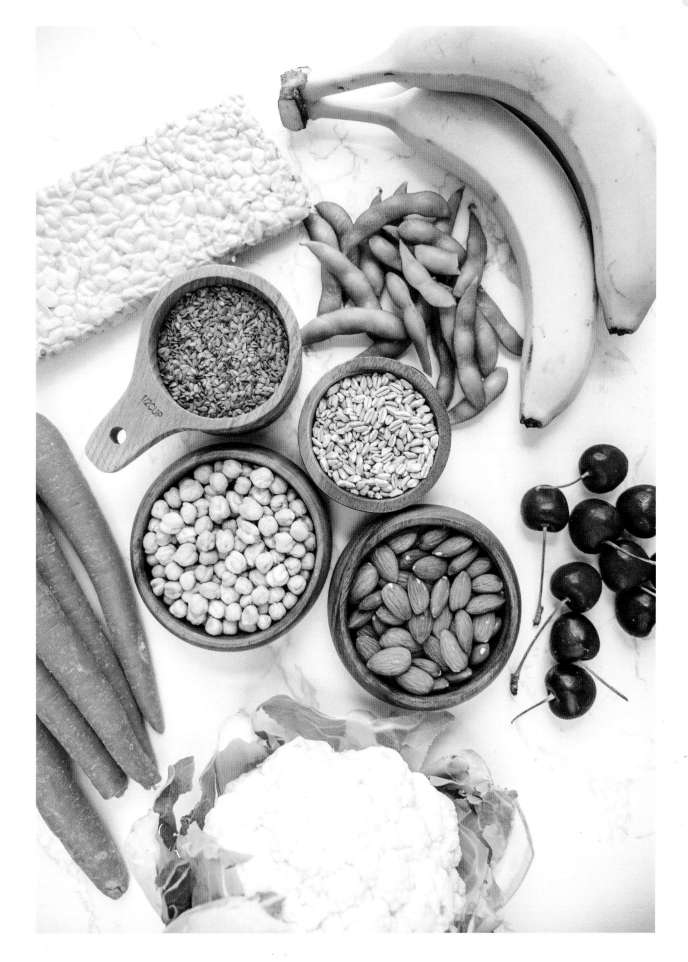

table of contents

introduction

Hi! I am thrilled that you've picked up *Mostly Plant-Based*. Before we dive in, allow me to introduce myself. My name is Mia Syn. I am a registered dietitian nutritionist with a master's degree in human nutrition from Columbia University, a national on-air nutrition expert, and a veggie lover (but I wasn't always that way).

I am so excited to be able to share with you my sustainable approach to nutrition rooted in science. It is intended to set you up for a lifetime of food freedom and give you the tools you need to make informed food choices and love what you eat, all while supporting energy, digestion, health, longevity, and so much more.

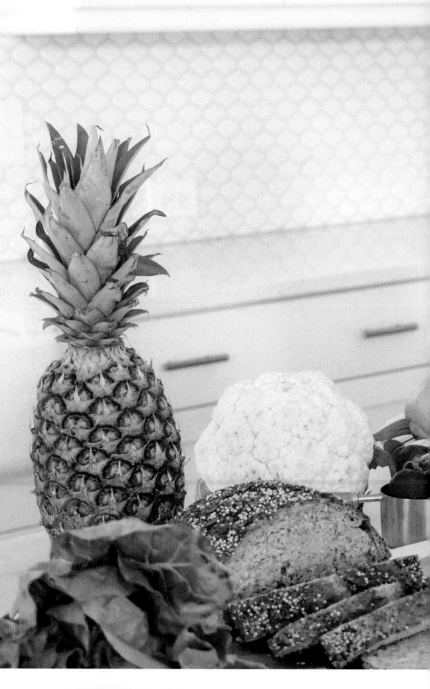

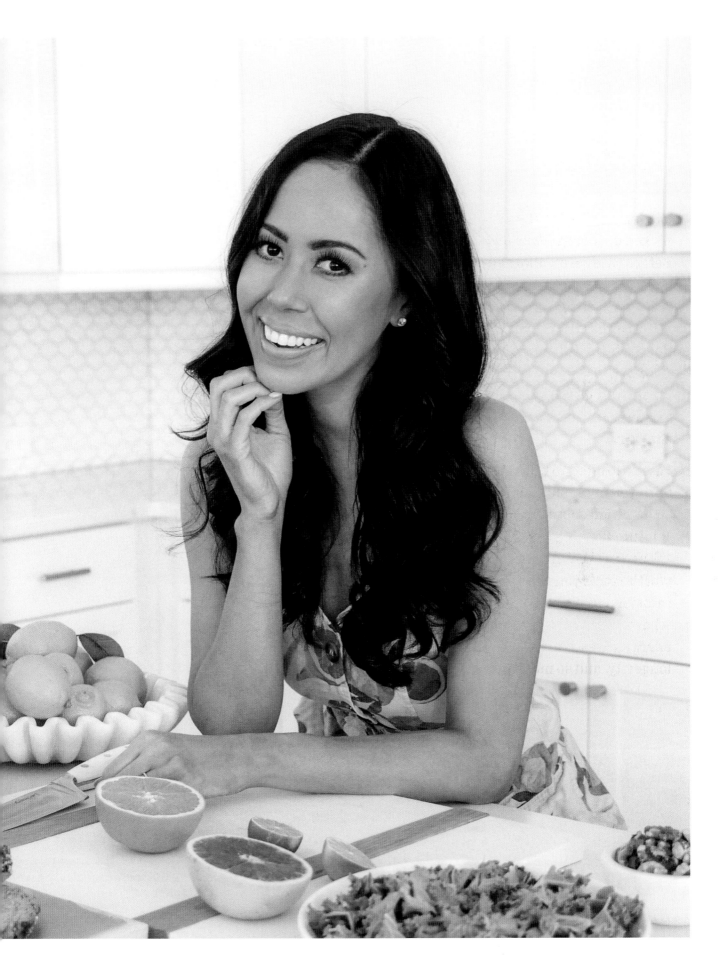

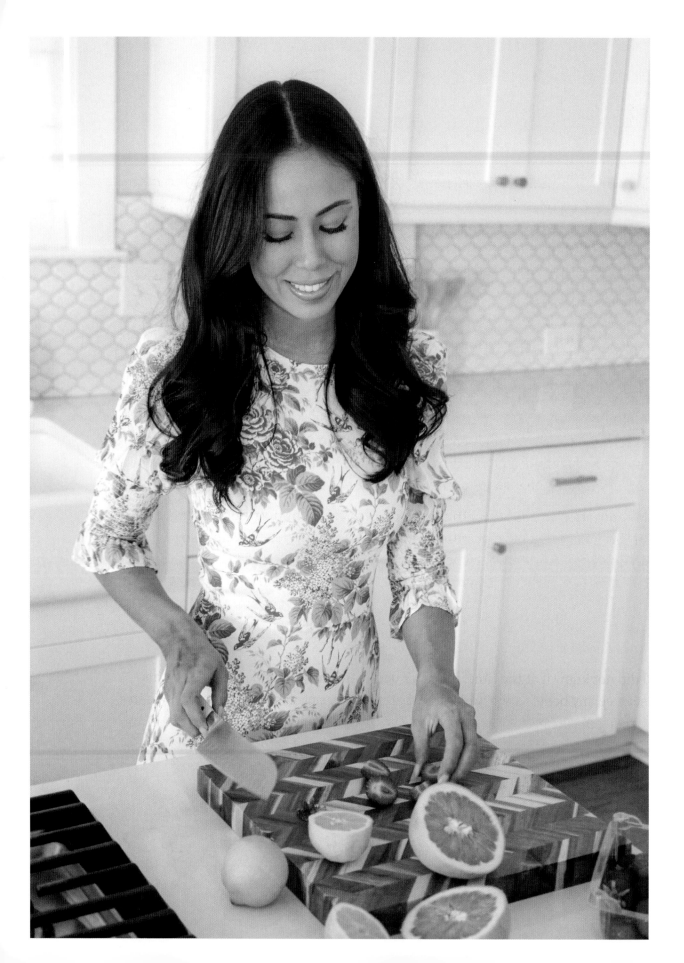

my story

My passion for nutritional science started in college at the University of California, Berkeley. I had somehow made it to the number one public university in the country fueled almost exclusively by processed refined carbohydrates—boxed breakfast cereal, sugary granola bars from the vending machine, and banana bread were my dietary staples by choice (I still love banana bread).

Despite growing up in a healthy household with two doctors for parents who always offered a vegetable with dinner, food to me was an afterthought. It never occurred to me that what I consumed daily was affecting my energy levels, my productivity, and even things like my hair, skin, and the way clothes fit.

It took a food journalism class with renowned author Michael Pollan to open my eyes to the world of food and nutrition. I couldn't believe that something each and every one of us does daily—eating—could be so intimately tied not only to our energy and body weight, but also to our overall health status, mood and memory, digestion, sleep quality, immunity, longevity, and so much more.

My education and career path since have been fueled by nutrition. After getting my bachelor's degree in nutritional sciences, physiology and metabolism, I completed my master of science in human nutrition at Columbia University's Institute of Human Nutrition at the College of Physicians and Surgeons, and I became a registered dietitian after completing the ten-month clinical internship at the Medical University of South Carolina and passing the national Commission on Dietetic Registration (CDR) exam.

I did not know it at the time, but after dedicating my professional years to this science, my beliefs align well with what my college professor so famously said in his *New York Times* bestselling book *The Omnivore's Dilemma:* "Eat food. Not too much. Mostly plants."

about this book

Mostly Plant-Based teaches you the science behind the food you eat and explains why eating plant-forward, while not entirely excluding animal-based foods, is the key to optimal health. In other words, it puts the focus on whole-food ingredients and rearranges the food pyramid that is etched in our brains—with plant foods at the base and animal products at the top.

This book helps you effortlessly transition to a plant-forward way of eating. You will find 100 *mostly* plant-based recipes designed for real life, each of which uses ten or fewer easy-to-source ingredients (not including basics like tap water, salt, pepper, and cooking spray) and requires only basic kitchen tools and appliances. This book is for those of you who don't want to (or don't have the time to) spend hours in the kitchen each week—but still want to eat in a way that makes you feel good and supports your health. Who doesn't want that? I wrote this book because I wholeheartedly believe plant-forward is the most realistic and sustainable way to eat for

- Health and longevity
- Energy
- Weight loss and maintenance
- Proper digestion and gut health
- Hair, skin, and nail health
- Having a healthy relationship with food and putting a stop to dieting

In the chapters to come, you will find

- The science behind what makes plant-based foods optimal for health…and why animal products shouldn't be discounted, and in fact play a small but essential role in supporting health because of their nutrient density and nutrient bioavailability.

- Sidebars that debunk common nutrition myths. I cover it all—including gluten, antinutrients, dairy, and more—using sound science.

- Simple plant-based swaps to boost nutrition without compromising taste. Like, did you ever think to add a serving of riced cauliflower to a smoothie? It bumps up the fiber and nutrient content while adding a thick and smooth creamy texture. Win-win!

- A 21-day meal plan with shopping lists to jump-start your veggie-loving journey, with three tiers to accommodate you wherever you are—whether you currently subsist on meat and potatoes or processed foods, or you are already starting to embrace the power of plants.

- A guide to stocking a plant-forward kitchen, including how to shop for the best ingredients and most helpful kitchen tools.

- Comfort food recipes with a veggie-forward twist, like lasagna made with zucchini noodles, pizza made with a cauliflower crust, and brownies made with sweet potatoes, to help turn even the pickiest eaters into veggie lovers.

- Recipes that include up to 12 customizable preparations, such as All-Day Energy Smoothie 6 Ways (page 146), Salad Jar 6 Ways (page 176), Sheet Pan Meal 6 Ways (page 246), and Adult Lunch Box 6 Ways (page 288).

- Options to customize most of the recipes to include or exclude meat, seafood, eggs, or dairy according to your preferences.

- Useful icons to identify quick recipes, recipes that require only one bowl/pot/pan/etc., and no-cook recipes (see below).

- Estimated nutrition facts for each recipe that include calories, carbohydrates, protein, and fat per serving, excluding optional ingredients listed (see page 352).

- A handy allergen chart to identify recipes free of meat, fish and shellfish, dairy, eggs, peanuts and tree nuts, gluten, soy, and sesame (see page 355).

Recipe can be prepared in 30 minutes or less.

Recipe requires only one pot/pan/baking dish/etc.

Recipe requires no cooking.

As with every three-minute TV segment I host, article I write, and recipe I create and share, my objectives for this book are the same: to make evidence-based nutrition information easy to understand and immediately implement into your life.

With that, I give you *Mostly Plant-Based*. Let's embrace the power of plant foods together.

why plants (and meat, too)?

defining
mostly plant-based

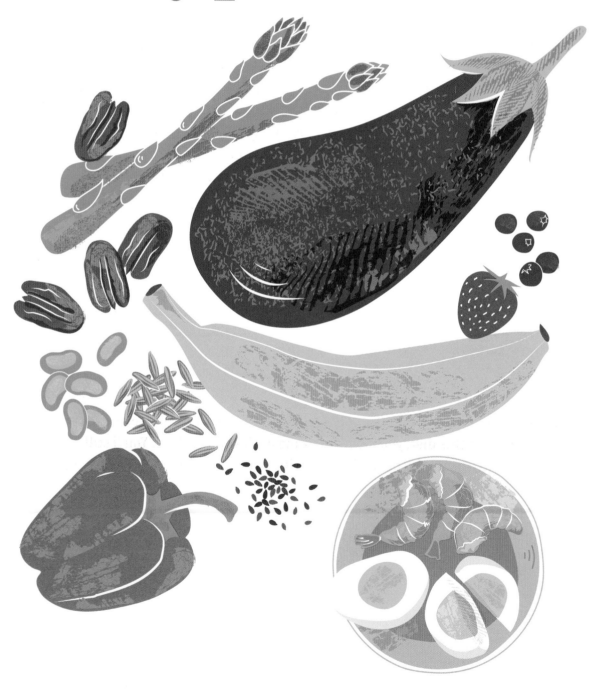

The prevalence of the term "plant-based" has skyrocketed in internet searches over the last five years, but there is a lot of confusion about what it really means. One article may describe it as a diet with a main objective of eliminating all animal products—dairy, eggs, and meat—whereas another article may describe it as a diet focused solely on plant-derived ingredients without regard to food quality (allowing for processed "plant-based" products such as alternative meats and snacks), and yet another may describe it as a diet that has a plant focus but also incorporates animal products in moderation. The truth is that there's no standard definition established by the FDA, so all these definitions could be correct.

People are drawn to plant-based diets for a variety of reasons, including health, weight loss, environmental concerns, and a desire to follow a celebrity-endorsed trend. I created the mostly plant-based diet because I've found it to be the best, most realistic approach to eating for energy, vibrancy, longevity, and so much more. As an added bonus, it's beneficial for the environment. My findings are supported by my time working one-on-one with clients in my private practice as a registered dietitian; my studies at Columbia University and the University of California, Berkeley; and my efforts to keep my finger on the pulse of where nutritional research is heading.

In this book, "plant-based" means a diet consisting primarily of plant-derived whole foods—focusing on nonstarchy vegetables—but not excluding animal products or discounting their important role in the healthiest way of eating. My definition of plant-based is not vegan or vegetarian, and it's not reliant on processed animal-free foods. Instead, it's focused on whole-food ingredients primarily consisting of plants.

The best part of eating mostly plant-based is that it not only supports you on a cellular level, but it's an exciting and fresh way to eat. You'll never get bored after you discover the power of plants. On this diet, you won't be eating boring desk salads. You'll still enjoy burgers, nachos, pizza, and brownies—all with a plant-powered twist, of course. I'll show you how plants can enhance overall nutrition without ever compromising taste.

how your health will improve

The greatest benefit that you will experience when following a mostly plant-based diet is that your health will undoubtedly improve. When you incorporate mostly plant-based whole foods into your diet, you naturally get more of the "good stuff" that supports overall health—namely fiber, essential vitamins and minerals, and phytonutrients—and less of the "bad stuff" that's linked to elevated chronic disease risk—namely saturated fat, trans fat, sodium, and added sugar.

Let's talk fiber. Fiber is one of the most underconsumed nutrients in the US, but it's arguably one of the most important. The recommended average daily intake for dietary fiber is 22 to 28 grams for adult women and 28 to 34 grams for adult men. These recommendations are based on levels observed to reduce the risk of coronary heart disease. The 2020–2025 USDA Dietary Guidelines for Americans estimate that a shocking 97 percent of men and 90 percent of women do not meet their recommended intakes for dietary fiber.[1] Fortunately, fiber is synonymous with plant foods. In fact, plant foods are the only natural sources of fiber, so when you adopt a mostly plant-based diet, you get plenty of fiber.

Fiber is a type of carbohydrate that your body can't break down for energy, so it passes through your body undigested. That quality makes fiber important for helping food move through the digestive system, and it promotes regularity and prevents constipation. It also may help lower blood cholesterol and thus supports heart health.

If you're looking to lose or help manage your weight, fiber is one of the key ingredients to success. It's one of the reasons my clients lose weight without counting calories. A study published in the *Annals of Internal Medicine* found that dieters who incorporated at least 30 grams of fiber per day without making any other dietary changes lost a significant amount of weight.[2] Fiber adds volume to meals and is the reason 3 cups of spinach (which is high in fiber) has only 21 calories, but 1 tablespoon of oil (which contains no fiber) has 120 calories. Fiber helps you feel full without adding calories, and it's the reason plant-based meals can be generously portioned.

Oh, and have I mentioned gut health? One particular type of fiber called prebiotics plays a powerful role in the health of your gut. Because fiber is indigestible, it moves to the colon to help selectively nourish the good bacteria and build a healthy microbiome. Gut

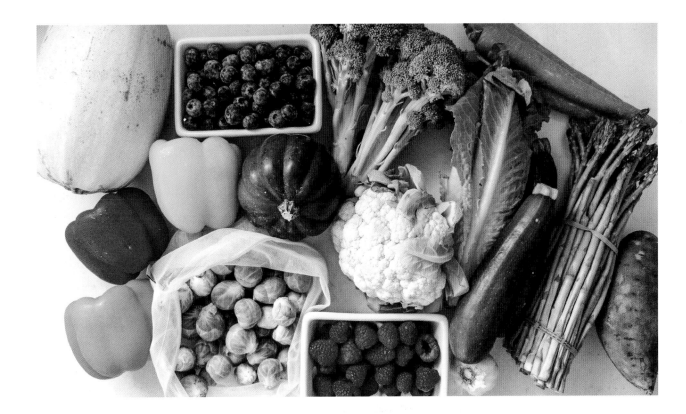

health is one of the hottest areas of research right now. A healthy gut has been linked to improved immune health, digestion, skin health, energy levels, and so much more.

Plant foods are nutrient-dense, meaning they provide a high level of vitamins and minerals relative to their calories. For example, one cup of kale offers 684 percent of the daily value (DV) of vitamin K, 206 percent DV of vitamin A, and 134 percent DV of vitamin C. Plant foods also offer beneficial plant compounds called phytonutrients, such as carotenoids, flavonoids, and polyphenols, to name a few, which research suggests benefit the body in hundreds of ways, from supporting immunity to slowing down aging to warding off chronic disease. It gives "food as medicine" a whole new meaning.

Of course, you'll be consuming *mostly* plant foods, and non-plant foods contribute good stuff, too. When you focus on high-quality animal products—meat, fish, poultry, eggs, and even dairy—you reap incredibly valuable bioavailable nutrients like DHA omega-3 fat and vitamin B12 that your body can readily absorb, utilize, and thrive on. Unfortunately, you can't get many of these nutrients from plants, and that's why I believe so strongly in a mostly plant-based diet that mindfully incorporates high-quality animal products in moderation for optimal health and well-being. I explain in Chapter 3 the importance of small amounts of quality animal products and how to treat them like "condiments" rather than the stars of your meals.

how mostly plant-based eating will change your life

The mostly plant-based way of eating is not a quick fix or a short-term approach to weight loss. It is a lifestyle. It is meant to provide you with tools to reframe the way you look at and prepare your food, with trickle-down effects that will transform the way you feel, look, think, and live. I can tell you ten ways (although there are probably many more) in which mostly plant-based eating will change your life.

You'll stop thinking about food all the time.

On a mostly plant-based diet, you consume foods that make you feel fuller longer and stabilize your blood sugar for steady energy. With this way of eating, you'll stop thinking about food all the time, release any guilt or anxiety you have about food, and free up energy and brainpower for living life instead of dieting. You'll stop counting calories, release the restrictive deprivation mindset associated with diets and weight loss, and gain a confident, relaxed approach to food and nutrition.

You'll lose weight (if that's your goal) and maintain a healthy weight.

We know that being overweight can increase the risk for heart disease, type 2 diabetes, and cancer. When you focus on mostly plant-based whole foods, you consume plenty of fiber, which increases satiety and means you'll eat less overall without trying. A mostly plant-based diet will help you lose unwanted pounds and reach your optimal weight.

You'll have more energy.

A mostly plant-based whole-food diet fuels your body with the bioavailable nutrition that it needs to thrive. Your body can efficiently break down whole foods, absorb the nutrition they provide, and utilize those nutrients. Everything starts working optimally. One of the first places you will notice a difference is in your energy levels.

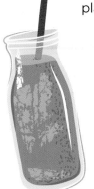
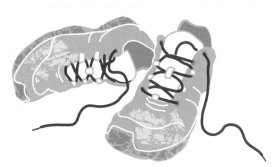

Your digestion and gut health will improve.

A diet focused on mostly plant-based whole foods like fruits, vegetables, legumes, whole grains, nuts, and seeds is naturally rich in fiber and supports digestion and gut health. You get three types of fiber on a mostly plant-based diet:

- **Soluble fiber** attracts water and turns to a gel to slow digestion, stabilize blood sugar for steady energy, and help you feel satiated longer. Soluble fiber may also help lower total blood cholesterol levels and thus support heart health.

- **Insoluble fiber** is responsible for adding bulk to stool. It helps food pass more quickly through the digestive tract and regulates bowel movements.

- **Resistant starch (prebiotics)** is an indigestible type of fiber that acts as food for selectively nourishing the good bacteria in the gut. As a result, both the diversity and number of good bacteria increase, which are two markers of a healthy gut.

Your blood pressure, cholesterol, and blood sugar will improve.

High blood pressure can increase the risk for myriad health issues, including heart disease, stroke, and type 2 diabetes. Although high blood pressure has a genetic component, it is also significantly affected by what you eat, with sodium being the main culprit.

The USDA Dietary Guidelines for Americans recommend keeping sodium intake to no more than 2,300 milligrams per day (about 1 teaspoon of salt), and the American Heart Association (AHA) recommends a daily limit of 1,500 milligrams for improved blood pressure and heart health.

Sodium is tricky because salty-tasting foods are not the only place it's found. In fact, it often goes undetected. The truth is that all foods contain sodium (yes, even vegetables). The foods lowest in sodium are those in their natural whole state, and the foods highest in sodium are those prepared outside the home—restaurant meals, fast food, processed foods, and frozen foods. Because sodium is found in all foods (naturally or added) and the daily limit is equivalent to 1 teaspoon of salt, following a mostly plant-based whole-food diet is the best way to stay below the recommended limit.

Your cholesterol levels will improve too. Nearly all plant foods (with a few unique exceptions, like coconut and palm oil) are free of saturated fat, which is directly linked to elevated cholesterol levels. High cholesterol can lead to fatty deposits in the blood that restrict blood flow and can eventually cause heart attack, stroke, or heart disease. Limiting saturated fat consumption can have a significant impact on cholesterol levels.

Additionally, your blood sugars will improve, and you'll reduce your risk of type 2 diabetes. Replacing processed foods and refined carbohydrates with plant-based whole foods and high-quality animal products can significantly reduce your risk of type 2 diabetes.

Your taste buds will be rewired.

Food addiction is a real thing. Scientists have looked at the brains of individuals following the consumption of hyperpalatable foods (those high in sugar, fat, and salt) and found that brain activity is comparable to what's seen in a person who's taken addictive drugs. So, there's a scientific explanation for why eating junk food can be a hard habit to kick!

When you follow a mostly plant-based whole-food diet, your taste buds will be rewired. A study published in the journal *Chemical Senses* found that repeated exposure to nutritious, less hyperpalatable foods like broccoli and leafy greens can change proteins in saliva to calm the initial distaste for bitter and other flavors.[3] Within weeks of starting a mostly plant-based diet, your taste buds will change, and you'll begin to lose interest in the nutrient-void foods you once desired and couldn't imagine life without.

Your skin will glow.

Science is continually unearthing the link between what we eat and the appearance of our skin, and one of the key contributors to dull, lifeless skin is an inflammatory diet that incorporates large amounts of fried food, sugar-sweetened beverages, refined carbohydrates, and processed meat. Conversely, plant-based whole foods are among those that may help prevent, and even reverse, the aging of skin.

Whole plant foods like vegetables, fruits, nuts, and seeds naturally contain polyphenols and antioxidants and have a direct impact on lowering inflammation in the body and, therefore, the skin.

You'll get sick less often and live longer.

Plant foods like bell peppers and almonds are rich in nutrients like vitamin C and vitamin E that play a role in supporting immune function. Furthermore, when you choose high-quality animal products like low-mercury seafood, pasture-raised eggs, and grass-fed beef, you get additional immune-supporting nutrients like bioavailable zinc and vitamin D. In Chapter 3, I explain how to choose high-quality animal products and the best ways to enjoy them.

Additionally, research shows that a diet rich in plant foods and low in sugar, salt, and processed meat may promote healthy cellular aging and reduce cardiovascular risk and overall mortality risk.[4]

You'll save money.

When clients begin working with me, they often have the misconception that following a healthy diet means a higher price tag. When you do things right, this is not true. Purchasing mostly plant-based whole-food ingredients like produce, grains, legumes, nuts, and seeds while limiting animal products and eliminating processed foods is bound to save you money month after month. In Chapter 4, I teach you how to shop smart for a mostly plant-based diet.

Additionally, because you get sick less often when you follow a mostly plant-based diet and you're warding off chronic disease, your healthcare costs will ultimately be lower.

You'll lower your carbon footprint.

For bonus points, a mostly plant-based diet is good for the planet. Plant foods have a lesser environmental impact than animal foods in all areas—land use, water supply, and greenhouse gas emissions.

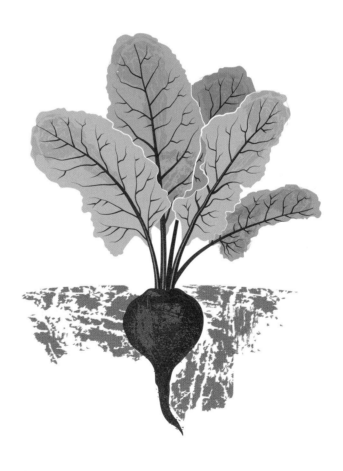

why all or nothing doesn't work

As a registered dietitian, I have to preface conversations with my clients, readers, and even everyday people I encounter that I am *not* the food police. And being a dietitian does not mean I always follow a "perfect" diet—after all, I'm human just like you. Yes, I am devoted to following a mostly plant-based diet every day to feel my best and optimize my health, but I also want to enjoy a mimosa at brunch with girlfriends on a Sunday or grab a chocolate chip walnut cookie from Levain Bakery when I'm in New York. The reality is that we don't live in a utopia that caters to eating "perfectly." A mostly plant-based lifestyle is designed to work in the real world.

Working with hundreds of clients has shown me that "all or nothing" does not work when it comes to diet. In fact, all-or-nothing eating can create an unhealthy relationship with food that can have long-term implications. This is what led me to design the mostly plant-based diet, which allows you to eat in a realistic way that preserves and promotes health and makes maintaining a healthy weight effortless.

I advocate for and live the "mostly" lifestyle. That means mostly healthy eating, whatever that looks like for you—six out of seven days of the week, or two out of three meals. We all start somewhere, and I am here to meet you where you are and to make the overall picture of eating one that supports you physically, energetically, and emotionally without denying you the joy that food brings. So, use this book as a guideline to a lifestyle of mostly plant-based eating. This isn't a one-week or one-month diet; it is meant to help guide your food choices for the rest of your life so that you can be your most vibrant self.

what a mostly plant-based plate looks like

It's time to revamp the food pyramid that you grew up with! Get ready to retrain your brain for the new pyramid and redesign your plate for a mostly plant-based diet.

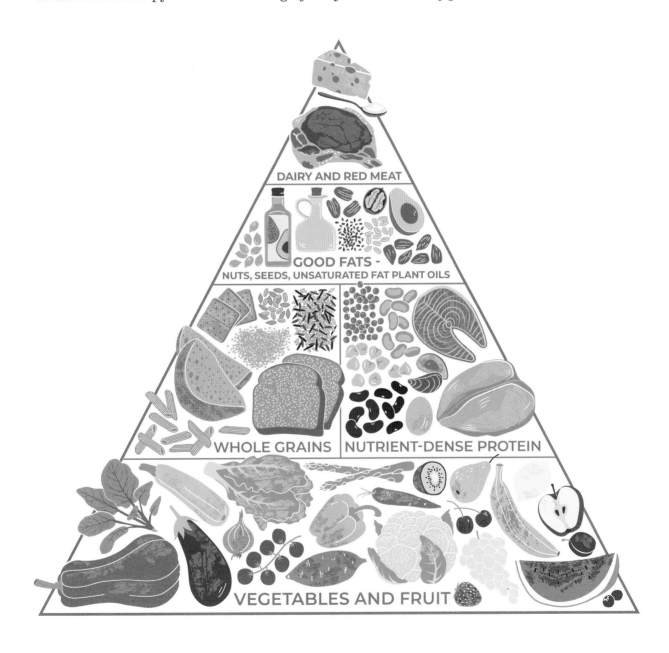

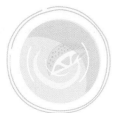

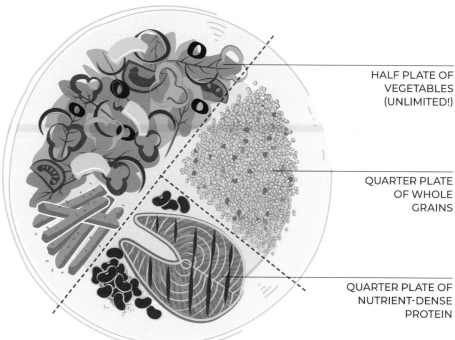

HALF PLATE OF
VEGETABLES
(UNLIMITED!)

QUARTER PLATE
OF WHOLE
GRAINS

QUARTER PLATE OF
NUTRIENT-DENSE
PROTEIN

ON THE SIDE:
fruit, good fats, dairy
and dairy substitutes

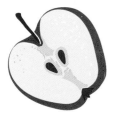

half plate of vegetables (unlimited!)

Half of your plate should be filled with veggies. The USDA recommends 2 to 3 cups of veggies per day, but on a mostly plant-based diet, you get unlimited veggies. Most of us simply do not eat enough vegetables. The 2020–2025 Dietary Guidelines for Americans reports that more than 85 percent of adults underconsume fruit, vegetables, and whole grains.[5]

Additionally, the veggies that Americans consume the most are among the least nutrient-dense: potatoes in the form of french fries and chips, tomatoes in the form of pizza sauce, iceberg lettuce, and corn.

To give your body the optimal nutrition it needs, eat a rainbow of produce. Colors are indicative of each food's unique phytochemicals, which offer different benefits—support for the immune system, the digestive system, circulation, and anti-aging, to name a few. Focus primarily on nonstarchy veggies, although you can sprinkle in starchy veggies like sweet potatoes and winter squash when desired.

MYTH BUSTING BOX

WHAT'S THE DEAL WITH STARCHY VEGGIES?

Starchy veggies provide an impressive amount of fiber, vitamins, minerals, and antioxidants (just like their nonstarchy counterparts do), but they're higher in carbohydrates with a higher glycemic index, meaning they raise blood sugar more quickly during digestion. That being said, you will never see me comparing a potato to a candy bar. Any veggies in your diet are good in my eyes. If you're starting with starchy veggies, slowly transition to more nonstarchy veggies, which give you more nutrition for your calorie buck.

quarter plate of whole grains

Whole grains are found in more foods than brown rice. They're also in whole-grain pastas; ancient grains like farro, quinoa, and teff; and sprouted whole-grain breads and tortillas. Whole grains are a good source of fiber, essential vitamins and minerals, and phytonutrients.

MYTH BUSTING BOX

WHAT ABOUT GLUTEN?

Gluten is a protein found in wheat, barley, and rye. A gluten-free diet has become trendy over the years. People with celiac disease, which is an autoimmune disease that affects about 1 percent of the population, and non-celiac gluten sensitivity, which is estimated to affect about 6 percent of the population, need to eliminate gluten from their diets. Otherwise, there is not enough data to recommend the elimination of gluten from a healthy diet. That being said, there are plenty of naturally gluten-free grains to add to your meal rotation if you choose to do so.

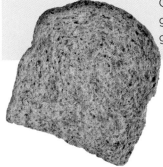 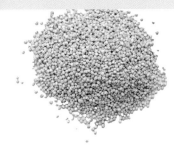 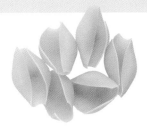

quarter plate of nutrient-dense protein

Protein is an essential part of the mostly plant-based plate. Not only is protein the most satiating of the three macronutrients, but it is the building block of every cell in your body. Here, you want to focus on plant-based sources of protein like beans and lentils along with high-quality animal-derived sources, such as low-mercury fish, grass-fed beef, and pasture-raised poultry and eggs.

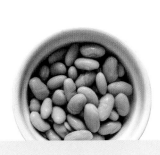 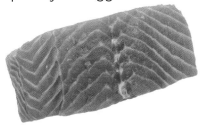

MYTH BUSTING BOX

ARE BEANS REALLY A GOOD SOURCE OF PROTEIN?

Beans and lentils are unique because they provide protein along with fiber and carbohydrates but zero fat. Animal proteins such as fish, beef, poultry, and eggs provide protein, fat, and zero carbohydrates. While beans and lentils may not be as rich in protein by weight, the truth is that you can easily meet your minimum protein need—which is only 0.8 gram per kilogram of body weight, or about 55 grams for a 150-pound person— by eating them. Note that your protein need increases as the amount of physical activity you do increases.

on the side

Although the following foods didn't make it onto the mostly plant-based plate, these "on the side" foods should not be overlooked. They still offer impressive nutrition to support overall health and well-being, but you just don't need them in significant quantities each day (with the exception of water!).

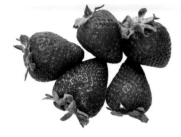

Fruit

Fruits and veggies are sister foods because they provide similar nutrition: fiber, vitamins, and minerals for few calories. The difference is that fruit is higher in naturally occurring sugar, which is why apples are sweeter than broccoli. Plus, fruits provide their own unique package of phytonutrients.

MYTH BUSTING BOX

SHOULD I WORRY ABOUT THE SUGAR IN FRUIT?

There is the added sugar you find in cakes and cookies, and then there is the naturally occurring sugar you find in fruit, dairy, and even vegetables. Added sugar is sugar in its isolated form that has been added to a food either for taste or as a preservative. Added sugar is essentially empty calories, which provide energy (carbohydrates) but no nutrition (vitamins and minerals). When it comes to fruit and dairy, both of which contain naturally occurring sugar, you are also getting a slew of essential nutrients like fiber, calcium, vitamin D, and protein. I tell my clients not to worry about the sugar in fruit because it is a nutrient-dense food.

Good fats

Fats are calorically dense, meaning a little goes a long way. For example, 1 tablespoon of oil provides around 120 calories. However, good fats are essential for overall well-being. Dietary fat helps your body absorb the fat-soluble vitamins A, D, E, and K.

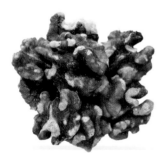

Good fat is found in oils such as avocado oil and olive oil. It's also available in whole foods like nuts, seeds, olives, and avocados. Stick to 1 tablespoon or less when portioning oil; a small handful of nuts, seeds, or olives; or one-third of a medium avocado.

MYTH BUSTING BOX

WHAT ABOUT ANTINUTRIENTS LIKE PHYTIC ACID?

Phytic acid, which is found in some nuts and seeds, can limit the absorption of certain vitamins and minerals. However, the amount is minimal and not enough to impact your overall nutritional status. Additionally, phytic acid can be significantly decreased by soaking raw nuts and seeds overnight before consuming them.

Dairy and dairy substitutes

Although dairy is not a mainstay of a mostly plant-based diet, it is not completely off-limits because it is a nutrient-dense food. When you're in the mood for some dairy, focus on kefir, unsweetened yogurt, and cheese. Kefir is fermented cow's milk and a good source of probiotics, which are beneficial bacteria that support gut health, digestion, and immunity. Flavored yogurts can pack as much sugar as a candy bar, so instead, opt for plain, unsweetened yogurt that you sweeten with fresh fruit at home. And many of us can't imagine life without cheese. If you're lactose intolerant, opt for hard cheeses like cheddar, Swiss, and Parmesan, which are naturally lower in lactose.

If you choose to ditch dairy completely, be mindful of dairy alternatives like almond milks and cashew yogurts, which can be highly processed with a laundry list of ingredients but a short list of nutrients. In Chapter 4, I teach you how to navigate dairy and dairy alternatives in the grocery store.

MYTH BUSTING BOX

IS DAIRY REALLY GOOD FOR US?

Dairy is a controversial part of a plant-based diet, but I think it gets a bad rap because it causes digestive discomfort for about 70 percent of people with reported sensitivities and intolerances. As we age, adults produce less lactase, the enzyme needed to break down lactose, the naturally occurring sugar in milk, which has deterred many health enthusiasts from including it in their diet. But the truth is that dairy foods are nutrient-dense, meaning they provide a high level of nutrition relative to their calories. For example, an 8-ounce glass of milk provides thirteen essential nutrients, including calcium, vitamin D, magnesium, and phosphorous.

Dairy-free substitutes are highly processed or do not come close to the nutritional profile of their dairy counterparts. A glass of cow's milk provides thirteen essential nutrients, only two of which are added (vitamins A and D), whereas a glass of almond "milk" made from ground almonds and water contains no significant naturally occurring nutrients. Instead, it's fortified with synthetic calcium and vitamins A, D, and E. So, overall, dairy is fine if you tolerate it; in fact, it has an impressive nutrition profile.

**IS WATER
REALLY THE
ONLY THING
I SHOULD BE
DRINKING?**

While plain ol' water is the smartest beverage option, there are plenty of other dietitian-approved beverages, such as herbal tea, sparkling water, homemade fruit and vegetable smoothies, and even fresh-squeezed 100 percent fruit juice in moderation (no added sugar). However, you should aim to get nearly all of your calories and nutrition from food rather than beverages, and stick to almost 100 percent water in your drinking glass.

water

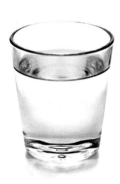

One of the first questions I ask my clients when assessing their diets is, "What are you drinking?" Sugar-sweetened beverages like soda, fruit juice, and alcohol are the number one contributors of empty calories, meaning they provide energy (carbohydrates) but no significant nutrition. Additionally, because they lack fiber, they are easy to overconsume because your brain does not signal that you are full or satiated. The US National Academies of Sciences, Engineering, and Medicine recommends an adequate intake of 2.7 to 3.7 liters of water per day, which can come from all fluids you drink as well as the food you eat (like a juicy piece of fruit, a salad, or even a bowl of yogurt). Staying sufficiently hydrated helps your body convert food to energy, deliver nutrients to your cells, and keep your organs functioning properly.

Now that you know what it means to eat mostly plant-based, it's time to unlock the power of plant foods.

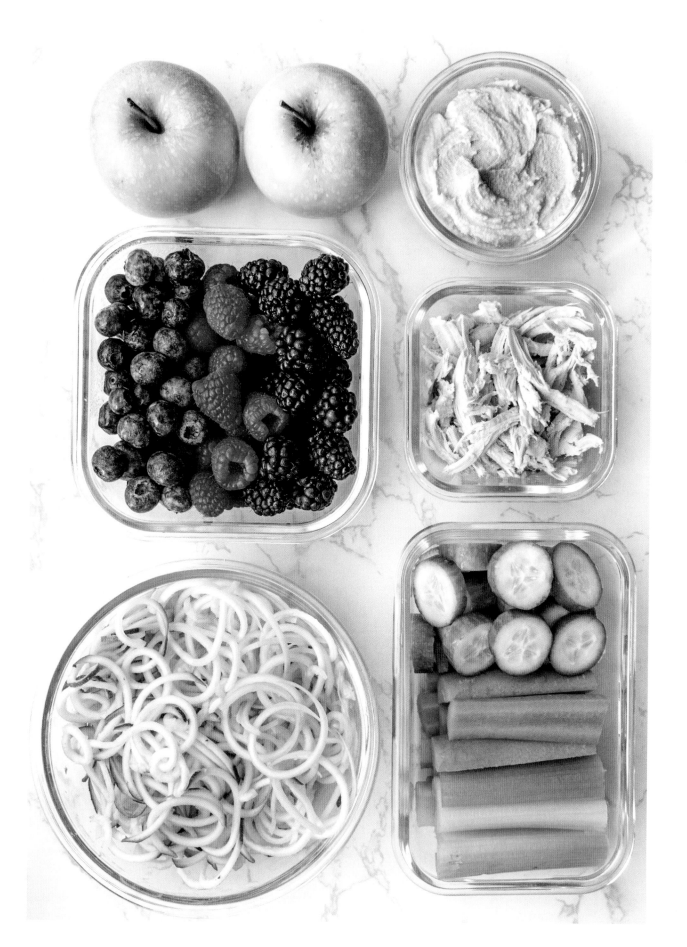

count colors, not calories

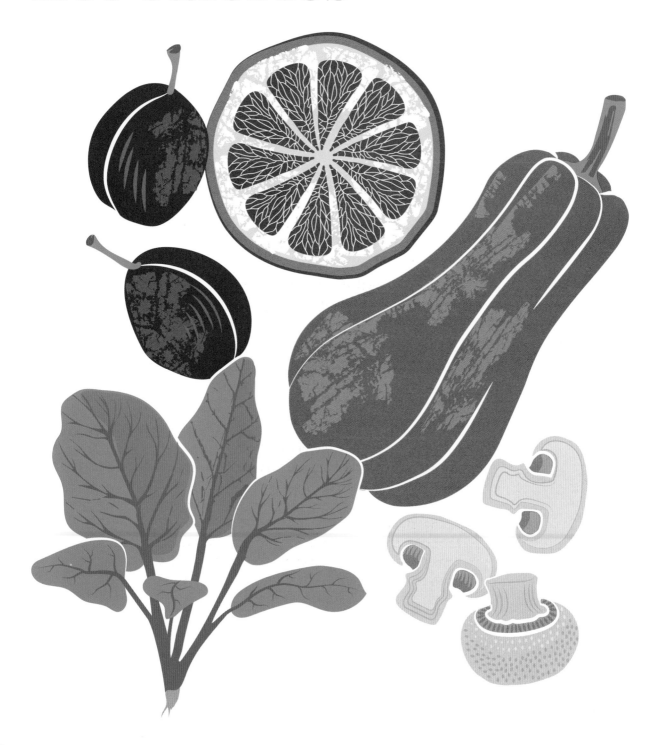

Food is more than just calories. Both plant and animal foods are made up of a complex system of carbohydrates, protein, fat, vitamins, minerals, fiber, prebiotics, probiotics, antioxidants, and phytonutrients, all of which dynamically influence your biology for better or worse with every bite you take. What you eat affects every aspect of your health—your muscles, bones, skin, energy levels, hormone balance, gut health, heart health, and more. Hippocrates was on to something when he said, "Let food be thy medicine," and in this chapter I am going to show you why he was right.

if food is medicine, then plants are the most powerful ones

The human body needs three essential categories of nutrients for survival, growth, disease prevention, and good health: macronutrients (fat, protein, and carbohydrates—including fiber), micronutrients (vitamins and minerals), and water.

Plant foods are nutrient-dense, meaning they provide a high level of nutrition relative to their calories. What they particularly have going for them is three main components: phytonutrients, micronutrients, and fiber.

phyto-nutrients

Phytonutrients, also known as phytochemicals, are not essential for survival, but they give you a major leg up in health. These nutrients are specific to plant foods such as vegetables, fruits, beans, and grains, with specific biological activities that support human health in myriad ways.[1] Proposed benefits include boosting immunity; warding off cancer; reducing inflammation; protecting against stroke, osteoporosis, and cardiovascular disease; and slowing the aging process. About 10,000 different phytonutrients have been identified, with experts estimating many left to be discovered.[2]

micro-nutrients

While macronutrients—carbohydrates, protein, and fat—make up the foundation of the human diet, micronutrients are where plant foods particularly shine. Micronutrients include vitamins and minerals that the body requires in smaller quantities to stay healthy and thrive. They play essential roles in a range of bodily functions, including energy production, immune function, the creation of neurotransmitters, and the protection of cells from potential free radical damage.

VITAMIN	ROLE IN THE BODY	PLANT-BASED FOOD SOURCES
Vitamin A (in the form of beta-carotene)*	Essential for vision, skin health, and immunity	Carrots, pumpkin, sweet potatoes, winter squash, spinach, mango
Vitamin B1 (thiamin)	Helps convert the food we eat into usable energy	Brown rice, soy milk, watermelon, acorn squash
Vitamin B2 (riboflavin)	Helps convert the food we eat into usable energy	Leafy green vegetables, whole and enriched grains and cereals
Vitamin B3 (niacin)	Helps convert the food we eat into usable energy	Whole grains, mushrooms, potatoes, peanut butter
Vitamin B5 (pantothenic acid)	Essential for building and breaking down fatty acids	Whole grains, broccoli, mushrooms, avocados, tomatoes
Vitamin B6 (pyridoxine)	Helps create red blood cells	Tofu and other soy products, potatoes, non-citrus fruits like bananas and watermelon
Vitamin B12 (cobalamin)*	Needed for red blood cell formation and proper nervous system and brain function	Fortified soy milk, fortified cereal, nutritional yeast
Biotin	Needed for healthy bones and hair	Whole grains
Vitamin B9 (folate)	Especially important for people who may become pregnant, as it helps prevent brain and spine defects in newborns; needed to make new cells daily	Fortified grains and cereals, asparagus, spinach, broccoli, legumes
Vitamin C (ascorbic acid)	Required for the production of collagen, the main protein in skin	Strawberries, oranges, bell peppers, kiwi
Vitamin D (calciferol)*	Essential for bone health and immunity	Fortified cereals (along with sunlight)
Vitamin E (alpha-tocopherol)	Acts as an antioxidant	Vegetable oil, nuts, seeds, whole grains, leafy green vegetables
Vitamin K* (phylloquinone)	Required for blood clotting, bone health, and heart health	Spinach, broccoli, sprouts, kale, other green vegetables

You'll notice that I have starred several vitamins and minerals in these charts, and for good reason. It is the basis of why I named this book *MOSTLY Plant-Based*. From a bioavailability standpoint, these starred nutrients are either simply *better* to get from animal foods, meaning our bodies can absorb and utilize them more easily and efficiently, are only or primarily found in animal foods naturally, or include forms that are only or primarily found in animal foods naturally. I go into depth about why that is in Chapter 3. But for now, let's continue to focus on the power of plants.

MINERAL	ROLE IN THE BODY	PLANT-BASED FOOD SOURCES
Calcium*	Builds and protects bones and teeth, assists in muscle function	Leafy green vegetables, tofu
Chloride	Helps maintain fluid balance and make digestive enzyme	Seaweed, salt, celery
Copper	Needed for normal brain and nervous system function	Whole grains, nuts, seeds, beans, prunes, cocoa powder, black pepper
Fluoride	Necessary for the development of bones and teeth	Water, tea
Iodine*	Part of the thyroid hormone, required during pregnancy for healthy fetal growth and cognitive development	Iodized salt
Iron*	Essential for carrying oxygen throughout the body	Fortified bread and grain products, green vegetables
Magnesium	Needed for over 300 chemical reactions in the body	Green vegetables, legumes, cashews, seeds, whole-grain bread
Manganese	Assists with carbohydrate, protein, and cholesterol metabolism	Nuts, legumes, whole grains, pineapple
Phosphorous	Part of bone and cell membrane structure	Green peas, broccoli, potatoes, almonds
Potassium	Helps with nerve transmission and muscle function	Fruit, vegetables, whole grains, legumes
Selenium	Important for thyroid health	Brazil nuts, whole grains
Sodium	Aids in fluid balance and blood pressure maintenance	Salt
Zinc*	Promotes immune function	Fortified cereals, beans, nuts

fiber & the gut microbiome

The third key thing that plants have going for them is fiber, which is found exclusively in plant foods. I touched on fiber in Chapter 1, but it's worth mentioning again—fiber is magical. For one, it fills you up for few calories without filling you out and is the key to weight loss and maintenance.

Fiber is also an essential ingredient in creating a healthy gut microbiome—the uniquely composed kingdom of trillions of microbes living within each of us that many experts suggest may just be the *most* important organ in the body.

The gut microbiome is composed of "good" microbes that support health and "bad" ones that can cause disease. Composition starts to take shape from the moment a baby passes through the mother's birth canal (and potentially in utero, studies are suggesting; babies born via Cesarean section may miss out on this benefit). As we grow, the gut microbiome begins to diversify and evolve. In fact, its composition is influenced by every bite of food we take.

Markers of gut health include microbe diversity and a proper balance of good to bad bacteria—the opposite of which is called gut dysbiosis. An unhealthy microbiome has been linked to digestive disorders such as irritable bowel syndrome and colitis, obesity, heart disease, diabetes, cancer, autoimmune disorders, dementia, allergies, asthma, skin disorders like eczema, and more.

Bad "bugs" grow in the gut for two reasons: not eating enough food that feed the good bacteria and eating too many gut-busting foods—namely sugar, processed foods, refined vegetable oils, and artificial sweeteners.

So, what fuels a balanced and diverse microbiome—markers of gut health? The answer is, for one, plants.

Good bacteria thrive on fiber, specifically a type called prebiotics, which are particularly prevalent in foods like apples, artichokes, asparagus, bananas, and oats.

Another way to support your gut health through plant foods is to consume foods that contain probiotics. Probiotics are beneficial bacteria found naturally in fermented foods such as sauerkraut, pickles, natto, and kimchi.

One study in particular resonates with me. Scientists mapped the gut microbial communities of herbivorous animals (plant eaters), carnivorous animals (meat eaters), and omnivorous animals (plant and meat eaters). The study determined not only the direct correlation between diet and gut microbiome composition but also the direct impact that plant foods have on gut microbiome diversity.[3]

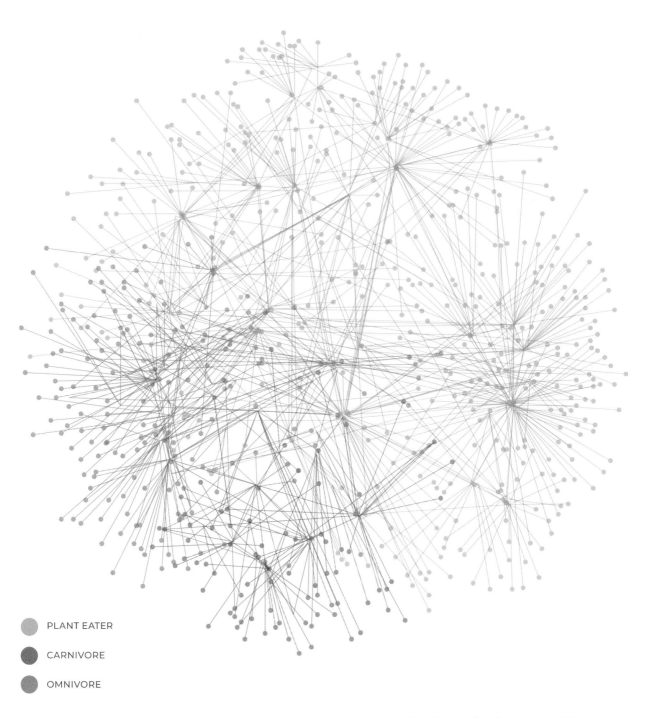

PLANT EATER

CARNIVORE

OMNIVORE

what plant foods don't have is just as important as what they do have

A healthy diet is just as much characterized by what it includes as what it doesn't include.

Low or zero saturated fat

Plant foods are low in or devoid of saturated fat, a type of dietary fat that should be limited for heart health to no more than 10 percent of total daily calories according to the Dietary Guidelines for Americans, or no more than 6 percent according to the American Heart Association. A few plant-based foods do contain saturated fat, including coconut and coconut oil, and I go into where they stand in Chapter 3.

Although decades of dietary recommendations have suggested that saturated fat is harmful, in recent years that notion has begun to evolve. New research is suggesting that dietary saturated fat may not increase the risk of cardiovascular disease or stroke as was once thought. However, until there is enough research to substantiate recommending changes to the dietary guidelines, the most elucidated link is that unsaturated fats like those found in plant foods remain the best for us.

No dietary cholesterol

Dietary cholesterol is found in animal foods, namely egg yolks, shrimp, beef, cheese, and butter, among others. Up until the 2015–2020 version, the Dietary Guidelines for Americans recommended restricting dietary cholesterol to 300 milligrams per day for heart health. However, that link may have been debunked recently; the current literature shows that dietary cholesterol itself isn't harmful and doesn't increase blood cholesterol levels.[4]

Today, there is no specific recommended limit for dietary cholesterol. But it is important to note that foods that are high in cholesterol also tend to be high in saturated fats—which, as mentioned above, should be monitored. Instead, the dietary guidelines recommend eating as little cholesterol as possible—something that is easy to do on a mostly plant-based diet.

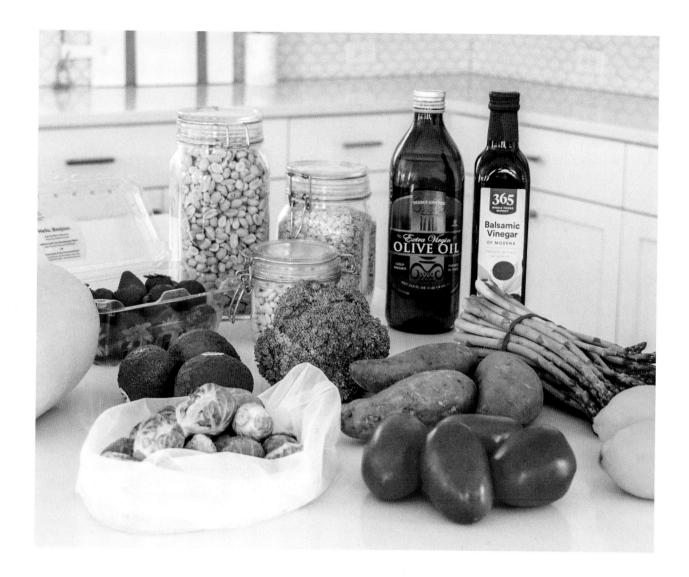

No added sugar

As with any whole-food ingredient, whole plant foods are free of added sugar. As touched upon in Chapter 1, added sugar should be treated differently than the natural sugars found in fruit and some vegetables because of the nutrition those foods provide. Foods that are high in added sugar include sugary beverages like soft drinks, sports drinks, and sugar-sweetened juice, desserts likes pies and cakes, and candy.

Very low sodium

As discussed in Chapter 1, all foods contain some sodium, a nutrient that should be monitored for health and is easily overconsumed, primarily from restaurant meals, fast food, processed foods, and frozen packaged foods. A benefit of whole plant-based foods is that they are among the lowest in sodium.

the foods that make up the mostly plant-based diet

It's time to dive into which foods make up the foundation of the mostly plant-based diet, what makes them nutritionally superior, and how to make them mainstays in your diet for life.

fruits & vegetables: reach for the rainbow

So, we know that fruits and veggies are good for you, but which ones are the best and why?

The USDA reports that the most commonly consumed vegetables are potatoes (often in the form of french fries and chips), tomatoes (often in the form of pizza sauce), onions, carrots, and head lettuce,[5] while apples, oranges, and bananas top the fruit chart.[6] Additionally, many of us stick to the same three or four fruits and vegetables in our shopping carts each week.

While any fruits and vegetables in your diet is better than none, on a mostly plant-based diet, you are encouraged to taste the rainbow—that is, to incorporate as many colored fruits and vegetables each week (and day) as possible. For example, start your day with a blueberry-strawberry smoothie (learn how to build a balanced smoothie on page 147), enjoy a packed salad with arugula, yellow bell peppers, and avocado at lunch, and eat a baked sweet potato with dinner. Let color be your guide.[7]

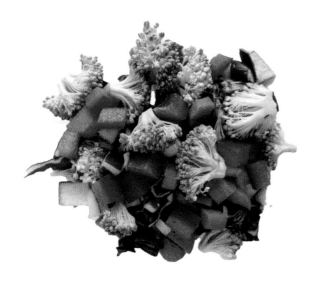

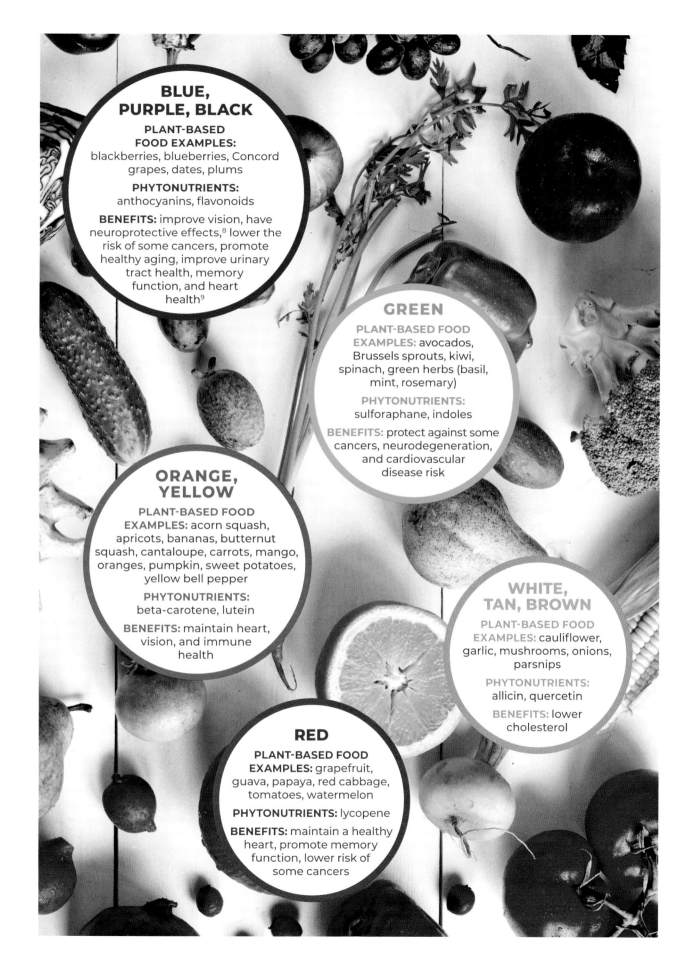

BLUE, PURPLE, BLACK

PLANT-BASED FOOD EXAMPLES: blackberries, blueberries, Concord grapes, dates, plums

PHYTONUTRIENTS: anthocyanins, flavonoids

BENEFITS: improve vision, have neuroprotective effects,[8] lower the risk of some cancers, promote healthy aging, improve urinary tract health, memory function, and heart health[9]

GREEN

PLANT-BASED FOOD EXAMPLES: avocados, Brussels sprouts, kiwi, spinach, green herbs (basil, mint, rosemary)

PHYTONUTRIENTS: sulforaphane, indoles

BENEFITS: protect against some cancers, neurodegeneration, and cardiovascular disease risk

ORANGE, YELLOW

PLANT-BASED FOOD EXAMPLES: acorn squash, apricots, bananas, butternut squash, cantaloupe, carrots, mango, oranges, pumpkin, sweet potatoes, yellow bell pepper

PHYTONUTRIENTS: beta-carotene, lutein

BENEFITS: maintain heart, vision, and immune health

WHITE, TAN, BROWN

PLANT-BASED FOOD EXAMPLES: cauliflower, garlic, mushrooms, onions, parsnips

PHYTONUTRIENTS: allicin, quercetin

BENEFITS: lower cholesterol

RED

PLANT-BASED FOOD EXAMPLES: grapefruit, guava, papaya, red cabbage, tomatoes, watermelon

PHYTONUTRIENTS: lycopene

BENEFITS: maintain a healthy heart, promote memory function, lower risk of some cancers

WAYS TO EAT MORE VEGETABLES

- Keep sliced raw veggies at eye level in the fridge for easy snacking.

- Keep bags of frozen vegetables on hand to easily incorporate into meals in a pinch.

- Roast a batch of veggies like broccoli, carrots, cauliflower, and Brussels sprouts each week to easily snack on and add to meals.

- Experiment with veggie noodles (see page 256) and veggie rice (see pages 192 and 240, for example).

- Tap into the magic of cauliflower in pizza crust (see page 254) and mashed "potatoes" (see page 310).

- Add chopped vegetables to omelets.

- Puree or finely chop spinach, carrots, onion, or bell peppers and add to sauces like All-Purpose No-Sugar Tomato Sauce (page 130).

- Blend mild-tasting vegetables like spinach and riced cauliflower into smoothies (see page 146).

- Combine ground meat with minced mushrooms (see page 132).

- Make veggie wraps with romaine or butter lettuce (see pages 190 and 266), veggie buns with portabella mushrooms (see page 252), and veggie toast with sweet potato slices (see page 152).

- Transform vegetables into oven-baked fries (see page 210) and air-fried chips.

- Incorporate veggies into baked goods like Zucchini Walnut Customizable Blender Oat Cups (see page 158).

- Add them to soups and stews.

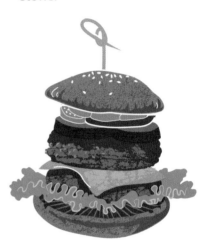

WAYS TO EAT MORE FRUIT

- Keep in-season fresh fruit sliced and at eye level in the fridge and whole fruit on the counter for easy snacking.

- Keep bags of frozen fruit on hand to easily incorporate into meals and snacks in a pinch.

- Add frozen fruit to smoothies (see page 146).

- Keep unsweetened dried fruit on hand for on-the-go snacking.

- Use dates (see page 332) or mashed bananas (see page 320) instead of refined sugar to sweeten baked goods.

- Freeze grapes for a cold and refreshing snack.

- Freeze leftover smoothies (see page 146) or pureed frozen fruit in ice pop molds.

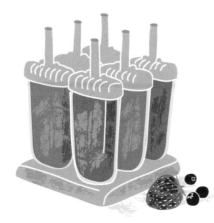

- Add a serving of fruit to a salad for a touch of sweetness (page 206).

- Puree frozen fruit into a fruit-only sorbet (see page 330) or a one-ingredient banana "ice cream."

- Make them the star of desserts like Any Berry Crumble Bars (page 322) and Single-Serve Cinnamon Apple Walnut Crisps (page 338).

- Cook fruits like pineapple, peaches, and nectarines on the grill at your next barbecue.

go with grains

For years, grains made up the bulk of the US Department of Agriculture's food pyramid—but how important are they? Not all grains are created equal, and the ones you want to focus on in a mostly plant-based diet are whole grains, as they are the most nutrient-rich. Whole grains include oats, quinoa, barley, bulgur, buckwheat, brown rice, and much more.

Whole grains, unlike refined grains, retain the entire kernel—the bran, germ, and endosperm—and therefore its fiber and key nutrients, such as iron and B vitamins. Refined grains, on the other hand, are stripped of the bran and germ, leaving only the nutrient-poor, starchy endosperm. Food manufacturers refine grains primarily to extend their shelf life and create finer-textured products. What's left is a highly processed grain of much lower nutritional quality.

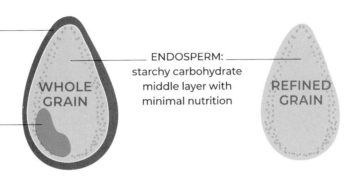

BRAN:
fiber-rich outer layer with B vitamins, iron, copper, zinc, magnesium, antioxidants, and phytonutrients

GERM:
nutrient-rich core with B vitamins, good fats, phytonutrients, and antioxidants

ENDOSPERM:
starchy carbohydrate middle layer with minimal nutrition

WHOLE GRAIN

REFINED GRAIN

While refined grains are often "enriched," meaning manufacturers add back those lost nutrients (fiber, iron, and B vitamins), I consider them inferior to their whole-grain counterparts because of my "stick to whole foods" philosophy (see the box on the next page).

Besides their nutrition-to-calorie ratio classifying them as a nutrient-dense food, research has linked whole-grain consumption to better health, including lower risk of cardiovascular disease, type 2 diabetes, cancer, and digestive disorders.

Buying whole-grain foods can be tricky, as marketing gimmicks have made it increasingly challenging. I go into how to do it properly in Chapter 4.

WHY IS IT IMPORTANT TO CONSUME "WHOLE" FOODS?

Nutritional science is rather new and ever evolving. In fact, the first *Dietary Guidelines for Americans* were released only about 40 years ago, when the link between food and disease was made evident. So, there is still a lot to be known about nutrition.

That being said, the research that does exist has consistently shown that a diet of minimally processed foods close to their natural state, predominantly plants, is unwaveringly associated with health promotion and disease prevention.[10] While fortified foods are an excellent manufacturing development to feed the masses and help prevent nutritional deficiencies, these foods don't address the way nutrients work synergistically in whole-food ingredients to influence health—an area of research that still needs work.

So, you will see me advocating for mostly minimally processed whole foods over their more processed counterparts. This could be as simple as choosing whole-grain oatmeal with berries over a fortified processed breakfast cereal, or air-popped popcorn (which is a whole grain!) over crackers.

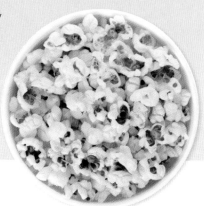

WAYS TO EAT MORE WHOLE GRAINS

· Start your day with stovetop oatmeal, baked oatmeal (see page 164), or overnight oats (see page 138).

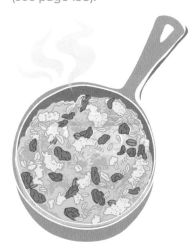

· Make simple swaps for the grains you are already eating, like sprouted whole-grain bread instead of white bread or whole-grain pasta instead of regular.

· Use whole-grain flours for baking.

· Cook a different batch of whole grains each week to easily add to meals like salads, soups, and Buddha bowls (see page 302).

· Snack on popcorn (3 cups of air-popped popcorn = 1 serving of whole grains).

· Pair whole-grain crackers with nutritious dips like guacamole (see page 118) and hummus (see page 120).

· Tap into the power of rolled oats in recipes other than oatmeal. Use them as a nutritious breading, add them to homemade veggie burgers, black bean "meatballs" (see page 312), and desserts, use them as the base for homemade granola bars (see page 242), or use them to thicken smoothies (see page 146).

nuts & seeds: small but mighty

In addition to being a significant source of key vitamins, minerals, fiber, and plant protein, nuts and seeds shine in the type of fats they provide. Research shows that the unsaturated fats found in nuts help lower low-density lipoprotein (LDL) or "bad" cholesterol and raise high-density lipoprotein (HDL) or "good" cholesterol. In fact, the US Food and Drug Administration (FDA) now allows some packaged nuts to carry the claim that "eating a diet that includes one ounce of nuts daily can reduce your risk of heart disease."

In one large study examining nuts and health, researchers analyzed data from over 210,000 health professionals followed for a period of up to 32 years and found that those who ate 1 ounce of nuts five or more times per week had a 14 percent lower risk of cardiovascular disease and a 20 percent lower risk of coronary heart disease compared to those who never or almost never ate nuts.[11]

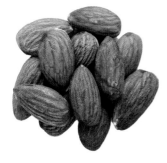

Nuts and seeds are nutritional powerhouses, but they are also calorically dense, meaning a little goes a long way. For example, a handful of 24 almonds clocks in at around 164 calories and 14 grams of fat (the good kind).

WAYS TO EAT MORE NUTS AND SEEDS

- Swap the butter on toast and in baked goods with nut or seed butter (see pages 320 and 340).

- Sprinkle a tablespoon of nuts or seeds onto a salad for nutrient-dense crunch.

- Make homemade pesto (see page 114).

- Bake with nut flours (such as in the bagels on page 162).

- Add nut milk and nut butter to smoothies (see page 146).

- Enjoy chia pudding for breakfast (see page 138).

- Try "cheesy" plant-based swaps for Parmesan (see page 124) and ricotta (see page 286) that tap into the power of cashews.

- Use nuts and seeds as a breading for lean proteins like chicken and fish.

- Add nuts and seeds to homemade granola (see page 150) and granola bars (see page 242).

- Use nut butter in sauces and dressings (see page 110 for my Peanut Dressing/Dip recipe).

- Use flax eggs as an egg replacement (see page 144).

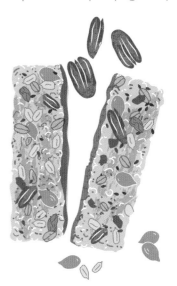

love your legumes

Legumes are a class of vegetables that includes beans, peas, and lentils. Not only do they come in a variety of colors and textures, making them versatile pantry staples, but they are an affordable source of nutrition: nearly devoid of fat, naturally cholesterol free, and rich in plant protein, phytonutrients, fiber, and important micronutrients, including B vitamins and potassium.

How to cook beans to avoid stomach discomfort

Many people avoid beans due to a fear of intestinal gas and stomach discomfort, so I feel it's important to address the subject here. When it comes to beans and other legumes, preparation is key. Research shows that responses to increased fiber intake vary from individual to individual. While I personally love and advocate for the convenience of canned beans, which are precooked, opting for dried beans gives you more control over the flavor, texture, and digestibility—and it's easy to do. Plus, you can cook a big batch and freeze them to have on hand.

To minimize gastrointestinal issues, I recommend buying dried legumes, picking them over, rinsing them under water, and then soaking them overnight in a bowl of water (with some exceptions, including lentils, split peas, black-eyed peas, and adzuki beans, which do not need soaking). Doing so helps reduce the cooking time and the gas-producing compounds while yielding more tender beans. Then simply cook them in a large pot covered with about 2 inches of water. Bring to a boil, reduce to a simmer, and cook for 30 to 120 minutes, depending on the type and size of legume.

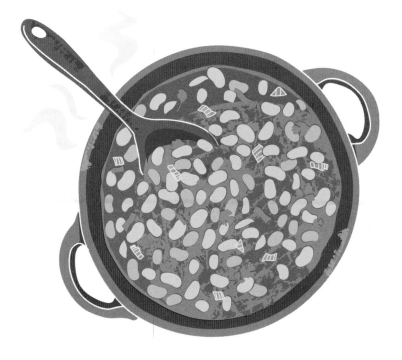

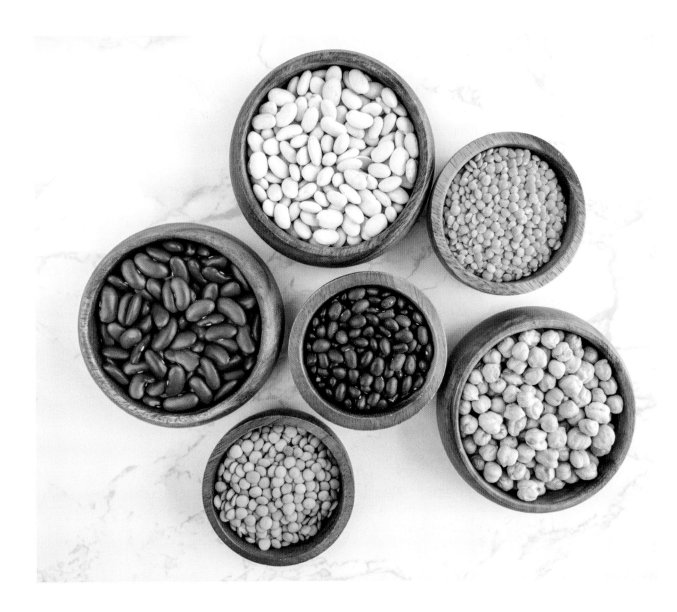

Here are some other tips for eating legumes:

- Increase beans in your diet slowly. The same goes with fiber in general. If your body is not used to consuming large amounts of fiber-rich foods, you should introduce them gradually to avoid stomach discomfort.

- Drink plenty of water when you consume beans. The fiber in beans acts as a sponge and needs water to plump up and pass through the intestines seamlessly.

- Consider adding a strip of kombu to the soaking water. Some research suggests that this seaweed helps soften beans and make them more digestible.

- Don't use the soaking water to cook the beans. If you continue to have digestive issues, you can try changing out the water several times during soaking. This water will have absorbed some of the gas-producing indigestible carbohydrate.

- Some legumes, such as lentils, adzuki beans, and black-eyed peas, may be easier to digest than others.

straight talk about soy

Soy is an often-misunderstood food. Soy foods are made from soybeans, a type of legume. For some, soy is exalted as a nutrient-dense source of plant-based protein (which it is), but others have written it off for fear that it can cause cancer. Yet research points to just the opposite—that soy may have cancer-preventing properties.

Soy contains phytoestrogens called isoflavones, which are naturally occurring compounds in plants and share a similar structure with estrogen. Increased estrogen levels have been linked to certain types of breast cancer; however, these plant estrogens function differently than the estrogen our bodies make. In fact, soy isoflavones are believed to be one of the main reasons behind the many health benefits of soy foods, including improved cardiovascular health, osteoporosis prevention, and even reduced breast cancer risk.[12] In a pooled analysis of three large prospective cohort studies, a soy isoflavone intake of at least 10 milligrams per day was associated with a 25 percent reduced risk of tumor recurrence in breast cancer survivors.[13]

Additionally, the American Cancer Society deems soy safe and healthy for consumption. As an excellent source of complete plant-based protein, fiber, polyunsaturated fat, phytonutrients, and other key nutrients, including B vitamins, calcium, and zinc, while also being naturally cholesterol-free and low in saturated fat, soy foods earn their spot in a mostly plant-based diet.

But it's important to note that not all soy is the same. As the second largest crop in the United States, it is often chemically altered and added to processed foods, which some studies suggest could be problematic—as may be the case with many processed ingredients. Instead, turn to whole soy foods where the benefits lie—like edamame (mature soybeans), soy milk (emulsified soybeans), tofu (soy milk curds), tempeh (fermented soybeans), and miso (fermented soybean paste).

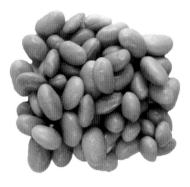

WAYS TO EAT MORE LEGUMES

- Enjoy hummus (see page 120) as a sandwich spread or a dip for crackers and sliced vegetables or thin it with water to make an easy salad dressing.

- Use blended white beans as the base for a low-fat salad dressing (see page 110).

- Toss cooked beans into a salad or use Chickpea Poppers (page 230) as a crunchy crouton swap.

- Use mashed chickpeas in place of tuna in Chickpea Tuna-Less Salad (page 260).

- Add a half-cup serving of beans to hearty soups, stews, and curries.

- Cook mashed beans and grated vegetables into fritters or burgers (see page 278).

- Toss legumes into pasta dishes.

- Add beans to frittatas and omelets.

- Serve beans out of a baked potato or sweet potato (see page 274).

- Add beans to enchiladas (see page 268), burritos and burrito bowls (see page 270), and taco filling (see page 282).

- Replace the butter in baked goods with mashed beans (see page 328).

- Use chickpeas in a Secret Ingredient Edible Cookie Dough (page 334).

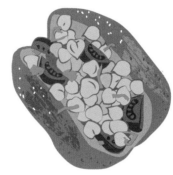
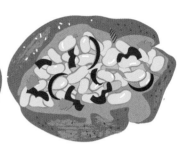

WAYS TO EAT MORE SOY

- Cook extra-firm tofu or tempeh on the grill.

- Puree silken tofu and add it to baked goods.

- Use tofu chunks or crumbled tempeh in place of chicken or ground beef in burrito bowls (see page 270) and tacos.

- Replace ricotta cheese in lasagna and stuffed shells with soft tofu blended with seasonings.

- Use pureed tofu in twice-baked potatoes.

- Blend silken tofu or soy milk into smoothies (see page 146).

- Make Tempeh Bacon (page 126) and add it to sandwiches, salads, and wraps.

- Use crumbled tofu instead of eggs in breakfast scrambles.

- Use soy milk in smoothies (see page 146), stovetop oatmeal, chia pudding, and overnight oats (see page 138).

- Add shelled edamame to salads (see page 178), noodle dishes (see page 256), Buddha bowls (see page 302), and more.

- Use miso to add flavor to dishes.

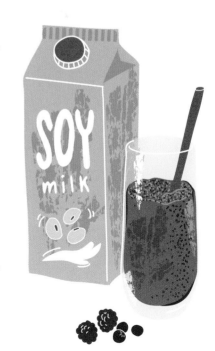

CHAPTER 3:

treat meat like a condiment

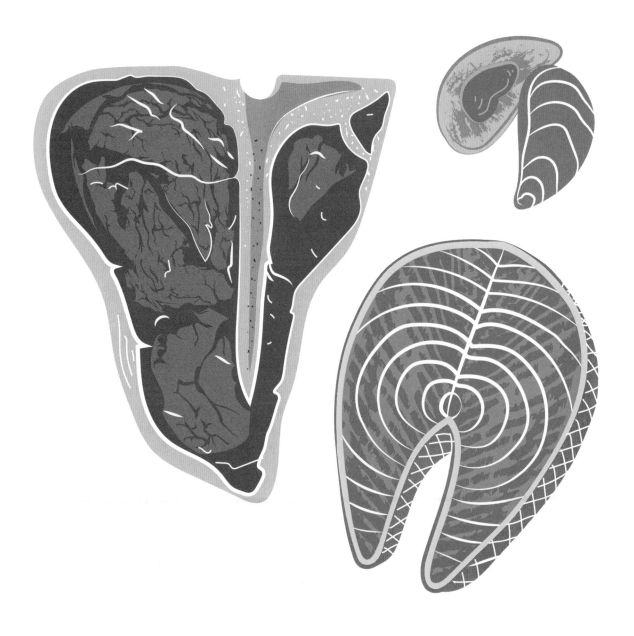

Animal products, particularly meat, are a controversial part of a plant-based diet. While many people choose to exclude them for reasons ranging from ethical and moral concerns to environmental and climate impacts, I am going to address them as a registered dietitian would—from a nutrition standpoint.

The truth is, animal foods such as meat, poultry, eggs, seafood, and dairy offer considerable nutrition when looked at on a molecular level, including complete protein and bioavailable vitamins and minerals—but also some drawbacks, such as saturated fat and a lack of fiber.

In my earlier chart of essential vitamins and minerals (see pages 32 and 33), I starred several and disclaimed that while plant foods are incredibly nutrient-dense and powerful, you are better off obtaining certain micronutrients from animal sources. In this chapter, I'm going to break down exactly why that is.

some animal food nutrients are more bioavailable

The term *bioavailability* refers to the proportion of a nutrient consumed in the diet that is absorbed and utilized by the body for normal metabolic and physiologic processes. Animal foods win by a landslide in the case of certain nutrients.[1] Bioavailability is influenced by several factors, including

- **A person's life stage:** Gastric acid, which is required for the digestion and absorption of several nutrients, including iron, calcium, and vitamin C, declines as we age. This means that healthy younger individuals can usually absorb micronutrients better than older individuals.

- **The chemical form of the nutrient:** For example, the heme iron found in animal foods is more readily available for absorption than the non-heme iron found in plants. In other words, consuming heme iron would result in considerably higher serum iron levels than consuming an equal amount of non-heme iron.

- **Interactions with other food compounds:** Some compounds found in plant foods, such as oxalic acid, phytate, and even fiber (a nutrient we otherwise love!), can bind to certain minerals, like calcium, iron, and zinc, and lower or prevent their absorption in the intestine.

nutrient face-off: plant vs. animal foods

Nutrition fact labels don't always present the whole picture when it comes to certain nutrients. While a plant and an animal food may list the same amount of a nutrient such as iron, only a fraction of that amount is absorbed, and the body ultimately prefers one form over the other—typically the animal form, which is more bioavailable. This is the case with a handful of nutrients, so it can be helpful to identify them on a mostly plant-based diet.

vitamin A: the immunity & skin-loving nutrient

BEST ANIMAL FOOD SOURCES: mackerel, salmon, tuna, trout, eggs, fortified dairy products

Vitamin A is a fat-soluble vitamin essential for normal vision, the immune system, and proper functioning of the heart, lungs, and kidneys. It is available in two forms in the human diet: pre-formed vitamin A found in animal foods and provitamin A carotenoids found in plant foods like yellow, orange, and red produce such as sweet potatoes and carrots. In order to use them, the body has to convert provitamin A carotenoids like beta-carotene to vitamin A, and that conversion process is largely inefficient. The equivalency for beta-carotene (found in plant foods) to vitamin A in animal foods is estimated to be 12:1, meaning you would have to consume 12 micrograms of beta-carotene to equal 1 microgram of vitamin A.[2]

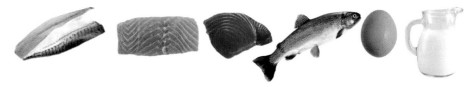

vitamin B12: for brain health & energy

BEST ANIMAL FOOD SOURCES: herring, tuna, salmon, eggs, dairy products

Vitamin B12 is a nutrient that helps keep the blood and nerve cells healthy and is essential for preventing megaloblastic anemia, a blood condition that makes people tired and weak. Inadequate B12 quantities in plant-based foods are one of the more widely known and acknowledged nutrient-related concerns for those who consume a primarily plant-based diet. This water-soluble vitamin is found naturally in foods of animal origin, while plant-based foods such as nutritional yeast and breakfast cereals are often fortified with it.

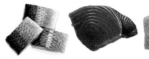

vitamin D3: the sunshine vitamin

BEST ANIMAL FOOD SOURCES: trout, salmon, tuna, sardines, eggs

Vitamin D is a fat-soluble vitamin essential for the health of our bones, muscles, immune system, and nervous system. We acquire vitamin D by two methods: from the sun's ultraviolet (UV) rays striking our skin and triggering vitamin D synthesis, and from the food we eat.

There are two forms of vitamin D: D3 (cholecalciferol) and D2 (ergocalciferol). In the body, both forms are converted to 25 hydroxyvitamin D (25(OH)D), which is used to measure vitamin D status in individuals. While both D2 and D3 are well absorbed by the gut, vitamin D3 increases serum 25(OH)D levels to a greater extent and maintains these high levels longer than D2. Because it is considerably more bioavailable, vitamin D3 is the form you find in most supplements.

Few foods are naturally rich in vitamin D3, and the ones that are, are animal derived. While some plant-based foods such as plant milks and cereals are fortified with vitamin D2, animal foods remain the only reliable naturally occurring food sources of D3.

You might have heard that mushrooms are a good source of vitamin D. Yes, some commercially grown mushrooms contain vitamin D because they have intentionally been exposed to high amounts of UV light—but it's primarily D2, not D3.

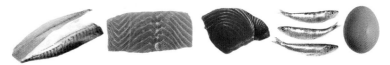

SHOULD I BE CONCERNED ABOUT MERCURY IN FISH?

While fish is an excellent source of protein, omega-3 fats, and key bioavailable nutrients, mercury remains a concern. Nearly all fish and shellfish contain traces of mercury, a metal found naturally in the air, water, and soil that in large amounts can cause serious health problems, including brain and heart effects. However, some seafood contains lesser amounts, namely small fish. As small fish are eaten by larger fish up the food chain, concentrations of mercury increase, so large predatory fish such as sharks, swordfish, tilefish, and king mackerel tend to contain the highest levels.

Experts agree that the health benefits of eating fish likely outweigh the risks as long as you limit your intake of high-mercury fish. Sticking to the recommendation of consuming seafood twice a week and focusing on small fish like shrimp, sardines, anchovies, and salmon can help you reap the nutritional benefits while keeping these risks at bay.

calcium: for more than just strong bones

Calcium is the most abundant mineral in the body. It is important not only for healthy bones and teeth, but also for helping muscles contract and helping nerves to carry messages between the brain and every other part of the body. It is available in both plant and animal foods, but in varying quantities and bioavailabilities.

The amount of calcium listed on a nutrition facts label of a food product is the measure of calcium in the food but does not necessarily reflect the amount the body will absorb. For example, spinach is renowned for being rich in calcium, but studies suggest only 5 percent of that is absorbed, compared to the 30 percent absorbed from dairy-based foods.[3] The key takeaway is not to avoid spinach, as it is a nutrient-dense food, but to avoid relying on it as a significant source of calcium.

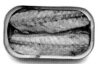

iron: the energy nutrient

Iron is an essential mineral used to make hemoglobin, a protein in red blood cells that carries oxygen from the lungs to all other parts of the body. The World Health Organization (WHO) describes iron deficiency as the most common cause of anemia in the world and notes that it is particularly prevalent in developing countries where diets are predominantly plant-based. This can pose a particular issue to those of childbearing age, whose iron needs are the highest because of menstruation.

Iron exists in two forms: heme iron found in animal foods and non-heme iron found in plant foods. Depending on an individual's iron stores, 15 to 35 percent of heme iron gets absorbed, compared to 2 to 20 percent of non-heme iron.[4] Meeting your iron needs is possible on a mostly plant-based diet.

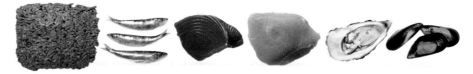

ASCORBIC ACID One dietary component can help enhance dietary iron absorption from plant-based foods. Ascorbic acid (vitamin C), when paired with iron-containing plant foods like spinach, beans, lentils, nuts, and seeds, can capture non-heme iron and store it in a form that's more easily absorbed by the body.[5]

zinc: for immunity

BEST ANIMAL FOOD SOURCES:
oysters, beef, crab, pork, chicken, yogurt

Zinc is a trace mineral—one needed in small amounts—yet it is necessary for almost 100 vital chemical reactions in the body, including supporting a healthy immune system and healing wounds. Zinc deficiency is now known to be a significant malnutrition problem worldwide, particularly in developing countries whose populations subsist on primarily plant-based diets. This is largely due not necessarily to diets low in zinc, but to diets that include zinc-containing foods with low bioavailability—namely plant foods.[6] Just like iron and calcium, phytates inhibit zinc absorption from plant-based foods. This is why the dietary reference intakes for zinc are nearly 50 percent higher for vegetarians.[7]

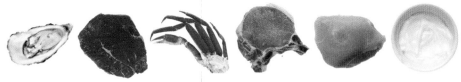

EPA and DHA omega-3 fatty acids: for brain & heart health

BEST ANIMAL FOOD SOURCES:
salmon, sardines, tuna, herring, trout, mackerel

Omega 3-fatty acids are essential, meaning our bodies cannot make them, so we need to consume them from the diet. These fats are an integral part of cell membranes throughout the body and particularly play a role in positively influencing cardiovascular risk factors, building brain and nerve cells, and warding off age-related mental decline.

The omega-3 fats found in plant foods differ from those found in animal foods. Eicosapentaenoic acid (EPA) and docosahexaenoic acid (DHA) are the forms found almost exclusively in animal foods (algae being a notable exception), and alpha-linoleic acid (ALA) is the form found in plant foods, including walnuts, chia seeds, and flaxseeds.

DHA and EPA appear to have more benefit to and use by the body. In fact, DHA is a key component of cell membranes and is found in abundance in the brain and retinas.[8] For reference, the brain is about 60 percent fat, and DHA makes up over 90 percent of the omega-3 fatty acids in the brain and up to 25 percent of its total fat content.[9] DHA also makes up an estimated 93 percent of the omega-3 fatty acids in the eyes.[10] The body uses EPA to produce signaling molecules called eicosanoids, which play many physiological roles, including lowering inflammation.[11]

The body can convert ALA to EPA and DHA, but the conversion efficiency is very low. Studies of ALA metabolism indicate that approximately 8 to 21 percent of dietary ALA is converted to EPA and 0 to 9 percent is converted to DHA in healthy young people.[12]

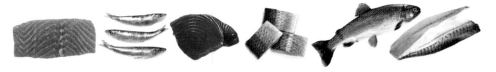

vitamin K2: the forgotten form of vitamin K

BEST ANIMAL FOOD SOURCES:
beef, chicken, eggs, cheese, grass-fed butter

Many people may not realize that just like omega-3 fats, vitamin K comes in multiple forms. Vitamin K1, needed primarily for blood clotting, is the form found in plant foods (think leafy greens). Vitamin K2 is just as important for different functions—namely integrating calcium into bones, which helps prevent blood vessel calcification that can be harmful to the heart. It is found primarily in animal foods—with natto (fermented soybeans) being the best plant-based source.

While a specific recommended intake has not yet been set for vitamin K2, it is a nutrient with undoubted benefits to the body, and I suspect it will be brought to greater light in the coming years.

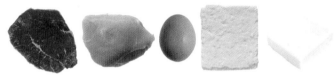

iodine: essential for metabolism

BEST ANIMAL FOOD SOURCES:
cod, oysters, shrimp, eggs, plain yogurt, cheese

Iodine is an essential trace mineral used by the thyroid gland to make thyroid hormones that control many functions in the body, including regulating metabolism. It is present naturally in some foods, namely animal proteins (with a notable plant-based exception—seaweed), and added to others, such as table salt.

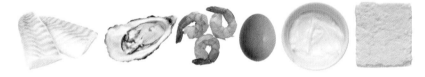

choline: to nourish your noggin

BEST ANIMAL FOOD SOURCES:
eggs, beef, chicken, turkey, cod, yogurt

Choline is an essential nutrient needed to produce acetylcholine, an important neurotransmitter for mood, memory, muscle control, and other brain and nervous system functions. The body also uses it to synthesize cell membranes. While our bodies can produce some choline, the amount produced is not sufficient to meet our needs; therefore, we must get it from the diet.

The best sources of choline are animal foods; plant foods such as beans, quinoa, broccoli, and Brussels sprouts provide lesser amounts.

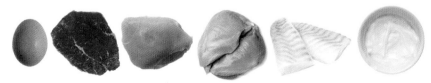

LET'S TALK SALT

Salt can make or break a dish, but what salt should you be using? While there are dozens of different types, these are four to consider for your pantry.

- **Table salt** is harvested from salt deposits underground, stripped of any minerals, processed into fine crystals, and treated with an anti-caking agent to prevent clumping. It is the only salt typically fortified with iodine. If you aren't regularly consuming iodine-containing foods, then using iodized salt could be beneficial.

- **Sea salt** is harvested from evaporating seawater. It is unrefined, so it is coarser-grained than table salt. It also contains minerals from where it is harvested, such as zinc, potassium, and iron, which give sea salt a more complex flavor.

- **Pink Himalayan salt** is sourced near the foothills of the Himalayan Mountains and gets its pink color from the minerals it contains, including iron, manganese, zinc, calcium, and potassium. It also has a slightly lower sodium content than table salt.

- **Kosher salt** is mined from salt deposits and has large, coarse grains. It is made solely of sodium chloride, with no trace minerals, additives, or iodine.

While I use pink Himalayan salt in the recipes throughout this book, feel free to use your salt of choice. (If you opt for table salt, you may need slightly less because it tastes saltier.) It is important to note that although sea salt and pink salt contain naturally occurring minerals, you would need to consume a large amount to make a meaningful contribution to your nutrient intake, which would provide excessive sodium and therefore potentially harmful effects. In other words, don't consume salt for the little nutrition it may provide, and remain mindful of how much salt you use—no matter the type.

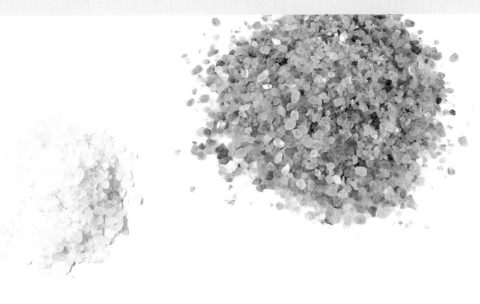

WHAT ABOUT PROTEIN?

Note that I didn't include protein in my roundup of nutrients. Protein is made up of building blocks called amino acids. Twenty amino acids are needed to make a protein in the body. Eleven of those amino acids our bodies can make, and nine are considered essential, meaning we need to get them from food.

It's true that animal proteins are considered complete proteins—meaning they contain all nine essential amino acids—while the vast majority of plant foods are considered incomplete proteins (with some exceptions, including quinoa, hemp seeds, and soy). So, what does the research say? As long as you are incorporating a variety of plant protein sources, including legumes, nuts, grains, and seeds, in large enough quantities, there is little reason to worry about getting too little complete protein on a mostly plant-based diet.[13]

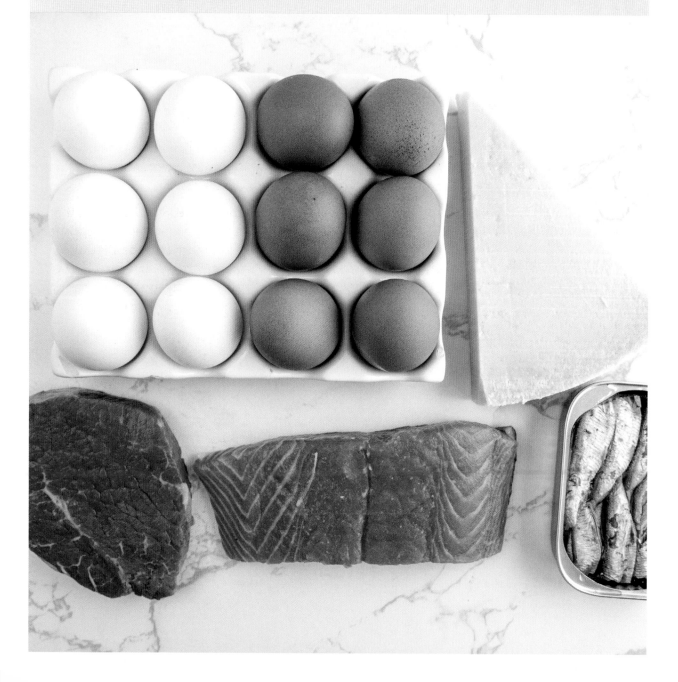

how do I know if I'm low in these nutrients?

The American food industry has done a good job of limiting nutritional deficiencies in the general population through fortifying foods and making food abundant and affordable. However, nutritional inadequacies still occur.

Nutritional inadequacies manifest themselves in a multitude of ways beyond those that can be objectively measured by blood tests. It may sound cliché, but listen to your body. I've seen countless clients who add back XYZ food to their exclusively plant-based diet, whether it's a palm-sized portion of red meat or a couple of eggs, and notice a world of difference in their energy levels, moods, hair, nails, and more.

Also remember that variety is the spice of life when it comes to optimal nutrition. One way to do that is by eating with the seasons—in-season produce is typically at its nutritional peak, tastes the best, and is most affordable. Switch up your legumes, grains, nuts, and seeds weekly, and experiment with new proteins.

And know that restriction is usually not the answer. Any approach that eliminates food groups can be detrimental in the long term, as each whole food offers its own unique package of nutrients. The Dietary Guidelines for Americans exist for a reason—to help ensure you meet your nutritional needs to support optimal health using the decades of research that exists in this still very new and ever-evolving science.

With the mostly plant-based diet, we aren't eliminating foods but rather shifting the ratios to put the emphasis on plants.

where animal foods fall short nutritionally

Of course, animal foods (like all foods to some degree) fall short in certain ways:

They are high in saturated fat.

Red meat, despite being rich in bioavailable key nutrients like B12, iron, and zinc, is particularly high in saturated fat, which the dietary guidelines recommend limiting to less than 10 percent of total daily calories. Many studies have linked high red meat consumption to increased health risks. However, the exact amounts for safe consumption are debated.

They contain cholesterol.

Dietary cholesterol is found only in animal products. While new research may have debunked the notion that dietary cholesterol negatively affects cholesterol levels in the body, the Dietary Guidelines for Americans still recommend consuming as little as possible without compromising the nutritional adequacy of your diet.

They provide no fiber.

Fiber, as covered in Chapters 1 and 2, is essential for digestion, regularity, heart health, and gut health. Fiber is exclusive to plant foods, so you won't find any in meat, dairy, poultry, or eggs.

They don't support beneficial gut bacteria.

Besides being devoid of fiber, meat, poultry, and eggs likely do not have a positive impact on the gut microbiome. For example, one study conducted in animals showed that consuming a large amount of meat helped a type of bacterium flourish that has been linked to inflammation and intestinal diseases.[14] Fermented dairy products that contain probiotics are an animal food exception—such as some yogurts and kefir.

Today's animal protein is often not what it's cut out to be.

Quality matters when it comes to choosing meat, dairy, poultry, and eggs, and it's becoming increasingly challenging to find good quality. Not all meat sold in grocery stores is the same—the products differ in terms of taste, nutrient density, and even phytonutrient content (affected by what the animals were fed).

For example, researchers have found that grass-fed meat is not only rich in phytonutrients but also higher in omega-3 fats and lower in saturated fat than its conventionally raised counterpart that often is given corn feed, resulting in nutritionally inferior meat.

I cover how to shop for the most nutritious animal products—meat, dairy, poultry, eggs, and fish—in Chapter 4.

How you cook animal protein matters too.

High-temperature cooking, such as grilling or frying, can produce toxic compounds such as advanced glycation end-products (AGEs) that, when accumulated in tissues, significantly increase the level of inflammation in the body, which has been associated with the development of certain cancers.[15] Roasting, baking, poaching, simmering, and stewing are healthier cooking methods; pan-frying and stir-frying at high heat for short periods are also fine.

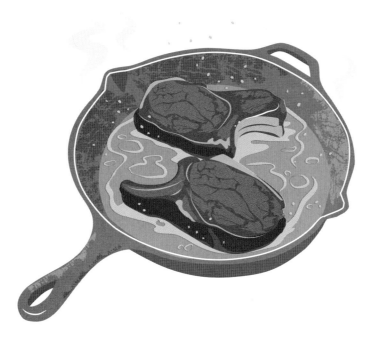

can I meet all my nutritional needs on an exclusively plant-based diet?

Yes—with proper meal planning and supplementation when needed. Additionally, it's worth reiterating that nutritional needs vary by life stage; children, people who are pregnant or breastfeeding, and older adults may require more or less of certain nutrients. It is best to work with a dietitian who can look at your diet to determine an eating and supplement plan that works for you and your unique needs and supports optimal health.

The following are some plant-based solutions to address those hard-to-get nutrients.

NUTRIENT	HOW TO ENSURE YOU GET ADEQUATE AMOUNTS
Calcium	Include fortified foods such as plant milks and plenty of calcium-containing foods such as leafy green vegetables, tofu, and tahini.
Choline	Red potatoes, kidney beans, quinoa, Brussels sprouts, and broccoli are sources.
Iodine	Seaweed, enriched bread and pasta, and iodized salt are plant-based sources.
Iron	Combine vitamin C–containing foods with plant-based iron-containing foods such as beans, whole grains, legumes, and tofu.
Omega-3 fats (EPA and DHA)	Seaweed, spirulina, and nori are among the only plant-based sources of EPA and DHA omega-3s. You can get ALA omega-3 fats that your body can somewhat convert to DHA and EPA from walnuts, flaxseeds, and chia seeds. Consider an algae-derived supplement.
Vitamin A	Focus on plenty of beta-carotene–containing foods, such as sweet potatoes, spinach, carrots, and red bell peppers, as well as fortified foods like plant milks.
Vitamin B12	Include fortified foods like plant milks, soy products, and nutritional yeast. Consider a supplement.
Vitamin D3	Get 15 minutes of daily sunlight exposure and incorporate fortified foods such as plant milks. Consider a supplement.
Vitamin K2	Incorporate fermented foods like natto, sauerkraut, and miso.
Zinc	Incorporate zinc-containing foods like beans, pumpkin seeds, cashews, oats, almonds, and kidney beans. Soak beans, grains, and seeds before preparing them to help increase bioavailability.

And to address protein: As mentioned in Chapter 1, we don't need nearly as much protein as is commonly preached to us. Americans easily meet their daily protein needs and can do so with exclusively plant protein or a mixture of both plant and animal foods.

A little goes a long way with animal foods thanks to their nutrient density and nutrient bioavailability.

think of animal foods as condiments rather than mainstays of your daily diet

A palm-sized portion of animal protein twice a day (grass-fed meat, pasture-raised poultry, eggs, or fish) is sufficient and, in my opinion, can be essential for optimal health.

Here's how to treat meat like a condiment:

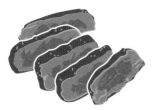

Turn a vegetable side dish into a satisfying main course with a little bit of flavorful animal protein like sliced grilled strip steak.

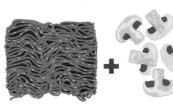

Use a 50/50 blend of ground meat and cooked minced mushrooms in tacos and in recipes like Cauliflower Potato Shepherd's Pie (page 310).

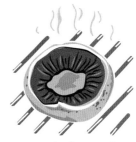

Throw portabella mushroom caps on the grill with steak or fish and enjoy a 50/50 blend over a mixed green salad with a whole-grain side dish.

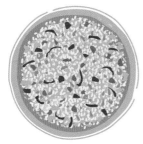

Make cauliflower fried rice (see page 240) into a satisfying veggie-packed meal with an egg for animal protein.

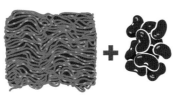

Go 50/50 with ground beef and beans for protein in tacos, burritos, and burrito bowls.

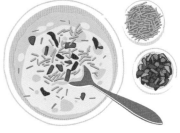

Prepare a plant-based dinner with an animal protein served on the side to add sparingly for flavor.

Go plant-based for two out of three meals per day. For example, you could have overnight oats (see page 138) for breakfast, Spaghetti Squash Lentil Bolognese Boats (page 258) for lunch, and Pesto Salmon Packets (page 314) for dinner.

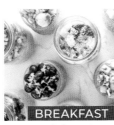

BREAKFAST
overnight oats

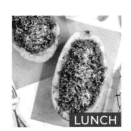

LUNCH
spaghetti squash lentil bolognese boats

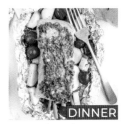

DINNER
pesto salmon packets

PART II:

how to go mostly plant-based

stock your mostly plant-based kitchen

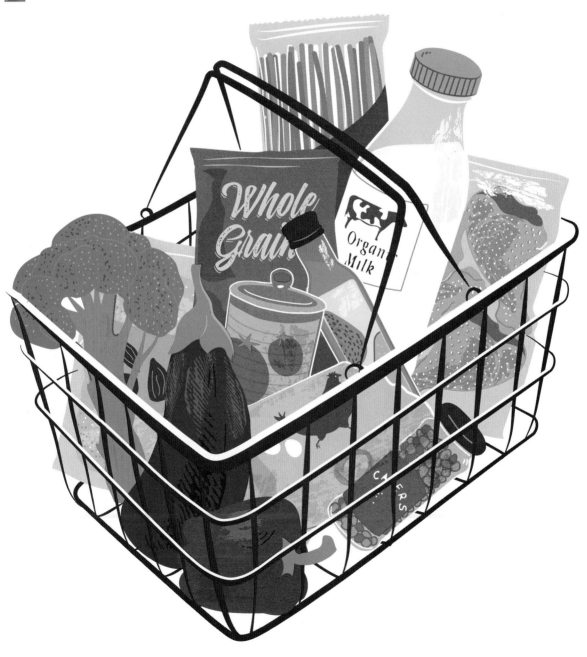

Navigating the grocery store can be overwhelming when you're starting out on your mostly plant-based journey. In this chapter, I take you through each major food category and outline what to look for and what constitutes a nutritious choice. I give you all the tools you need to make informed decisions about purchasing each and every ingredient.

Even if you don't make a single recipe in this book, you can use these simple tips and strategies to tackle your grocery shopping, plan your meals, and set yourself up for success. It all starts with ingredients.

shopping for vegetables and fruit

The perimeter of the grocery store is a great place to start your shopping, as this is where stores typically keep the bulk of their fresh foods. Not surprisingly, produce makes up the foundation of a mostly plant-based diet, and while some produce is nutritionally superior to others, any vegetable or fruit is a good choice.

organic vs. conventional

The US Department of Agriculture defines organic crops as those that are grown on farms that have not used most synthetic fertilizers and pesticides for three years prior to harvest. On average, organic foods cost 10 to 40 percent more than their conventionally produced counterparts.[1] So how do they stack up nutritionally? Research says, virtually the same.

The main difference is that conventional produce is produced using pesticides, which, though safe for human consumption according to FDA regulations, may pose health risks in vulnerable periods of development according to new research, such as infancy, childhood, and pregnancy.

The answer? Buy organic when you can, and wash your produce thoroughly before consuming it to limit your exposure to pesticides. Additionally, the Environmental Working Group (EWG) puts out "Dirty Dozen" and "Clean Fifteen" lists each year, which can be helpful guides to buying organic when it counts. The lists for 2022 are shown on the following page.

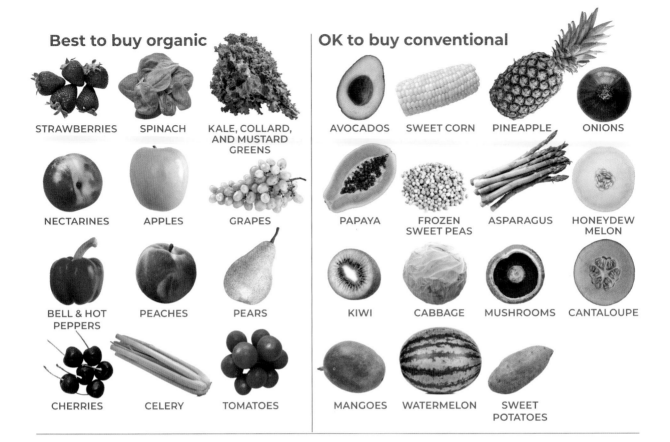

Best to buy organic

STRAWBERRIES

SPINACH

KALE, COLLARD, AND MUSTARD GREENS

NECTARINES

APPLES

GRAPES

BELL & HOT PEPPERS

PEACHES

PEARS

CHERRIES

CELERY

TOMATOES

OK to buy conventional

AVOCADOS

SWEET CORN

PINEAPPLE

ONIONS

PAPAYA

FROZEN SWEET PEAS

ASPARAGUS

HONEYDEW MELON

KIWI

CABBAGE

MUSHROOMS

CANTALOUPE

MANGOES

WATERMELON

SWEET POTATOES

frozen & canned produce

Frozen produce has many advantages over fresh, including typically being more affordable and lasting much longer (8 to 12 months), thus reducing potential food waste. Additionally, many of the fruits and vegetables you find in the frozen food aisles are picked at the peak of ripeness (when they are freshest and most nutritious) and flash-frozen soon after, which helps lock in their vitamins, minerals, and phytonutrients. Nutritionally speaking, fresh and frozen produce stack up comparably.

Canned fruits and vegetables are usually canned within hours of picking, which helps preserve their nutrition and flavor. For the most part, the amounts of fat-soluble vitamins, minerals, protein, fat, and carbohydrate remain relatively unchanged. However, because the canning process requires high heat, canned foods may contain less heat-sensitive vitamins such as vitamin C and B vitamins. On the other hand, the canning process increases the amount of lycopene in tomatoes.

While their long shelf life of one to five years makes canned foods a convenient and affordable way to incorporate more fruits and vegetables into your diet, it is important to choose fruit canned in water or its own juices rather than syrup (added sugar), and vegetables canned without added salt. Draining and rinsing canned vegetables can reduce the sodium content.

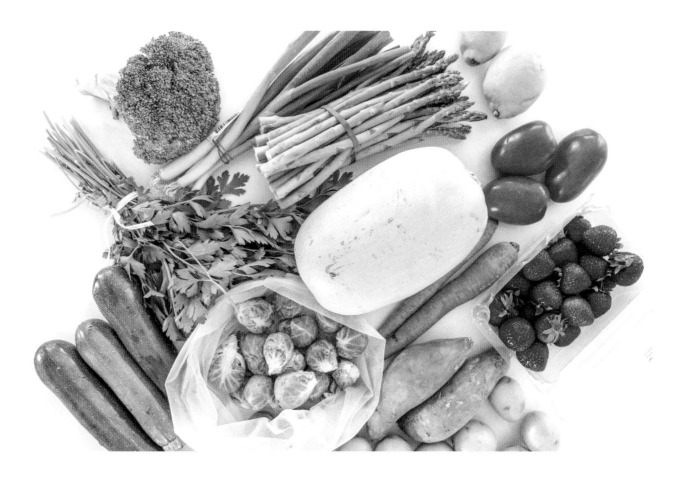

The verdict? Keep a variety of all types on hand—like frozen berries for smoothies, frozen riced cauliflower for stir-fries, canned tomatoes for pasta dishes, and canned pumpkin for waffles, along with fresh in-season options that you plan to eat that week.

fresh in-season produce

Produce that is in season can essentially grow on its own without requiring excess labor, transportation, or other resources. These ideal conditions result in cheaper, tastier, and more nutritious produce. For example, broccoli grown during peak season is found to be higher in vitamin C than broccoli grown out of season. Produce that is out of season locally may have been imported from overseas and must be picked before it's fully ripe and chilled during transport, which reduces its flavor.

While grocery stores often offer specials on in-season produce, saving you money, another way to eat with the seasons is to purchase locally grown fruits and vegetables from a farmers market or get fresh, in-season produce delivered right to your door by your local agriculture association, often known as community-supported agriculture (CSA).

Use this table as a guide to shopping with the seasons so you get the most flavor and nutrition for your buck.

Typical seasons for common produce

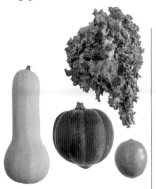
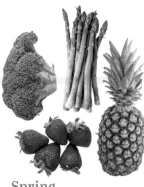
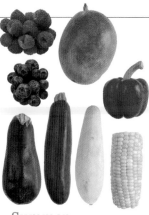
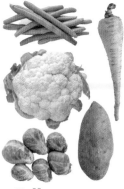

Winter

AVOCADOS

BEETS

COLLARD GREENS

GRAPEFRUIT

KALE

LEEKS

LEMONS

LIMES

RUTABAGA

SWISS CHARD

TURNIPS

WINTER SQUASH

Spring

APRICOTS

ASPARAGUS

BANANAS

BROCCOLI

CARROTS

CELERY

KIWIFRUIT

MUSHROOMS

PEAS

PINEAPPLE

RADISHES

SPINACH

STRAWBERRIES

Summer

BELL PEPPERS

BLACKBERRIES

BLUEBERRIES

CANTALOUPE

CHERRIES

CORN

CUCUMBERS

EGGPLANT

HONEYDEW MELON

MANGOES

OKRA

PEACHES

PLUMS

RASPBERRIES

SUMMER SQUASH

TOMATOES

WATERMELON

ZUCCHINI

Fall

APPLES

BRUSSELS SPROUTS

CABBAGE

CAULIFLOWER

CRANBERRIES

GRAPES

GREEN BEANS

PARSNIPS

PEARS

PEAS

POTATOES

PUMPKIN

RUTABAGA

SWEET POTATOES

Some produce is considered in-season year-round thanks to different growing regions in the US, greenhouses, and imports, including apples, avocados, bananas, cabbage, carrots, celery, cherry tomatoes, lemons, onions, and potatoes.

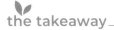 the takeaway

All produce is a good choice! Organic and conventional produce stack up similarly in the nutrition department. Frozen and canned produce are nutritious, affordable, and convenient options that are long-lasting. When it comes to fresh produce, shop with the seasons to reap benefits in nutrition and taste while also lowering your carbon footprint and saving money.

shopping for grains

Type matters when it comes to grains and health. Eating whole grains instead of refined grains has a plethora of benefits, including reduced risk of heart disease and type 2 diabetes and better weight management. I encourage you to cook with whole grains, and many types are listed in the table below; you can also choose breads and pastas made from whole grains for convenience.

Intact whole grains: Switch up your intact whole grains each week! Just like produce, each whole grain offers its own unique package of vitamins, minerals, antioxidants, protein, and fiber that work synergistically to support health. Oats, brown rice, and quinoa are great choices that I use in recipes throughout this book, but I encourage you to branch out into other types. Intact whole grains should have just one ingredient listed—the grain itself.

Bread: The bread aisle can be confusing. Just because a bread is brown instead of white doesn't automatically make it a healthy whole-grain choice. The best bread for health has whole grains listed as the first ingredient—whole wheat, quinoa, brown rice, wheatberries, or oats, for example.

My favorite bread is sprouted, which I buy frozen. Sprouted grains make the bread higher in protein and fiber and lower in carbohydrates while ensuring that the vitamins and minerals it contains are bioavailable, or easier for our bodies to digest, absorb, and utilize.

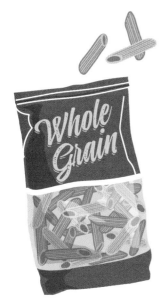

Pasta: Traditional pastas are made from refined grains that have been stripped of their nutrition, leaving only the starchy endosperm (carbohydrate), and then enriched with vitamins, minerals, and fiber. While this pasta has the taste and texture that many of us crave, I prefer 100 percent whole-grain pasta from a nutritional standpoint, as the grain retains its natural package of nutrition. Whole-wheat pasta is the most common type you'll find on grocery store shelves, but other varieties, such as brown rice pasta, buckwheat pasta, quinoa pasta, and teff pasta, are becoming more widely available. Look for those made with just one ingredient—the whole grain itself. While not made with whole grains, bean pasta and edamame pasta are also good options when you need a pasta fix that packs more protein.

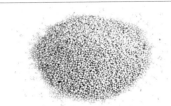

Amaranth

Similar to buckwheat and quinoa, amaranth is considered a pseudograin but is listed as a grain because of its similar nutritional profile and uses. It has a peppery taste, and is among the grains highest in protein (roughly 13 to 14 percent).

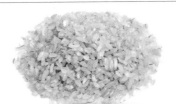

Bulgur*

Bulgur is made by boiling wheat and drying and cracking it into various sizes to turn it into a quick-cooking grain.

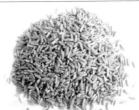

Kamut*

This rich, buttery-tasting whole grain is higher in protein than wheat and has more vitamin E.

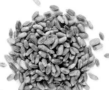

Barley*

Look for whole barley, hulled barley, or hull-less barley as opposed to lightly pearled barley, which is not considered whole because some of its bran layer has been removed.

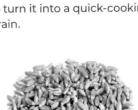

Farro*

This ancient grain has a nutty flavor and chewy texture and is among the highest-fiber whole grains.

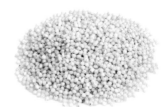

Millet

This whole grain has a delicate flavor that can be enhanced by toasting the dry grains before cooking.

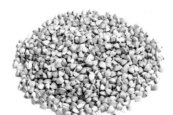

Buckwheat

Buckwheat is a cousin of rhubarb (a vegetable) and technically not a grain, but because it has a similar nutrition profile and appearance, it is classified as such. Besides being served as a side dish, it is used in pancake mixes as well as soba noodles.

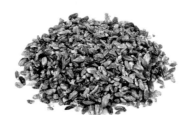

Freekeh*

Freekeh is harvested when young and green and then roasted, which gives it a smoky, earthy flavor. It is often sold cracked into smaller, quicker-cooking pieces.

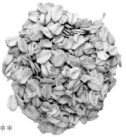

Oats**

Oats almost never have their bran and germ layers removed in processing, so if you see oats or oat flour on a label, it's almost guaranteed to be a whole grain. Oats contain a unique fiber called beta-glucan found to be especially effective in lowering cholesterol.

GLUTEN-CONTAINING GRAINS

The starred grains in the table contain gluten, which, as described in Chapter 1, is a protein best avoided by those with celiac disease, an autoimmune disease that affects about 1 percent of the population, and those with non-celiac gluten sensitivity, estimated to affect about 6 percent of the population.

**Oats are unique because although they are inherently gluten-free, they are frequently contaminated with wheat (a gluten-containing grain) during growing and harvesting. Certified gluten-free oats are required to have fewer than 20 parts per million of gluten, so they may be a safer option for those with celiac disease or non-celiac gluten sensitivity.*

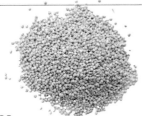

Quinoa

Quinoa is a botanical relative of beets and Swiss chard but is classified as a whole grain due to its comparable nutrition, taste, and uses. This light and fluffy grain is one of the only plant-based sources of complete protein. Rinsing quinoa before cooking removes some of the bitter saponin residue, a natural plant defense that helps ward off insects.

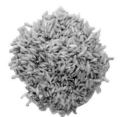

Rice

While white rice is a refined grain, whole-grain rice comes in a variety of colors in addition to brown, such as black, red, and purple. Wild rice is another whole-grain option.

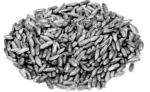

Rye*

Because of the high level of fiber in its endosperm (in addition to bran), rye generally has a relatively low glycemic index, meaning it will keep you satiated for longer. *Note:* When purchasing rye bread, look for "whole rye" or "rye berries" in the ingredients list to guarantee it's a whole-grain option.

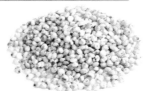

Sorghum

This naturally gluten-free grain has an impressive mix of phytonutrients and a high antioxidant level.

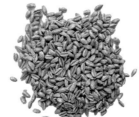

Spelt*

Spelt is a variety of wheat with a relatively high protein content and a mild taste. On the packaging, look for "whole spelt."

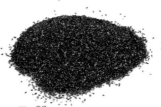

Teff

This type of millet has a sweet, molasseslike flavor. Cook this fine grain into porridge or grind it into flour to use in baked goods or pancakes.

grains

LEARN the labels

ENRICHED Nutrients have been added to the product. This is often done with foods like white bread or pasta that have been stripped of their nutrition in the first place. When given the option, opt for whole foods that still contain their natural package of nutrition.

MULTIGRAIN While these products sound good for you, this term simply indicates that the product is made with more than one type of grain—which can be a combination of several whole grains, several refined grains, or a mix of both.

WHEAT VS. WHOLE WHEAT The word "wheat" appears on both whole-grain and refined-grain foods; the difference is the inclusion of the word "whole." Look for "whole wheat" when identifying whole-grain foods.

the takeaway

Just like produce, switch up your whole-grain foods each week to get a new range of vitamins, minerals, and phytonutrients. Read ingredient lists to ensure that you are buying whole-grain foods instead of relying on front-of-package labels, which can be deceiving.

shopping for legumes

Legumes such as beans and lentils are an essential part of a mostly plant-based diet. Not only are they naturally fat-free and rich in plant protein, fiber, vitamins, minerals, and phytonutrients, but they count as both a protein and a vegetable, so you get the best of both worlds. For 10 cents a serving on average, they are both convenient and affordable. Aim for at least a half-cup per day to reap their benefits. Just like produce and whole grains, aim for variety to get a range of nutrients into your diet.

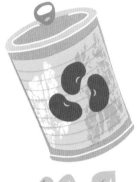

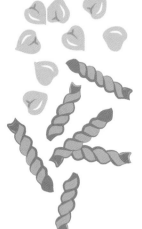

Canned beans beat the dried variety in the convenience department even though they cost three times more per serving (albeit are still very affordable!). Like many canned foods, canned beans can be sodium bombs, so look for those with no salt added or drain and rinse them well, which rids them of about half their sodium.

Dried legumes are superior in affordability. While they take much longer to cook, you can control the flavor, texture, digestibility, and salt content. The great part? You can cook up batches and freeze them. Refer to page 44 for the best way to cook dried beans.

Legume pastas have taken over supermarket shelves. Get your pasta fix and a serving of legume goodness at the same time with pastas made from chickpeas, red lentils, black beans, and more. While they typically have a chewier texture than traditional wheat pasta, they are a convenient way to bump up the protein on pasta night. Look for options made with just legumes—thankfully, there are many to choose from.

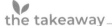

the takeaway

Make legumes a daily half-cup habit. No-salt-added canned beans that are drained and rinsed well are a convenient choice. For an even more affordable option where you control the flavor, texture, and digestibility, opt for dried legumes, and cook them in batches to freeze for future use.

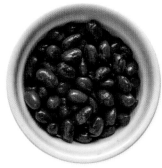

Black beans
Colored beans, including red and black, possess greater antioxidant activity than white beans.

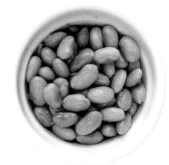

Pinto beans
The pinto bean is the most widely produced dry bean in the United States. These soft, creamy, earthy-flavored beans are perfect for burritos, burrito bowls, and tacos.

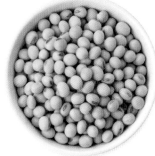

Soybeans
Soybeans are rich in isoflavones, which may help fight certain types of cancer (see page 46). They are also the only legume considered a complete protein.

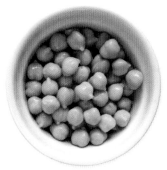

Garbanzo beans
Garbanzo beans, aka chickpeas, can be added whole to salads, soups, and stews; mashed and used in baked goods as a replacement for flour; roasted for a crunchy snack; or blended into homemade hummus.

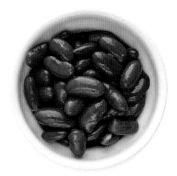

Red kidney beans
The firm texture of red kidney beans allows them to hold up well in soups, stews, and other dishes that cook for a long time. They also work well in cold bean salads.

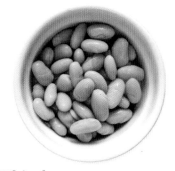

White beans
The term "white beans" is often used to describe navy beans, Great Northern beans, and cannellini beans. While these types vary slightly in flavor and size, they can often be used interchangeably because of their similar delicate flavor.

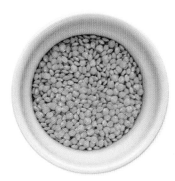

Lentils
Lentils pack more protein than most legumes with an average of 12 grams per ½-cup serving. They are also a good source of plant-based iron and folate.

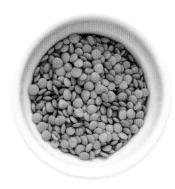

shopping for eggs

Eggs are a convenient source of complete protein on a mostly plant-based diet, and they offer an impressive package of bioavailable nutrients—but not all eggs in the grocery store are the same.

egg shell color—does it matter?

The first thing many people look at when shopping for eggs is the color. Are brown eggs better than white eggs, or vice versa? The answer is that egg nutrition has nothing to do with shell color; rather, it depends on how the hens are raised and what they are fed.

Generally speaking, brown-shelled eggs are laid by brown-feathered hens, while white-shelled eggs come from hens with white feathers. The reason brown eggs tend to cost more is that the hens that lay brown eggs are typically larger and eat more food. The recipes in this book call for large eggs, which are available from both brown-feathered and white-feathered hens.

While the most nutritious egg you can buy is pasture-raised, as explained in the box on the opposite page, all eggs from the grocery store offer valuable nutrition. Eggs are the lowest-cost animal source of protein, vitamin A, iron, vitamin B12, riboflavin, and choline.[2]

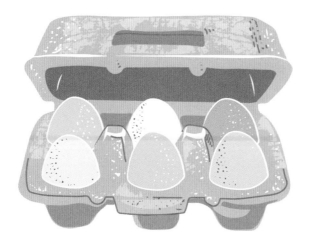

eggs

CAGE-FREE These eggs come from hens not confined to cages but allowed to roam in a room or open area, typically a barn or poultry house. They are not required to have access to the outdoors.

FREE-RANGE These eggs come from cage-free hens housed in a building, room, or area that allows continuous access to the outdoors during their laying cycle with at least 2 square feet of outdoor access on grass per hen. There is no specific dietary implication.

ORGANIC Organic eggs are laid by cage-free hens that are free to roam in their houses and have access to the outdoors. They are fed a diet of organic feed produced without conventional pesticides or fertilizers.

VEGETARIAN-FED

These eggs are laid by hens that are fed a vegetarian diet. The hens are kept in cages or in pens indoors and do not peck bugs or worms. Hens are natural omnivores, so a vegetarian diet isn't necessarily better.

OMEGA-3 ENRICHED

These eggs are laid by hens whose diets include things like flaxseed, algae, and fish oils to boost their omega-3 content from 30 milligrams per egg to 100 to 200-plus milligrams per egg. Most omega-3 enriched eggs also contain slightly less saturated fat.

PASTURE-RAISED

Pasture-raised is not yet a USDA-regulated term. However, if the egg label also includes "Certified Humane" and/or "Animal Welfare Approved" stamps, it means that each hen was given 108 square feet of outdoor space as well as barn space indoors. Because these hens can forage on grass and bugs in addition to commercial organic feed, their eggs tend to be the richest in certain nutrients, including vitamin E, vitamin A, and omega-3 fats, while being the lowest in saturated fat.

100% NATURAL OR ALL-NATURAL

All eggs must meet this criterion, so it is not a necessary label. It simply means that nothing was added to the egg, like flavoring or coloring.

NO ADDED HORMONES

Poultry producers are not allowed to give hormones to chickens, ever. If this language is used on a label, it must be accompanied by a statement making it clear that federal regulations ban the use of hormones.

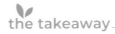

the takeaway

Brown and white eggs stack up similarly from a nutrition standpoint; they just come from different types of hens. While pasture-raised eggs are likely to be the most nutritious variety, all eggs offer valuable nutrition. On a mostly plant-based diet, you can be picky about your non–plant-based protein since it makes up a small part of your overall diet.

shopping for meat, poultry, and seafood

As discussed in Chapter 3, meat is treated more like a condiment than a mainstay on a mostly plant-based diet, but that doesn't mean you shouldn't be mindful of your choices. Here's how to pick the healthiest meat, poultry, and fish.

beef, bison, goat, lamb, pork & game meat

Choose lean and extra-lean cuts: While meat consumed mindfully can be a nutritious addition to a mostly plant-based diet because of its high-quality protein and bioavailable nutrients, opting for lean or extra-lean cuts will help keep your saturated fat intake in check. Choose cuts with minimal visible fat and those that contain the words "round," "loin," or "sirloin" on the package. Additionally, cuts graded "choice" or "select" tend to have less fat than "prime" cuts.

Fresh and frozen: Fresh and frozen meat are both smart options. Keep in mind that fresh beef, lamb, and pork steaks, chops, and roasts have a shelf life of 3 to 5 days in the refrigerator, and ground meat lasts 1 to 2 days. On the other hand, frozen beef, veal, lamb, and pork steaks, chops, and roasts have a shelf life of 4 to 12 months, and frozen ground meat lasts 3 to 4 months.[3]

Take quality into account: While the most nutritious meat you can buy is grass-fed (for beef and other ruminant meats) or pasture-raised (for pork), as explained below, it is not always feasible due to availability and/or cost. Know that all meat options offer valuable nutrition, including high-quality complete protein and bioavailable nutrients that are harder to get from plant foods, such as iron and zinc.

poultry— chicken, duck, turkey & game birds

Choose fresh poultry without skin: Poultry is a nutritious source of lean protein and one of the most popular animal proteins in the US (which is why I've included several recipes for it). Opt for skinless cuts and white (breast) meat over dark to limit your saturated fat intake.

Fresh and frozen: Fresh and frozen poultry are both smart options. Keep in mind that fresh ground poultry, whole poultry, and poultry pieces last for 1 to 2 days in the refrigerator. On the other hand, frozen ground poultry lasts for 3 to 4 months, and frozen whole poultry and poultry pieces last for 1 year and 9 months, respectively.[4]

meat

GRASS-FED Grass-fed cows (along with goats and lambs) are fed grass and forage (like hay) for the length of their life, which ultimately has an impact on the meat. Generally, grass-fed animal protein has more omega-3 fats and less saturated fat than grain-fed animal protein, as well as more vitamins A and E.

ORGANIC Animals are raised in living conditions that accommodate natural behaviors such as grazing on pasture, fed 100 percent organic feed and forage, and not administered antibiotics or hormones.

PASTURE-RAISED

Pork that is pasture-raised comes from pigs kept on pastures with the freedom to roam and forage outdoors instead of being confined indoors in a barn or feedlot. This results in nutritionally superior animal protein compared to its conventionally raised counterpart, just like grass-fed beef. Pasture-raised pork generally has more omega-3 fats and less saturated fat, as well as a higher level of vitamin D and antioxidants including vitamin E and selenium.

poultry

NATURAL The product contains no artificial ingredients or added color and is only minimally processed, meaning it was processed in a manner that does not fundamentally alter the product.[5]

ORGANIC The hens must be raised on 100 percent certified organic feed on pasture or roughages used as bedding that is also certified organic.

FREE-RANGE The hens are allowed access to the outdoors, the extent of which is unclear.

NO ADDED HORMONES

Growth hormones are banned from all poultry production, so there is no reason to put this language on a label.

PASTURE-RAISED

A pasture-raised chicken is given 108 square feet of outdoor space as well as barn space indoors. Because these hens forage on grass and eat bugs in addition to commercial organic feed, their meat is typically more nutritious with higher levels of omega-3 fatty acids.

fish and seafood

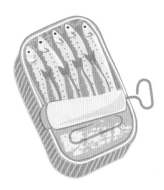

LEARN **the** labels

WILD-CAUGHT VS. FARMED

Wild-caught seafood is caught from a natural habitat such as a lake, ocean, or river, whereas farmed seafood is raised in large tanks. The nutrition quality of seafood is largely dependent on what the fish eats.

Fish in the wild eat a natural diet and tend to be slightly lower in saturated fat than their farm-raised counterparts. Farmed fish, on the other hand, can be slightly higher in omega-3 fatty acids due to the farms' fortified feed—so there may be advantages to both types. Wild-caught seafood is typically more expensive than farmed. Frozen and canned are more budget-friendly options than fresh.

fish & seafood

Incorporate lower methylmercury fish twice per week: Stick to mostly lower-mercury seafood such as scallops, clams, shrimp, oysters, sardines, tilapia, anchovies, and salmon. High-mercury fish that should be limited include king mackerel, ahi tuna, swordfish, tilefish, marlin, grouper, and Chilean sea bass.[6]

Fresh, frozen, and canned: Fresh, frozen, and canned fish are all smart options. Fin fish such as salmon, tuna, cod, halibut, sole, and trout have a shelf life of 1 to 3 days in the refrigerator or 2 to 8 months in the freezer, depending on the species. Shellfish like shrimp last for 3 to 5 days in the refrigerator or 6 to 18 months in the freezer. Canned fish is convenient, affordable, and just as nutritious as fresh and frozen and can last for up to 5 years in the pantry.

the takeaway

Incorporate fresh, frozen, or canned low-mercury seafood twice a week, and opt for lean cuts of meat and poultry. Studies suggest that grass-fed meat and pasture-raised poultry and pork may be better options from a nutritional standpoint than conventional varieties. Because grass-fed and pasture-raised options are not always readily available or affordable, know that all animal protein provides high-quality protein along with bioavailable nutrients such as zinc and iron.

shopping for dairy and nondairy swaps

As mentioned in Chapter 1, dairy is not off-limits on a mostly plant-based diet for those who choose to incorporate it mindfully and tolerate it well. Dairy foods provide three of the four nutrients of public health concern for the general US population—calcium, potassium, and vitamin D (dietary fiber is the fourth)—in addition to protein, vitamin B12, phosphorous, riboflavin, zinc, choline, magnesium, selenium, and other nutrients.

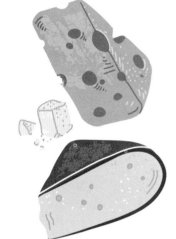

Cheese: All cheeses contain protein and calcium in addition to vitamins A and B12 and other nutrients. Because most types are high in saturated fat, cheeses should be consumed mindfully. Choose natural cheeses over processed, and opt for whatever types you enjoy. Aged hard cheeses tend to be lower in lactose (the sugar in milk that some people have trouble digesting) than fresh, soft cheeses.

Dairy and nondairy milks: Dairy milk provides 13 essential nutrients, including high-quality complete protein, calcium, phosphorus, and vitamins A and D. If you are lactose intolerant, opt for lactose-free milk, which is real dairy milk, so it offers the same nutrition. Additionally, emerging research suggests that the A1 protein in milk may be a cause of digestive discomfort for some people. A2 milk offers the same nutrition as real dairy milk but contains only the A2 protein and no A1 protein, so it may be easier to digest. Like meat, dairy is a source of saturated fat, so opting for lower-fat varieties will help you limit your intake.

LEARN the labels

dairy

ORGANIC Organic cattle must have access to grazing and consume grain on land that has not been treated with prohibited pesticides or fertilizers. Organic farmers are not allowed to administer antibiotics or hormones.

LACTOSE-FREE This dairy is free of lactose, the naturally occurring sugar found in milk that may be the cause of digestive discomfort in some people.

GRASS-FED Grass-fed dairy comes from cows that are fed a nearly 100 percent forage-based diet, which, like eggs and meat, results in milk that is higher in omega-3 fats.

A2 Regular cow's milk contains both the A1 and A2 proteins. A2 milk comes from cows that naturally produce only the A2 protein. Some research suggests that it may be easier for some people to digest.

That being said, if you aren't a dairy milk drinker, nondairy milks like oat, almond, and coconut can play the same role in meals and recipes. However, they don't offer the same nutrition as cow's milk. For example, while cow's milk offers 13 nutrients, two of which are added—vitamin A and vitamin D—store-bought almond milk contains four nutrients, calcium, vitamin A, vitamin D, and vitamin E, all of which are synthetic and added.

Nut milks like almond milk should be made with just two ingredients: nuts and water. However, this is not the case with most store-bought nondairy milks, which typically contain thickeners and stabilizers. If you can't make your own nondairy milks at home, look for unsweetened varieties with short ingredient lists.

For the recipes in this book that call for milk, you have the option to use dairy milk or the unsweetened nut milk of your choice.

Plain unsweetened kefir: This fermented cow's milk may be easier to digest than regular milk thanks to its naturally occurring probiotics and lower lactose content.

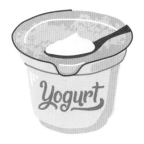
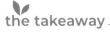

Plain unsweetened yogurt: Like dairy milk, opt for lower-fat yogurt to help you limit your saturated fat intake. Sweetened varieties can pack as much sugar as a candy bar, so plain unsweetened yogurt is the best option; you can naturally sweeten it yourself with fresh fruit.

the takeaway

Dairy foods offer significant nutrition and can be incorporated mindfully if you choose to and tolerate them well. Since you treat dairy as more of a condiment than a mainstay when following a mostly plant-based diet, choose dairy products that you enjoy and do well with.

shopping for pantry items

Having a well-stocked pantry makes cooking simpler, faster, and tastier. This section outlines some key ingredients.

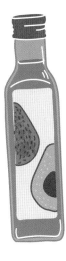

Oils and vinegars: Oils are fats that are liquid at room temperature. While oils are not a food group, they are a source of important nutrients such as unsaturated fats and vitamin E. Choosing unsaturated fat in place of saturated fat can reduce your risk of heart disease and improve "good" HDL cholesterol levels. In this book, I recommend and use avocado oil and extra-virgin olive oil because of their neutral taste, relatively high smoke points, and favorable nutritional profiles. Vinegars like apple cider, balsamic, red wine, and unseasoned rice can brighten up the flavor of food and add balance to a rich dish for anywhere from 2 to 15 calories per tablespoon.

Nuts, seeds, and nut and seed butters: Nut and seed butters often have the unnecessary addition of sugar and oils. Instead, look for one-ingredient butters. The same goes for whole nuts and seeds—opt for unsalted raw or dry roasted when possible.

MYTH BUSTING BOX

COCONUT OIL: SHOULD WE OR SHOULDN'T WE CONSUME IT?

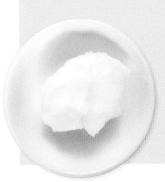

Coconut oil and other tropical oils, such as palm oil and palm kernel oil, are unique plant oils because they are considered solid fats like butter, lard, and shortening, which come from animals. One tablespoon of coconut oil has over 11 grams of saturated fat, which is close to the daily limit of 13 grams recommended by the American Heart Association for heart health.

However, in recent years, numerous studies have linked medium-chain triglycerides (MCTs), a type of saturated fat found in coconut oil, to potential benefits, such as weight loss and appetite control. However, most of the coconut oils sold in grocery stores have only 13 to 14 percent MCTs.

Despite these findings, the Dietary Guidelines for Americans and American Heart Association still advise limiting intake of all forms of saturated fat coupled with a higher intake of unsaturated fats, the type produced from plant foods such as nuts and seeds, until enough research shows otherwise.

Go nuts for nuts and seeds

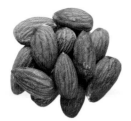

Almonds
Almonds are one of the highest-fiber nuts, which may contribute to their ability to reduce bad (LDL) cholesterol, thus mitigating coronary heart disease risk.

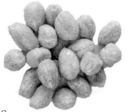

Peanuts
Botanically a legume but often classified as a nut, peanuts are the highest in protein in this list with 7 grams per 1-ounce serving.

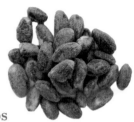

Pistachios
Pistachios are a complete plant protein with 6 grams per 1-ounce serving. Cracking open pistachio shells may slow you down during snack time and promote mindful eating.

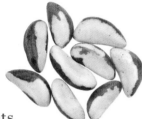

Brazil nuts
Think of Brazil nuts as your real-food daily selenium "supplement." With about 96 micrograms of selenium per nut, just 1 Brazil nut meets your entire daily need.

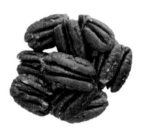

Pecans
This naturally sweet and buttery-tasting nut is among the highest in fat (the good kind) and lowest in carbohydrates.

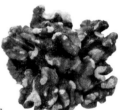

Walnuts
Walnuts are one of the few nuts that provide plant-based ALA omega-3 fatty acids.

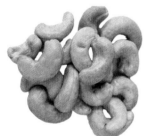

Cashews
Cashews are among the lowest-fat nuts and the highest in copper, an essential mineral that plays a role in a wide range of physiological processes, including iron utilization and fighting free radicals. When soaked and blended with water, they make a creamy, nutritious cheeselike sauce or filling (see page 286) without the dairy.

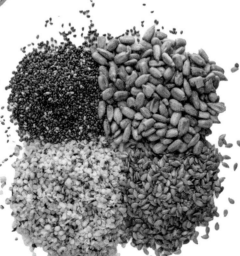

Chia seeds
Chia seeds are a fiber powerhouse with 10 grams per 1-ounce serving. These unique seeds can expand up to 10 times their weight in liquid, which makes them perfect for puddings (see page 138).

Hemp hearts
Though small, hemp hearts offer nearly 10 grams of plant-based protein per 3-tablespoon serving.

Sunflower seeds
Sunflower seeds are an excellent source of vitamin E, an essential nutrient and antioxidant that helps fight free radicals. Allergic to peanuts or tree nuts? Sunflower seed butter may be a suitable alternative.

Flaxseeds
Similar to walnuts, flaxseeds are a source of plant-based omega-3 fats. Ground flaxseed is easier to digest than the whole variety and can even make a plant-based "egg" replacement when combined with 3 parts water.

MYTH BUSTING BOX

WHAT ABOUT OMEGA-6 TO OMEGA-3 RATIO?

Most nuts and seeds are rich in omega-6 fats, with exceptions like walnuts, flaxseeds, hemp seeds, and chia seeds providing plant-based omega-3 fats (ALA). Both omega-6 and omega-3 fats are essential, meaning we need to get them from foods.

However, some experts argue that Western diets are too high in omega-6 fats and too low in omega-3s (largely due to the refined oils used to make processed and fried foods), with a ratio as high as 16.7:1. Studies suggest that this high ratio may promote the pathogenesis of many diseases, including cardiovascular disease, cancer, and inflammatory and autoimmune diseases, whereas increased levels of omega-3 fats (a low omega-6 to omega-3 ratio) may exert suppressive effects.[8]

The verdict? Since omega-3 fats are harder to come by in the diet, pay special attention to them daily, whether it means changing your cooking oil, aiming to meet your two servings of fish per week, or snacking on omega-3–containing nuts and seeds such as walnuts.

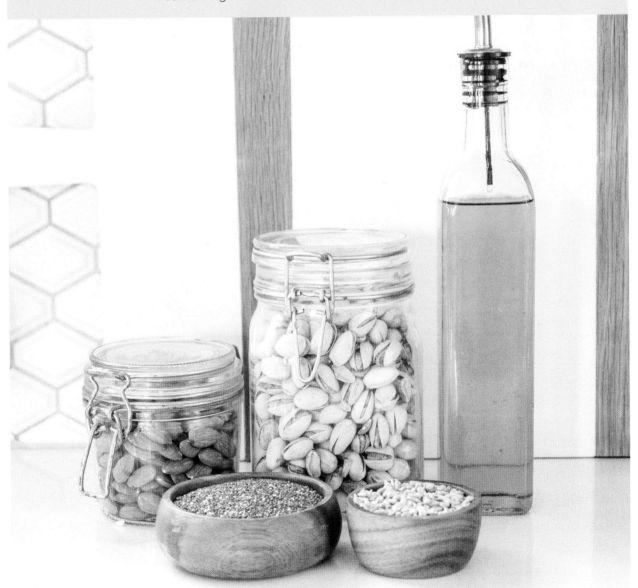

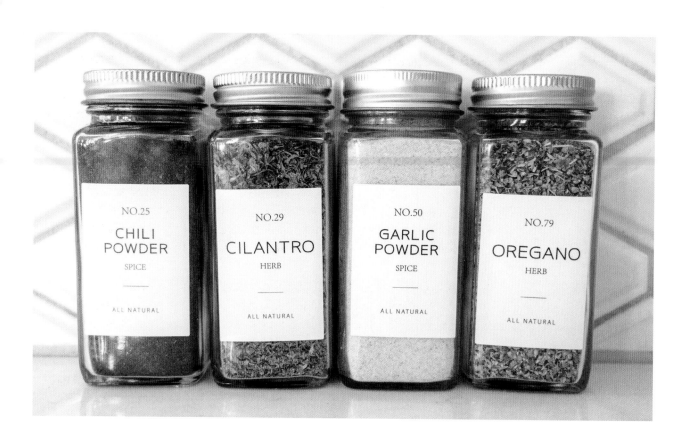

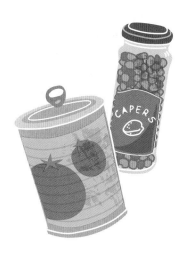

Canned and jarred foods: Nothing beats the convenience of jarred and canned foods such as canned diced tomatoes, olives, capers, and pumpkin puree. Stick to those with minimal additives, including salt and sugar.

Dressings, dips, sauces, and condiments: Finding healthy options that aren't packed with refined oils, artificial flavors, and added sugar is not nearly as difficult as it once was. Look for products made with real-food ingredients and nutritious oils like extra-virgin olive oil and avocado oil. For just a small investment of time, you can also make your own salad dressings (see page 110), pesto (see page 114), tzatziki (see page 128), and other basics.

Dried herbs, spices, and seasonings: Dried herbs and spices can jazz up meals and snacks for virtually zero calories. While most herbs and spices are nutritious options, be sure to read the labels of seasoning blends since they can contain added sugar, high sodium, and additives. Some of my favorite blends are no-sugar-added taco seasoning, Italian seasoning, everything bagel seasoning, and all-purpose seasoning. Dried herb and spice staples include black peppercorns, ground cinnamon, ground cumin, garlic powder, dried oregano, and dried thyme. I use ground pink Himalayan salt for general seasoning.

Nutritional yeast: This pantry staple adds a savory, umami flavor to recipes and is often used as a plant-based cheese substitute. This powdered product is the inactivated version of the same type of yeast used to bake bread and brew beer. It offers a wide array of vitamins, minerals, and antioxidants, including vitamin B12—a nutrient that's hard to get on a plant-based diet.

Broth: Besides adding flavor and depth to soups and stews, broths such as vegetable, chicken, and beef are easy ways to add flavor to cooked grains for little calories. Look for broth that is made with real-food ingredients and is low in sodium (with little to no added salt).

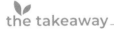

Flours: Naturally gluten-free flour options such as almond flour and coconut flour offer more whole-food-nutrition bang for your buck than refined white flour. Plus, because they have more protein and fiber, they won't spike your blood sugar as quickly or significantly. Whole-grain flours like buckwheat, oat, and quinoa are also nutritious options. Almond flour, coconut flour, and oat flour are used in recipes throughout this book.

Sweeteners: While sugar is sugar no matter what form it takes and should be limited for overall health and weight management, I like to stick to better-for-you options that I refer to as "sweeteners with benefits." In other words, they add the sweetness you want (to baked goods or oatmeal, for example) along with a sprinkling of vitamins, minerals, and antioxidants—not a reason to eat them regularly, but a bonus when you do. These are dates (or 100 percent date syrup), pure maple syrup, coconut sugar, and raw manuka honey.

the takeaway _____

Stock up on plant-based oils like olive and avocado and vinegars like balsamic and rice to make cooking nutritious meals at home simpler. Switch up your unsalted raw and dry roasted nuts and seeds weekly. When it comes to pantry items such as condiments, seasonings, broth, and nut butters, it's important to read labels and look for whole-food ingredients with little to no added salt and sugar. For baking, opt for nut flours, whole-grain flours such as oat, and "sweeteners with benefits" such as dates.

simple plant-based swaps to boost your nutrition

There are plenty of simple ways to boost nutrition without completely overhauling your diet. In fact, you can use these swaps to transform meals you may already be eating on a daily basis, without compromising flavor.

instead of this ➡ try this

BOXED BREAKFAST CEREAL ➡ Overnight oats or chia pudding (page 138)

GROUND BEEF ➡ Minced mushrooms or 50/50 Mushroom Meat (page 132)

REFINED WHITE FLOUR PIZZA CRUST ➡ Cauliflower pizza crust (page 254)

BUTTER IN BAKED GOODS ➡ Mashed avocado or cooked and pureed chickpeas (see page 328), black beans, or white beans

MASHED POTATOES ➡ Cauliflower Parsnip Mash (page 310)

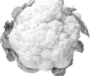

REFINED WHITE FLOUR HAMBURGER BUNS ➡ Portabella mushroom buns (page 252)

FRUIT SMOOTHIES ➡ All-Day Energy Smoothies (page 146) with mild-tasting vegetables like riced cauliflower and spinach, fruit, protein like Greek yogurt or plant-based protein powder, and nutritious mix-ins like oats, spirulina, or turmeric

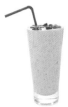

POTATO CHIPS ➡ Chickpea Poppers (page 230)

REFINED WHITE RICE ➡ Cauliflower rice (page 270)

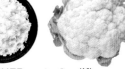

REFINED WHITE FLOUR ➡ Almond or oat flour

SODA ➡ Kombucha, prebiotic soda, or sparkling water with fresh fruit and herbs

SPAGHETTI ➡ Spiralized veggie noodles like zucchini or sweet potato, or spaghetti squash

helpful tools and equipment

The recipes in this book do not require many special tools beyond the basics, like mixing bowls, measuring cups and spoons, pots, pans, and baking sheets. However, there are a few specialty items that I think are worth the investment when eating mostly plant-based:

Air fryer: The latest and greatest tool to make its way into health-conscious kitchens, an air fryer helps you achieve that crunchy "fried" texture without the need for much or any oil, thus lowering the calories and fat. If you have an air fryer, you can use it to make several of the recipes in this book, including Plant Bacon (page 126), Baked Veggie Fries (page 210), Protein Pasta Chips (page 218), and Chickpea Poppers (page 230).

Blender: A high-powered blender not only is essential for smoothies, which can pack a boatload of nutrition (learn how to build an All-Day Energy Smoothie on page 146), but also comes in handy for fine grinding and pureeing soups, sauces, and dressings.

Food processor: Though they perform similar tasks, a food processor is better than a blender for shredding, slicing, finely chopping, and mincing foods.

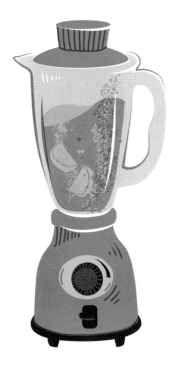

Salad spinner: When you eat mostly plant-based, you learn to love your veggies, including loaded everything-but-the-kitchen-sink salads. While a salad spinner takes up a lot of cabinet space, it is worth the real estate because it washes and dries your greens while keeping them fresh and crisp.

Spiralizer: If you love noodles, a spiralizer will be your best friend in a mostly plant-based kitchen. It transforms vegetables such as beets, carrots, sweet potatoes, yellow squash, and zucchini into a mild-tasting, naturally lower-calorie, fiber- and antioxidant-rich base for your favorite pasta fixings. Plus, it pays for itself in a week if you enjoy veggie noodles as much as I do; prespiralized options from the grocery store cost a lot more.

Waffle maker: A handy waffle maker can be used for more than just your standard boxed waffle mix. In addition to my Savory Zucchini Waffle Minis (page 144), you can quickly cook up hash browns, omelets, and more.

CHAPTER 5

21 days to mostly plant-based

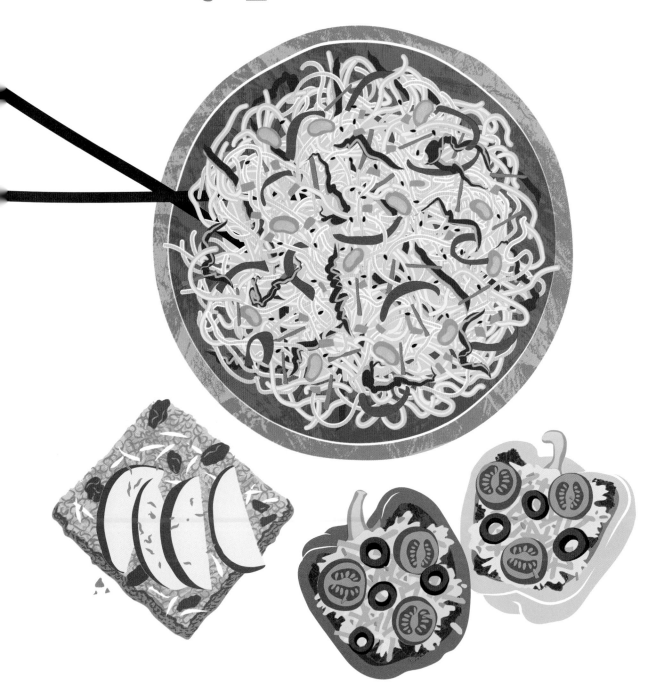

Now that you have the evidence-based reasons to follow a mostly plant-based diet and the tools to do so, it's time to dive into it in a realistic way that will set you up for a lifetime of success. This chapter gives you an easy-to-follow 21-day meal plan, complete with shopping lists. Here is what you can expect on this plan:

- The weeks progress from most animal protein–heavy to least (with every week being veggie-heavy) to help you ease into a mostly plant-based lifestyle. You can also treat the weeks like levels:
  - If you currently rely heavily on animal protein in your diet, then start with Week 1.
  - If you enjoy plant-based meals from time to time but want to strike a better balance between plant and animal foods, start with Week 2.
  - If you consider yourself a mostly plant-based eater and are looking to add more variety to your weekly meals or are wanting a reset after a vacation or holiday weekend, you can head to Week 3.

- Each week's meal plan is designed to serve two people. Recipes that yield four to six servings set you up to cook once and eat that dish two or three times that week. If you are following the plan on your own or you need to feed a family, feel free to halve or double the recipes.

- Keep in mind that meals are not necessarily portioned to your unique nutrition and energy needs, which are influenced by a range of factors, including your age, sex, weight, health status, and activity level. Instead, allow each week's plan to serve as a template for your meals, and feel free to increase or decrease the portion sizes as needed. An easy way to do so is to add or subtract from carbohydrate or protein portions. Additionally, rolling over leftover vegetables from the week before and serving them steamed or roasted is always welcome (and encouraged).

- I've set up these meal plans to include breakfast, lunch, and dinner, but I encourage you to have one or two snacks as well to help meet your daily energy and nutrition needs. Each week includes five snack ideas to choose from that you can enjoy between meals to help keep your energy levels up throughout the day.

- Some of the ingredients included in the shopping lists can be made from scratch using basic recipes from Chapter 6, such as pesto, pico de gallo, and tomato sauce. I've starred these ingredients for reference. If you choose to make them, be sure to add the ingredients to the week's shopping list. However, don't feel like you have to shy away from store-bought options for health reasons, as there are many products available made with high-quality whole-food ingredients. See pages 346 to 348 for my recommendations.

- The idea that you will have 21 uninterrupted days to follow this plan to a "T" may not be realistic for you. Use dining out and social gatherings as an opportunity to implement the mostly plant-based principles into your food choices. After all, this isn't a quick fix; it's a lifestyle choice. At the end of this chapter, you'll find tips for navigating menus at popular types of restaurants.

- Finally, think progress, not perfection. If this meal plan encourages you to add riced cauliflower to smoothies or try Meaty Mushroom Grounds (page 132) over beef once a week, then consider it a nutritional win.

Without further ado, I give you Week 1 of 21 days to mostly plant-based.

WEEK 1 easing into a mostly plant-based lifestyle

Start here if:

you currently rely heavily on animal foods such as meat, eggs, and dairy in your diet but want to experience the power of plants.

This week you will

- **Learn to love veggies.** Vegetables are so much more than steamed broccoli or wilted spinach. Once you learn how to prepare them in unique ways, such as turning them into waffles, pizza, and smoothies paired with other fresh and flavorful ingredients, you will find that they are actually the *most* exciting food group. And the best part—you will discover that eating more veggies makes you feel great.

- **Learn how to treat plants like meat.** You'll find that with the right marinating, seasoning, and cooking preparations, you can transform "meaty" plant-based ingredients such as mushrooms, eggplant, and lentils into what tastes like the real deal.

- **Learn that mostly plant-based doesn't have to be boring.** Eating mostly plant foods doesn't look like boring desk salads. In fact, it's the complete opposite. You can seamlessly transform vegetables into your favorite classic comfort foods, as you'll discover this week and in the weeks to come.

snack ideas

The week's meal plan does not include snacks, so be sure to add them to your grocery list. Pair fiber-rich fruit, vegetables, or whole grains with a protein or healthy fat source to build a satisfying snack with staying power. Here are five mostly plant-based snacks to help fuel you between meals this week:

- Customizable No-Bake Granola Bars (page 242)

- Sliced apple with natural nut or seed butter

- Sliced natural cheese with almond flour crackers (see page 236 for my recipe, or buy boxed crackers)

- Celery or mini bell peppers stuffed with cream cheese (regular or dairy-free) and topped with everything bagel seasoning

- Plain low-fat Greek yogurt with fresh berries

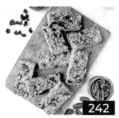

242

customizable
no-bake
granola bars

meal plan

	BREAKFAST	LUNCH	DINNER
MONDAY	basic breakfast burrito — 156	cauliflower potato shepherd's pie — 310	easy rotisserie chicken enchiladas — 268
TUESDAY	basic breakfast burrito — leftover	easy rotisserie chicken enchiladas — leftover	cauliflower potato shepherd's pie — leftover
WEDNESDAY	savory zucchini waffle minis — 144	avocado chicken salad — 190	easy taco soup — 204
THURSDAY	savory zucchini waffle minis — leftover	easy taco soup — leftover	baked feta vegetable pasta — 280
FRIDAY	brain booster avo toast — 166	pizza-stuffed peppers — 292	baked feta vegetable pasta — leftover
SATURDAY	berry blast smoothie — 146	baked feta vegetable pasta — leftover	pizza-stuffed peppers — leftover
SUNDAY	berry blast smoothie — leftover	BBQ chicken all-in-one loaded sweet potato meal — 274	greek salmon sheet pan meal — 246

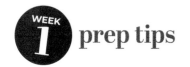

prep tips

The weekend before:

- Before grocery shopping, take inventory of the items you already have. Keep in mind that some ingredients from this week will carry over to Week 2.

- If you're going to make any of the starred items on the shopping list from scratch, make sure to add those ingredients to the list.

- To keep the proteins fresh, shred the rotisserie chicken and freeze 6 ounces, along with the chicken breasts, 2 pounds of ground beef, and the salmon. *Note:* If you prefer to buy these ingredients shortly before using them, you can do so on the following schedule:

  - The weekend before: Purchase the bacon, 1 pound of ground beef, and the rotisserie chicken.

  - Tuesday or Wednesday: Buy 8 ounces of chicken breasts and 1 pound of ground beef.

  - Thursday or Friday: Purchase 1 pound of ground beef.

  - Saturday or Sunday: Buy two 4-ounce salmon fillets.

- Slice four bananas, place in a freezer bag, and store in the freezer for the Berry Blast Smoothies on Saturday and Sunday.

- Make and freeze the Basic Breakfast Burritos to enjoy on Monday and Tuesday.

tip

Save your leftover ingredients! Use leftover vegetables before they go bad—steam or roast them and add them to meals throughout the week.

During the week:

TUESDAY	WEDNESDAY	THURSDAY	FRIDAY	SATURDAY
Defrost the chicken breasts and 1 pound of beef to be used tomorrow in the Avocado Chicken Salad and the Easy Taco Soup.		Defrost 1 pound of beef to be used tomorrow in the Pizza-Stuffed Peppers.		Defrost the 6 ounces of shredded rotisserie chicken and the salmon to be used tomorrow in the BBQ Chicken All-in-One Loaded Sweet Potato Meal and the Greek Salmon Sheet Pan Meal.

shopping list

Fresh produce:

Avocados, 3 medium

Bananas, 4 medium

Basil, 1 small bunch

Bell peppers, any color, 3 large

Cauliflower, 1 small head

Cherry tomatoes, 3 pints

Cilantro, 1 small bunch

Coleslaw mix, 1 (16-ounce) bag

Eggplant, 1 small

Garlic, 1 head

Lemons, 2

Lime, 1

Parsley, Italian, 1 small bunch

Pico de gallo, ½ cup*

Potatoes, baby, 1 pound

Potatoes, russet, 2 large

Potatoes, Yukon Gold, 2 medium (about 12 ounces)

Red onion, 1 medium

Spinach, 1 (10-ounce) bag

Sweet potatoes, 2 medium

Yellow onions, 2 medium

Yellow squash, 1 large

Zucchinis, 3 medium and 1 large

Frozen foods:

Berries, mixed, 2 (16-ounce) bags

Corn, 1 (12-ounce) bag

Mixed vegetables, such as peas, corn, and carrots, 1 (12-ounce) bag

Riced cauliflower, 1 (10-ounce) bag

Meat, poultry & seafood:

Bacon, 1 (8-ounce) package

Chicken breasts, boneless, skinless, 8 ounces

Ground beef, lean, 3 pounds

Rotisserie chicken, plain, 1

Salmon, skin-on, 2 (4-ounce) fillets

Sardines in water, 1 (3.75-ounce) can

Dairy, nondairy substitutes & eggs:

Cheddar cheese, sharp, 1 cup shredded

Eggs, 6 large

Feta cheese, 1 (8-ounce) block

Greek yogurt, plain, 1 (24-ounce) container

Mozzarella cheese, ⅔ cup shredded

Nut milk of choice, unsweetened, 2 quarts*

Parmesan cheese, grated, 1 (8-ounce) container

Pantry items:

Almond flour, blanched, 1 (16-ounce) bag

BBQ sauce, no added sugar, 1 (8.5-ounce) jar

Beef broth, low sodium, 1 (32-ounce) carton

Black beans, no salt added, 2 (15-ounce) cans

Black olives, sliced, 1 (2.25-ounce) can

Celery seeds, 1 jar

Chickpea rotini or other pasta of choice, 1 (14.5-ounce) box

Dijon mustard, 1 (8-ounce) jar

Greek seasoning, 1 jar

Marinara sauce, 1 (24-ounce) jar*

Pinto beans, no salt added, 1 (15-ounce) can

Sprouted bread, whole-grain, 1 loaf

Thyme, ground dried, 1 jar

Tomato paste, 2 (6-ounce) cans

Tomatoes, fire-roasted diced, 1 (14.5-ounce) can

Tortillas, whole grain, 10 (10-inch)

Pantry staples:

Avocado oil

Avocado oil mayonnaise

Baking powder

Black peppercorns

Chia seeds

Cinnamon, ground

Cumin, ground

Extra-virgin olive oil

Himalayan pink salt, finely ground

Honey

Italian seasoning

Maple syrup, 100% pure

Taco seasoning

Vanilla extract, pure

These ingredients will be used throughout the three weeks of the meal plan, so I suggest you purchase them (if you don't already have them on hand) along with the items you'll need for Week 1. These items aren't listed in the weekly grocery lists.

finding your mostly plant-based balance

Start here if:
you enjoy plant-based meals from time to time but want to strike a better balance between plant and animal foods.

This week you will

- **Realize you don't need animal protein at every meal to feel satisfied.** You will be incorporating one fully plant-based meal per day. Notice how this affects how you feel, your energy levels, and your meal satisfaction.

- **Reframe your approach to taco, pasta, and burger night.** You'll learn how to make over your weekly staple meals with a plant-forward twist.

- **Expand your plant-based recipe repertoire.** By this week, you will have tried a range of recipes that utilize plant-based ingredients in new and exciting ways intended to spark ideas for creative applications of ingredients you know and love.

snack ideas

The week's meal plan does not include snacks, so be sure to add them to your grocery list. Pairing fiber-rich fruit, vegetables, or whole grains with a protein or healthy fat source is the way to build a satisfying snack with staying power. Here are five mostly plant-based snacks to help fuel you between meals this week:

- Energy Bites 4 Ways (page 220)

- Sliced carrots with white bean hummus (see my recipe on page 120, or buy premade hummus)

- Whole in-season fruit like an apple, orange, or peach with a handful of raw or dry-roasted nuts

- Half a ripe avocado with almond flour crackers (see my recipe on page 236, or buy boxed crackers)

- Air-popped popcorn with a sprinkle of nutritional yeast

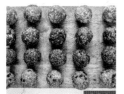

220

energy bites 4 ways

meal plan

	BREAKFAST	LUNCH	DINNER
MONDAY	morning glory baked oatmeal — 164	taco-stuffed zucchini boats — 282	rainbow veggie noodles — 256
TUESDAY	morning glory baked oatmeal — left-over	rainbow veggie noodles — left-over	italian spaghetti squash casserole — 298
WEDNESDAY	peanut butter cup smoothie — 146	italian spaghetti squash casserole — left-over	pesto salmon packets — 314
THURSDAY	peanut butter cup smoothie — left-over	pesto salmon packets — left-over	one-skillet greek chicken and veggies — 264
FRIDAY	grown-up pb&j overnight oats — 138	one-skillet greek chicken and veggies — left-over	summer shrimp sheet pan meal — 246
SATURDAY	grown-up pb&j overnight oats — left-over	everyday quinoa salad — 184	portabella bun double smash burgers — 252
SUNDAY	very veggie shakshuka — 154	portabella bun double smash burgers — left-over	everyday quinoa salad — left-over

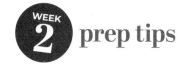

The weekend before:

- Before grocery shopping, take inventory of the items you already have. You should have some ingredients left over from Week 1. Keep in mind that some ingredients from this week will carry over to Week 3.

- If you're going to make any of the starred items on the shopping list from scratch, make sure to add those ingredients to the list.

- Slice four bananas, place in a freezer bag, and store in the freezer for the Peanut Butter Cup Smoothies on Wednesday and Thursday.

🌱
tip_____

Save your leftover ingredients! Use leftover vegetables before they go bad—you can steam or roast them and add them to meals throughout the week.

- To keep the proteins fresh, freeze the chicken breasts, the ground beef, and the salmon. *Note:* If you prefer to buy these ingredients shortly before using them, you can do so on the following schedule:

  - The weekend before: Purchase the ground turkey and the rotisserie chicken.
  - Tuesday or Wednesday: Buy the salmon.
  - Wednesday or Thursday: Purchase the chicken breasts.
  - Friday or Saturday: Buy the ground beef.

- Make the Morning Glory Baked Oatmeal and store in the fridge to enjoy for breakfast on Monday and Tuesday.

During the week:

MONDAY	TUESDAY	WEDNESDAY	THURSDAY	FRIDAY
	Defrost the salmon to be used tomorrow in the Pesto Salmon Packets.	Defrost the chicken breasts to be used tomorrow in the One-Skillet Greek Chicken and Veggies.	Prep four servings of Grown-Up PB&J Overnight Oats and place in the fridge to enjoy for breakfast on Friday and Saturday.	Defrost the beef to be used tomorrow in the Portabella Bun Double Smash Burgers.

shopping list

Fresh produce:

Apple, 1 medium

Asparagus, 2 pounds

Bananas, 4 medium

Basil, 1 small bunch

Bell peppers, red, 2 medium

Carrots, 1 pound

Cherry tomatoes, 2 pints

Corn, 2 ears

English cucumber, 1 small

Garlic, 2 heads

Green onions, 1 small bunch

Lemons, 2

Medjool dates, soft pitted, 4

Parsley, flat-leaf, 1 small bunch

Portabella mushrooms, about 4 inches in diameter, 9

Raspberries, 1 quart

Red cabbage, 1 small head

Red onion, 1 small

Spaghetti squash, 1 medium (about 3 pounds)

Spinach, 1 (10-ounce) bag

Yellow onions, 3

Yellow squash, 1 medium

Zucchini noodles, 3 cups

Zucchinis, 6 medium

Frozen foods:

Edamame, shelled, 1 (12-ounce) bag

Riced cauliflower, 1 (10-ounce) bag

Shrimp, large, peeled and deveined, 8 ounces

Meat, poultry & seafood:

Chicken breasts, boneless, skinless, 1 pound

Ground beef, lean, 1 pound

Ground turkey, lean, 1½ pounds

Rotisserie chicken, plain, 1

Salmon, skin-on, 1 (1-pound) fillet

Dairy, nondairy substitutes & eggs:

Almond milk, unsweetened, 1 gallon

Cheddar cheese, shredded, 1 (8-ounce) bag

Eggs, 4 large

Greek yogurt, plain, nonfat, 1 pint

Mozzarella cheese, shredded, 1 (8-ounce) bag

Pantry items:

All-purpose seasoning, 1 jar

Applesauce, unsweetened, 1 (4-ounce) single-serving cup

Artichoke hearts, quartered, 1 (14-ounce) can

Balsamic vinegar, 1 (16-ounce) bottle

Black beans, no salt added, 1 (15-ounce) can

Chickpeas, 1 (15-ounce) can

Chocolate plant-based protein powder, 1 tub

Cocoa powder, unsweetened, 1 (8-ounce) container

Dill relish, 1 small jar

Kalamata olives, sliced, 1 (12.3-ounce) jar

Marinara sauce, 1 (24-ounce) jar*

Mustard, spicy brown, 1 (8-ounce) jar

Orzo, 1 (16-ounce) bag

Paprika, 1 jar

Peanut butter, creamy, natural, 1 (12-ounce) jar

Peanut sauce, 1 (11-ounce) jar*

Peanuts, roasted, ¼ cup

Pesto, 1 (6-ounce) jar*

Quinoa, any color, 1 (16-ounce) bag

Raisins, 1 (12-ounce) box

Rolled oats, 1 (18-ounce) carton

Shredded coconut, unsweetened, 1 (12-ounce) bag

Tomatoes, crushed, 1 (28-ounce) can

Tomatoes, fire-roasted, 1 (14.5-ounce) can

WEEK 3 mostly plant-based for life

Start here if:

you consider yourself a mostly plant-based eater and are looking to add more variety to your weekly meals or wanting a reset after a vacation or holiday weekend.

This week you will

- **Realize you can feel satiated and energized on mostly plant-based foods.** You will realize that you don't need animal protein to be included in every meal to feel full. You'll harness the power of plant fiber, plant protein, and good fats.

- **Learn to live with less dairy.** Dairy foods can be hard to limit—especially cheese, which is a mainstay of classic comfort foods like pizza, tacos, and pasta dishes. Of course, on a mostly plant-based diet, dairy is fine in moderation. But this week, you will learn some plant-based subs for classic dairy ingredients.

- **Gain kitchen confidence and momentum to live mostly plant-based.** By this week, you should feel excited and confident about incorporating more plant-based foods into your diet because of the taste, variety, and the way it makes you feel.

snack ideas

The week's meal plan does not include snacks, so be sure to add them to your grocery list. Pairing fiber-rich fruit, vegetables, or whole grains with a protein or healthy fat source is the way to build a satisfying snack with staying power. Here are five mostly plant-based snacks to help fuel you between meals this week:

- Chickpea Poppers 6 Ways (page 230)

- Edamame with a piece of in-season fruit such as an apple, peach, or mango

- Mini bell peppers or endive leaves stuffed with white bean hummus (see my recipe on page 120, or buy premade hummus)

- Frozen grapes and a handful of raw or dry-roasted nuts

- Olive, cherry tomato, and basil bites (simply skewer with toothpicks)

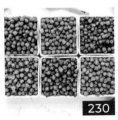

chickpea poppers
6 ways

meal plan

	BREAKFAST	LUNCH	DINNER
MONDAY	naturally sweetened banana oat pancakes — 142	hummus and veggie no-bread wrap — 266	chipotle burrito bowl with cauliflower rice — 270
TUESDAY	naturally sweetened banana oat pancakes (leftover)	mediterranean medley salad jar — 176	cauliflower cashew ricotta–stuffed shells — 286
WEDNESDAY	apple cinnamon chia pudding — 138	cauliflower cashew ricotta–stuffed shells (leftover)	burrito all-in-one loaded sweet potato meal — 274
THURSDAY	apple cinnamon chia pudding (leftover)	chickpea tuna-less salad — 260	chicken fajitas sheet pan meal — 246
FRIDAY	blueberry almond customizable blender oat cups — 158	chickpea tuna-less salad (leftover)	veggie chili — 188
SATURDAY	blueberry almond customizable blender oat cups (leftover)	zucchini noodle lasagna — 272	veggie chili (leftover)
SUNDAY	blueberry almond customizable blender oat cups (leftover)	veggie chili (leftover)	zucchini noodle lasagna (leftover)

The weekend before:

- Before grocery shopping, take inventory of the items you already have. You should have some ingredients left over from Week 2.

- If you're going to make any of the starred items on the shopping list from scratch, make sure to add those ingredients to the list.

- To keep the proteins fresh, freeze the beef in one 1-pound portion and one 6-ounce portion, and freeze 8 ounces of the chicken. *Note:* If you prefer to buy these ingredients shortly before using them, you can do so on the following schedule:

  - The weekend before: Purchase 6 ounces of chicken breasts.
  - Tuesday or Wednesday: Purchase 6 ounces of ground beef.
  - Wednesday or Thursday: Purchase 8 ounces of chicken breasts.
  - Friday or Saturday: Buy 1 pound of ground beef.

🌱
tip_____

Save your leftover ingredients! Use leftover vegetables before they go bad—you can steam or roast them and add them to meals throughout the week.

During the week:

MONDAY	TUESDAY	WEDNESDAY	THURSDAY	FRIDAY
Prep four servings of Apple Cinnamon Chia Pudding and place in the fridge to enjoy for breakfast on Wednesday and Thursday.	Defrost the 6-ounce portion of beef to be used tomorrow in the Burrito All-in-One Loaded Sweet Potato Meal.	Defrost the chicken to be used tomorrow in the Chicken Fajitas Sheet Pan Meal.		Defrost the 1-pound portion of beef to be used tomorrow in the Zucchini Noodle Lasagna.

shopping list

Fresh produce:

Apples, 2 medium

Arugula, 1 (10-ounce) bag

Bananas, 2 medium

Basil, 1 small bunch

Bell pepper, red, 1 medium

Bell peppers, any color, 2

Bell peppers, green, 2 medium

Carrots, shredded or julienned, 1 (10-ounce) bag

Cauliflower, 1 medium head and 1 large head

Celery, 1 small bunch

Cherry tomatoes, 1 pint

Cilantro, 1 small bunch

Cucumbers, Persian, 1 pound

Garlic, 1 head

Guacamole, 1 (10-ounce) container*

Hummus, roasted red pepper, 1 (10-ounce) container*

Lettuce, romaine, 2 heads

Lime, 1

Microgreens, 1 (8-ounce) container

Parsley, flat-leaf, 1 small bunch

Pico de gallo, 1 (14-ounce) tub*

Red onions, 3

Roma tomatoes, 2

Romaine lettuce, 2 heads

Sweet potatoes, 2 medium

Yellow onions, 2 medium

Zucchinis, 4 large

Frozen foods:

Blueberries, 1 (16-ounce) bag

Corn, 1 (12-ounce) bag

Meat, poultry & seafood:

Chicken breasts, boneless, skinless, 14 ounces

Ground beef, lean, 1 pound 6 ounces

Dairy, nondairy substitutes & eggs:

Almond milk, unsweetened, 2 quarts

Eggs, 3 large

Feta cheese, crumbled, 1 (6-ounce) container

Mozzarella cheese, shredded, 1 (8-ounce) bag

Plant-based parmesan, ¼ cup*

Ricotta cheese, part skim, 1 (15-ounce) container

Pantry items:

Almonds, sliced, ¼ cup

Applesauce, unsweetened, 2 (4-ounce) single-serving cups

Balsamic vinaigrette, 1 (16-ounce) bottle*

Black beans, no salt added, 1 (15-ounce) can

Cashews, raw, 1 cup

Chickpeas, no salt added, 2 (15-ounce) cans

Chili powder, 1 jar

Chipotle powder, 1 jar

Coconut oil, 1 (14-ounce) jar

Dill relish, 1 small jar

Farro, 1 (24-ounce) bag

Flaxseed meal, 1 (16-ounce) bag

Jumbo pasta shells, 1 (12-ounce) box

Kalamata olives, whole, pitted, 1 (12.3-ounce) jar

Kidney beans, no salt added, 1 (15-ounce) can

Marinara sauce, 2 (24-ounce) jars*

Nutritional yeast, 1 (4.5-ounce) container

Onion powder, 1 jar

Pecans, raw, 1 (4-ounce) bag

Pinto beans, no salt added, 1 (15-ounce) can

Rolled oats, 1 (18-ounce) carton

Tomatoes, fire-roasted, 1 (14.5-ounce) can

Tortillas, corn, 4 (6-inch)

beyond the 21 days

If there is one takeaway after these 21 days, it is this: think plants first. I call it my "crowding-out principle" because when you add enough of the good stuff (plant-based ingredients), you crowd out the "bad stuff." Let this principle guide the way you plan meals, cook, and order out. When you choose plant foods first and incorporate animal protein mindfully, plant foods naturally crowd out the rest.

dining out

Dining out can be challenging when you want to make good choices for your health. But let's face it, many of us don't have the time or the energy to cook every meal from scratch. Thankfully, there are nutrient-forward ways to order meals that allow you to enjoy what that cuisine is known for (like smoky pulled pork at a BBQ joint, or a juicy burger at an American restaurant) but still get the nourishment your body needs while not feeling deprived.

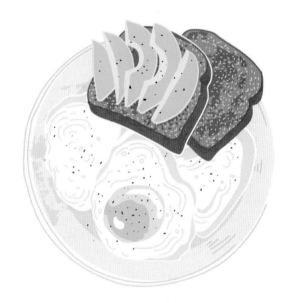

- **American:** Grass-fed (if available) burger wrapped in a lettuce "bun" with extra vegetable toppings (tomatoes, onions, pickles, lettuce) and sauce on the side, served with a house salad, dressing on the side. Order a side of sweet potato (or regular) fries to share with the table, if desired.

- **BBQ:** Pulled pork, smoked turkey, white-meat chicken, or naked brisket, no bun, with sauce on the side, served with a side of a vinegar-based coleslaw or cucumber onion salad, sautéed collard greens, or green beans.

- **Brazilian BBQ:** Start the meal at the salad bar and load up on the deliciously prepared vegetable and grain options, which will fill you up on the good stuff first. End the meal with a modest meat portion.

- **Breakfast/brunch diner:** Omelet made with one whole egg + two egg whites, vegetables, and cheese (for taste, if desired), with a side of whole-grain toast or home fries. Or swap the omelet for one over-easy egg + two egg whites and a side of avocado.

- **Chinese:** Stir-fried chicken or shrimp with broccoli and other mixed vegetables. Or enjoy half a serving of your favorite protein dish such as orange chicken, kung pao chicken, or Mongolian beef with a side of sautéed mixed vegetables and steamed brown rice.

- **Coffee shop:** Oatmeal with fresh fruit and nuts, whole-grain avocado toast (if available), or plain yogurt with a side of fresh fruit.

- **Deli:** Choose a lean cut of meat such as turkey or chicken breast and whole-grain bread. Pile on the vegetables, like spinach, pickles, tomatoes, cucumbers, bell peppers, and onions. Ask for hummus instead of mayonnaise or avocado instead of cheese, if available.

- **Greek/Middle Eastern:** Deconstructed gyro over a Greek salad, with dressing on the side. Tabbouleh, hummus, tzatziki, and baba ghanoush are nutritious dip options.

- **Italian:** Pasta primavera (cheese on the side), eggplant Parmigiana, minestrone, grilled calamari, or fresh fish with steamed vegetables.

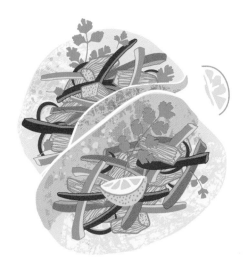

- **Mexican (sit-down):** Chicken fajitas with corn tortillas and extra vegetables instead of rice, or a chicken taco salad with dressing on the side.

- **Mexican (takeout):** Burrito bowl with brown rice and a lettuce base, including all available vegetable toppings (fajita vegetables, corn salsa, fresh tomato salsa), guacamole, and chicken, if desired.

- **Pizzeria:** Veggie lover's pizza on cauliflower crust (if available), whole-wheat crust (if available), or regular thin crust.

- **Steakhouse:** Choose one of the lean cuts (which typically contain the words "round," "loin," or "sirloin"), plus a side salad with vinaigrette on the side and a baked sweet potato.

- **Sushi:** Salmon avocado roll or sashimi with low-sodium soy sauce and a side of steamed brown rice. Miso soup and edamame are nutritious starters.

- **Thai:** Summer rolls, chicken satay, tom yum soup, chicken larb, or a stir-fry.

- **Vietnamese:** Fresh spring rolls, shrimp salad, or chicken or vegetable pho.

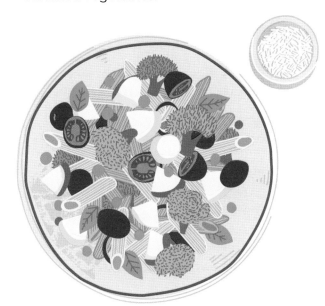

travel foods

Eating well while you're traveling can be tricky too. Here are some tips for making nutritious mostly plant-based choices on the go.

Airports snacks/road trip convenience stores:

- Air-popped popcorn
- Apples
- Bananas
- Dark chocolate
- Hummus with whole-grain pita or sliced veggies
- Pickles
- Plain Greek yogurt
- Raw or dry-roasted nuts
- String cheese
- Unsweetened dried fruit

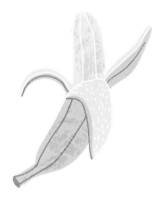

Some recipes from this book that travel well in a small cooler:

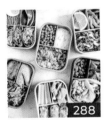 **288**

adult lunch box
6 ways

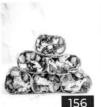 **156**

basic breakfast
burritos

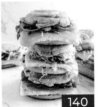 **140**

customizable
make-ahead
freezer breakfast
sandwiches

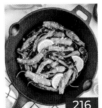 **216**

lemony blistered
shishitos

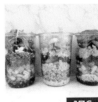 **176**

salad jars 6 ways

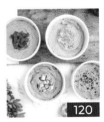 **120**

white bean
hummus
4 ways with
sliced veggies

Some recipes from this book that travel well without a cooler:

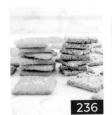 **236**

3-ingredient
almond flour
crackers 2 ways

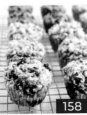 **158**

customizable
blender oat cups
6 ways

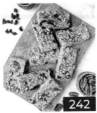 **242**

customizable
no-bake
granola bars

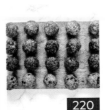 **220**

energy bites
4 ways

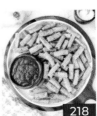 **218**

protein pasta
chips

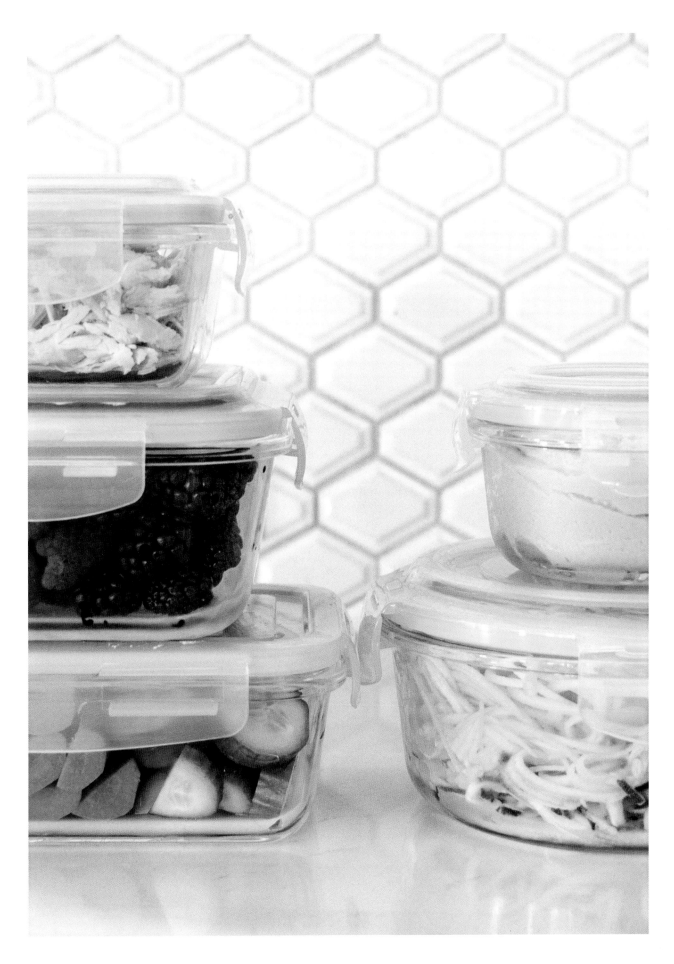

10-ingredient or less mostly plant-based recipes

CHAPTER 6:

basics

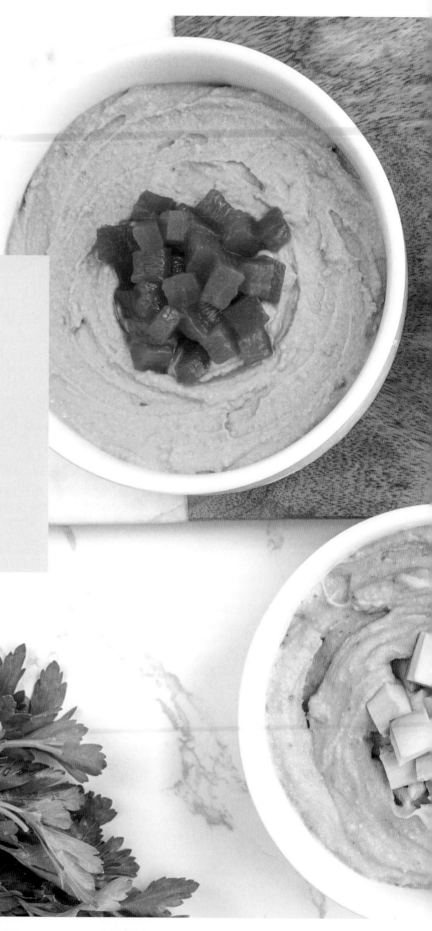

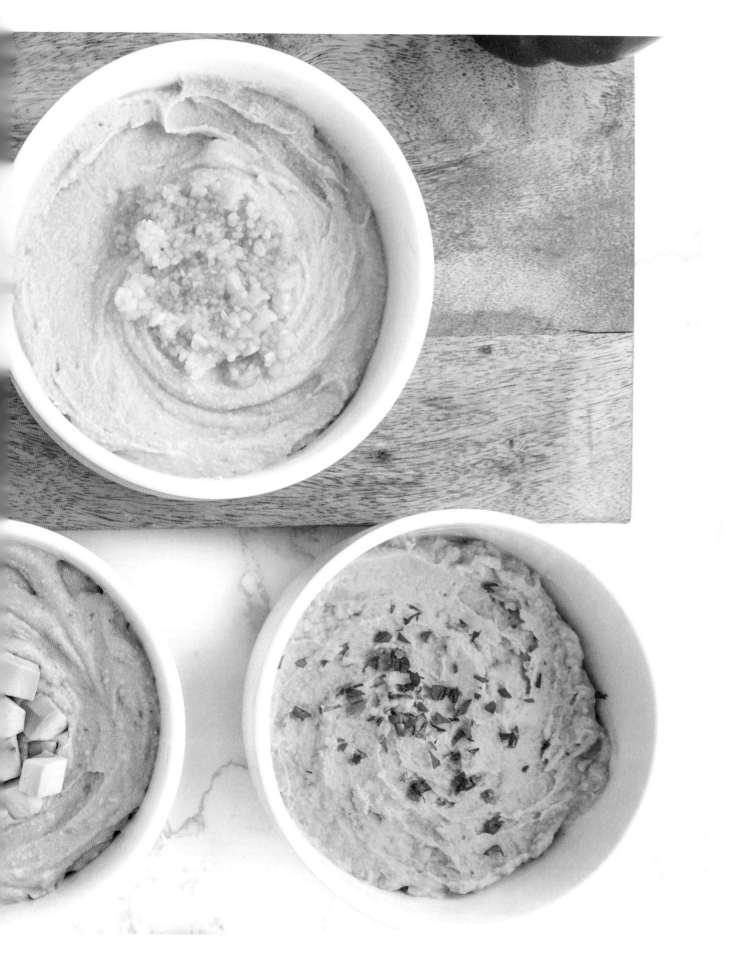

6 everyday dressings/dips

yield: 1 cup (2 tablespoons per serving)   prep time: 5 minutes

A fresh and flavorful dressing can go a long way toward making eating vegetables exciting. Store-bought dressings are often high in added sugar and fat, while the healthier options are typically accompanied by a premium price tag. The good news is that dressings are easy to make at home using staple ingredients.

balsamic vinaigrette:

⅓ cup extra-virgin olive oil

3 tablespoons balsamic vinegar

1 clove garlic, minced

1 teaspoon Dijon mustard

⅛ teaspoon ground black pepper

Finely ground Himalayan pink salt

fat-free honey dijon dressing:

½ cup cooked white beans (see page 44)

¼ cup Dijon mustard

¼ cup water

1 tablespoon apple cider vinegar

1 tablespoon raw manuka honey

⅛ teaspoon ground black pepper

Finely ground Himalayan pink salt

peanut dressing/dip:

¼ cup natural creamy peanut butter

1 tablespoon unseasoned rice vinegar

1 tablespoon lime juice

1 tablespoon toasted sesame oil

1 tablespoon raw manuka honey

1 clove garlic, minced

¼ teaspoon red pepper flakes

⅛ teaspoon ginger powder

2 tablespoons water

Finely ground Himalayan pink salt

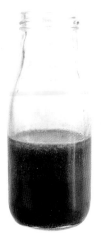 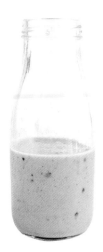 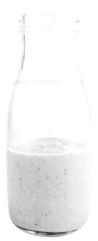

plant-based avocado green goddess dressing:

1 cup loosely packed fresh flat-leaf parsley leaves

½ cup fresh basil leaves

½ cup fresh dill fronds

2 cloves garlic, peeled

2 teaspoons capers

1 large ripe avocado

2 tablespoons avocado oil

1 tablespoon lemon juice

1 tablespoon apple cider vinegar

¼ cup water

Finely ground Himalayan pink salt

plant-based caesar dressing:

½ cup tahini

2 tablespoons extra-virgin olive oil

2 tablespoons lemon juice

2 cloves garlic, minced

2 teaspoons capers plus 2 teaspoons caper brine

2 teaspoons Dijon mustard

¼ teaspoon ground black pepper

¼ cup water

Finely ground Himalayan pink salt

yogurt ranch dressing:

1 cup plain 2% Greek yogurt

2 cloves garlic, minced

½ teaspoon onion powder

½ teaspoon ground black pepper

1 teaspoon dried dill weed

2 tablespoons water

2 teaspoons lemon juice

Finely ground Himalayan pink salt

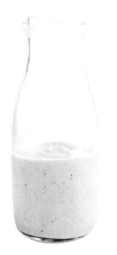

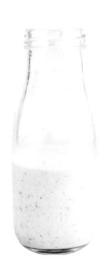

note _____

For a dairy-free ranch dressing: Replace the yogurt with ¼ cup of lemon juice and ¼ cup of tahini.

1. Place all of the ingredients, except the salt, in a blender or food processor and blend until smooth. Add more water 1 teaspoon at a time to thin the dressing to the desired consistency. Season with salt to taste.

2. Store the dressing in a sealed container in the refrigerator for up to 5 days.

oat milk

yield: **3 cups (1 cup per serving)**   prep time: **5 minutes**

Love oat milk but not the premium price tags or long lists of ingredients of the store-bought varieties? Make your own with just a few simple ingredients. This homemade version is silky-smooth and creamy—perfect for adding to coffee, oatmeal, and baked goods.

1 cup rolled oats

3 cups cold water

1 teaspoon pure vanilla extract

Pinch of finely ground Himalayan pink salt

1 soft pitted medjool date, for sweetness (optional)

1. Place all of the ingredients in a blender and blend just until you can't see the oats anymore, 20 to 30 seconds. Do not overblend.

2. Place a nut milk bag, fine-mesh strainer, or clean kitchen towel over a large bowl and strain the milk.

3. Strain once more. This will help ensure the milk is super smooth and creamy.

4. Store in a sealed jar in the refrigerator for up to 2 weeks.

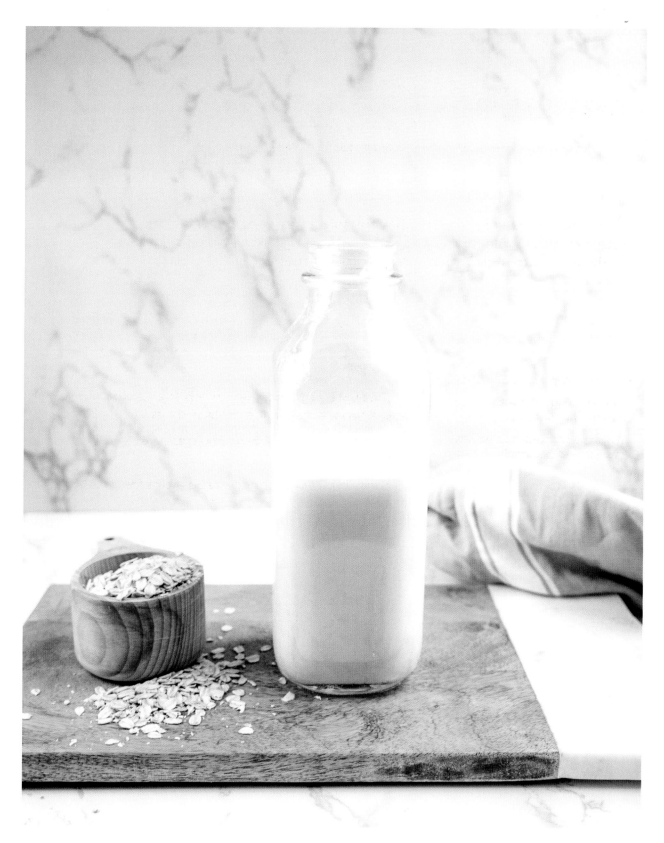

any greens basil pesto

yield: 1 cup (2 tablespoons per serving)   prep time: 10 minutes

Add earthy flavor to roasted vegetables, grilled proteins, and pasta dishes with this "any greens" basil pesto. It has all the makings of a traditional pesto with your chance to customize using whatever leafy green you have in the fridge.

⅓ cup pine nuts, lightly toasted

2 cloves garlic, peeled

1 cup packed fresh basil leaves

1 cup packed leafy greens of choice, such as baby kale, spinach, or arugula

⅓ cup grated Parmesan cheese or plant-based parmesan, store-bought or homemade (page 124)

¼ cup extra-virgin olive oil

Juice of ½ lemon

¼ teaspoon finely ground Himalayan pink salt

1. Put the pine nuts and garlic in a food processor and pulse until coarsely chopped, about 10 seconds.

2. Add the basil and greens and pulse until relatively smooth, about 30 seconds.

3. Add the cheese, oil, lemon juice, and salt and process until smooth. If the pesto is too thick, add water 1 teaspoon at a time to thin it to the desired consistency.

4. Store in a sealed container in the refrigerator for up to a week. You can also freeze the pesto in an ice cube tray. Once frozen, store the cubes in a freezer bag or other freezer-safe container for up to 4 months.

note _____

No pine nuts, no problem! Replace them with an equal amount of coarsely chopped almonds, walnuts, pistachios, or cashews.

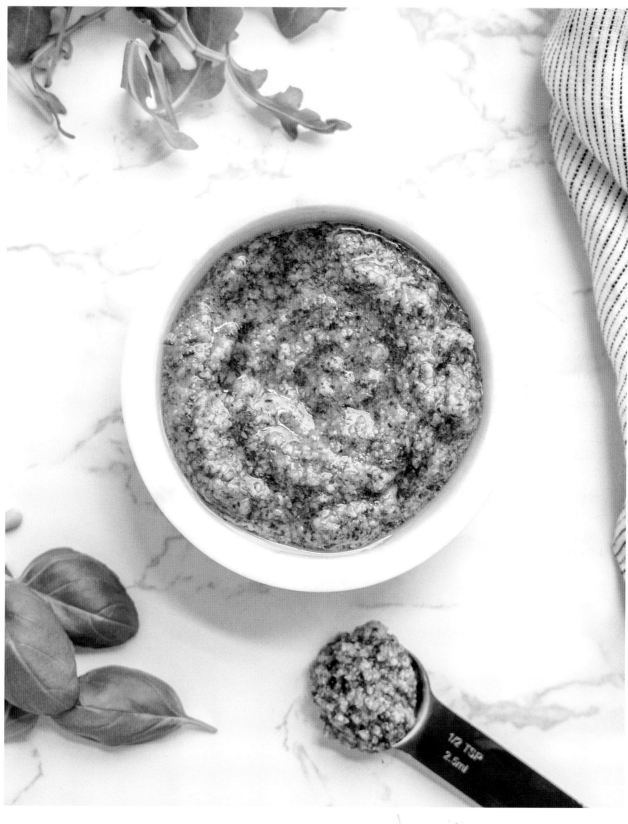

quick pico de gallo

yield: 2 cups (¼ cup per serving)   prep time: 15 minutes

Add fresh, low-calorie flavor to tortilla chips, burrito bowls, scrambled eggs, and more with a quick and flavorful homemade pico de gallo. Unlike traditional salsa, which has more liquid and is often cooked, pico de gallo is made with raw ingredients.

4 Roma tomatoes, diced

1 clove garlic, minced

½ medium red onion, diced

¼ cup chopped fresh cilantro

2 tablespoons lime juice

1 teaspoon diced jalapeño pepper (optional)

Finely ground Himalayan pink salt

Combine the tomatoes, garlic, onion, cilantro, lime juice, and jalapeño, if using, in a medium bowl. Season with salt to taste. Serve immediately, or, for best flavor, chill the pico in the fridge for a few hours before serving. Store in a sealed container in the refrigerator for up to 3 days.

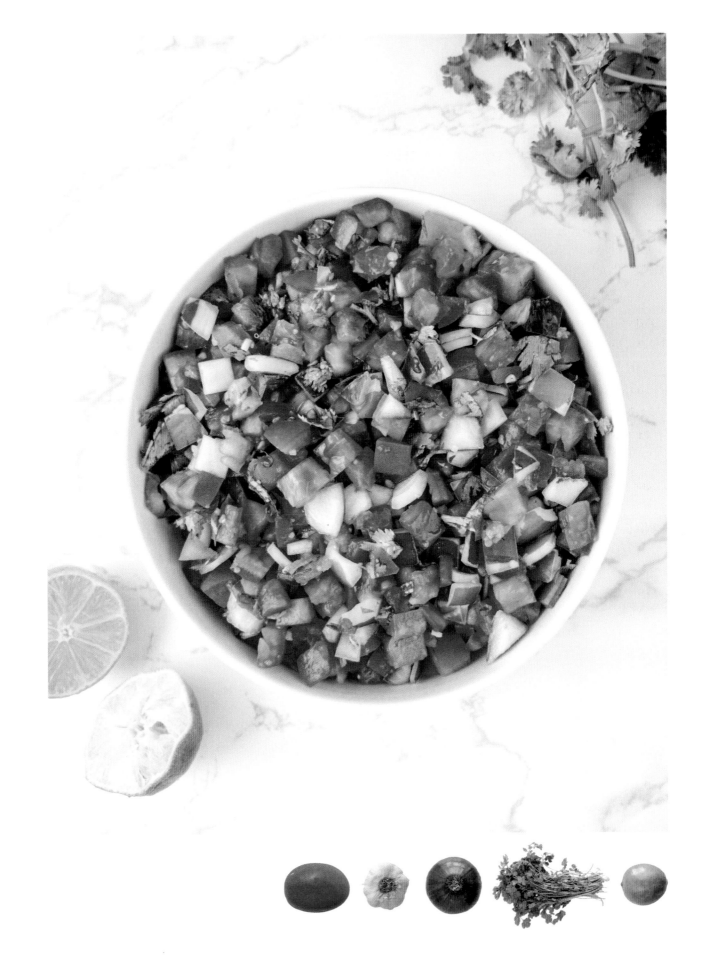

basic guacamole

yield: 1½ cups (¼ cup per serving)   prep time: 15 minutes

Guacamole is for more than just tortilla chips. Use it as a nutritious topping for Loaded Cauliflower "Chip" Sheet Pan Nachos (page 262), or as a dip for sliced veggies and Everything Bagel Almond Flour Crackers (page 236). Avocados are high in fat, but it's the good kind. The unsaturated fats found in avocados can act as a nutrient booster by helping to increase the absorption of fat-soluble vitamins A, D, E, and K—yet another reason to pair this creamy guac with your favorite meals and savory snacks.

3 large ripe avocados

½ small red onion, finely diced

¼ cup finely chopped fresh cilantro

2 cloves garlic, minced

Juice of ½ lime

1 teaspoon finely ground Himalayan pink salt

1. Take an avocado and carefully slice it open by running a knife all around the exterior, cutting through to the pit in the center. Twist the two halves to open. Remove the pit and scoop the flesh into a medium bowl. Repeat with the remaining two avocados.

2. Mash the avocado flesh using a potato masher or fork until mostly broken down and only smaller chunks remain.

3. Stir in the onion, cilantro, garlic, lime juice, and salt. Serve immediately for maximum freshness.

4. When stored properly, guacamole can last up to 3 days in the refrigerator. To store, place it in a bowl that has a tight-fitting lid. Pack the guacamole tightly in the bowl and press out any air bubbles with the back of a spoon. Pour a thin layer of water over the entire surface of the guacamole, secure the lid, and refrigerate for up to 3 days.

 notes _____

If you don't have a lime on hand, you can use a small lemon. Not only does the citrus help balance the richness of the avocado, but the citric acid it contains will help delay the avocados from browning (oxidizing).

For some heat, add ½ to 1 seeded and finely diced jalapeño pepper in Step 3.

You can also add diced tomatoes.

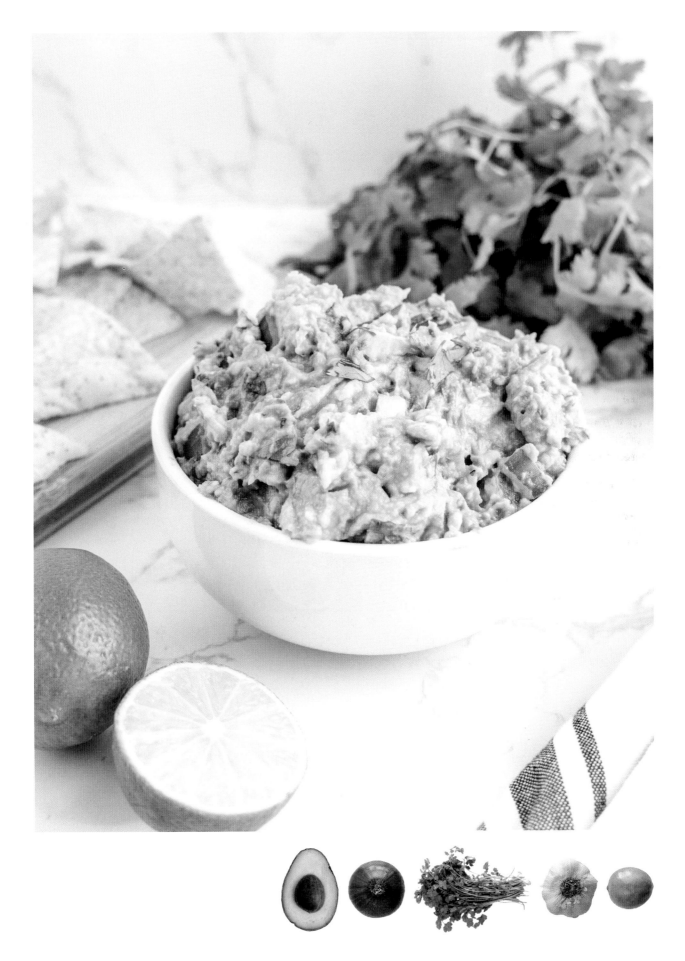

white bean hummus

yield: ¾ cup to 1 cup, depending on flavor (2 tablespoons per serving) prep time: 10 minutes
cook time: 0 to 60 minutes, depending on flavor

Hummus is the perfect creamy accompaniment to sliced fresh veggies and whole-grain pitas, makeshift salad dressing or pasta sauce, topping for toast... and the list goes on. While this Middle Eastern dip is traditionally made with a base of chickpeas, white beans produce an even creamier result and a mild-tasting canvas for these four unique flavor profiles. *Tip:* Looking for a no-cook recipe that comes together super fast? Use canned beans and opt for the avocado flavor.

base:

1 (15-ounce) can no-salt-added white beans, drained and rinsed well, or 1½ cups cooked white beans (see page 44)

3 tablespoons water

1 tablespoon tahini

1 tablespoon extra-virgin olive oil

Juice of ½ lemon

¼ teaspoon finely ground Himalayan pink salt

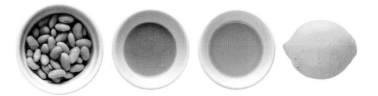

sweet potato white bean flavor:

1 large sweet potato (about 8 ounces), scrubbed

½ teaspoon ground cinnamon (optional)

Minced fresh cilantro, for garnish (optional)

Preheat the oven to 400°F. Place the sweet potato on a sheet pan and prick all over with a fork. Roast until tender, 50 minutes to 1 hour. Once cool enough to handle, cut into chunks and put in a food processor. Add the cinnamon, if using, and process until smooth, then transfer to a serving bowl. Garnish with cilantro, if desired.

roasted red pepper white bean flavor:

2 large red bell peppers, or 1 (16-ounce) jar roasted red peppers, drained

1 large clove garlic, minced

¼ teaspoon ground cumin

First, roast the bell peppers; skip this step if using jarred roasted peppers. To roast the peppers, place an oven rack just below the broiler and set the oven to broil. Remove the stems, cores, and seeds from the peppers, then slice into large chunks and arrange, skin side up, on a sheet pan in a single layer. Broil until the skin is charred, 5 to 10 minutes. Allow the peppers to cool, then remove the charred skin using your hands and discard. Reserve 1 to 2 pieces of roasted pepper for topping at the end. Place the roasted pepper and the remaining ingredients for this flavor in a food processor. Add the base ingredients, process until smooth, and transfer to a serving bowl. Dice the reserved roasted bell pepper pieces and scatter across the top.

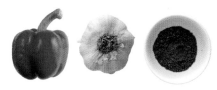

avocado white bean flavor:

1 large ripe avocado, pitted and peeled

½ cup fresh cilantro leaves

2 large cloves garlic, minced

Diced avocado, for garnish (optional)

Put the base ingredients and avocado hummus ingredients in a food processor and process until smooth. Transfer to a serving bowl. Garnish with avocado, if desired.

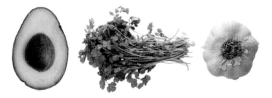

roasted garlic white bean flavor:

1 head garlic

1 teaspoon extra-virgin olive oil, for drizzling

Minced garlic, for garnish (optional)

Preheat the oven to 375°F. Cut off the top of the head of garlic so that the tops of the cloves are exposed. Set the garlic head on a sheet of foil, drizzle the exposed cloves with the oil, and wrap in foil to seal. Roast for 1 hour. Allow to cool and squeeze the roasted garlic out of each clove into a food processor. Add the base ingredients and blend until smooth, then transfer to a serving bowl. Garnish with minced garlic, if desired.

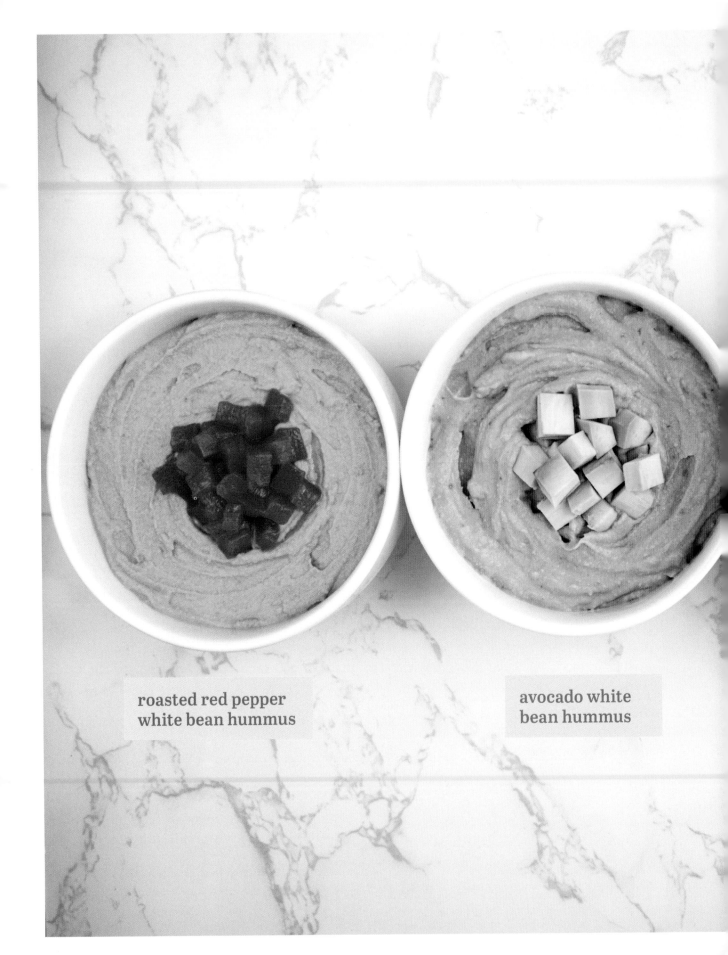

roasted red pepper
white bean hummus

avocado white
bean hummus

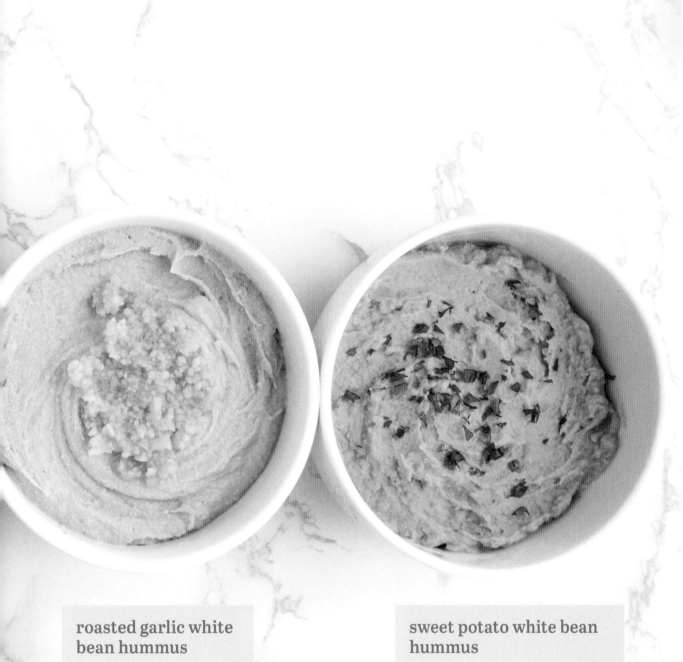

roasted garlic white
bean hummus

sweet potato white bean
hummus

plant-based parm

yield: 1 cup (2 tablespoons per serving)   prep time: 5 minutes

If you love cheese but not the dairy, this plant-based parm will become a staple in your fridge. It's made with a base of cashews and seasonings and the queen of "cheeze" in the plant-based world: nutritional yeast. Use this parmesan for pizza, pasta dishes, and just about any other savory dish you want to add some cheezy goodness to.

1 cup raw cashews

¼ cup nutritional yeast

½ teaspoon garlic powder

¼ teaspoon onion powder

¼ teaspoon finely ground Himalayan pink salt

Put all of the ingredients in a food processor and process until crumbly and combined. Store in a sealed container in the refrigerator for up to 1 month.

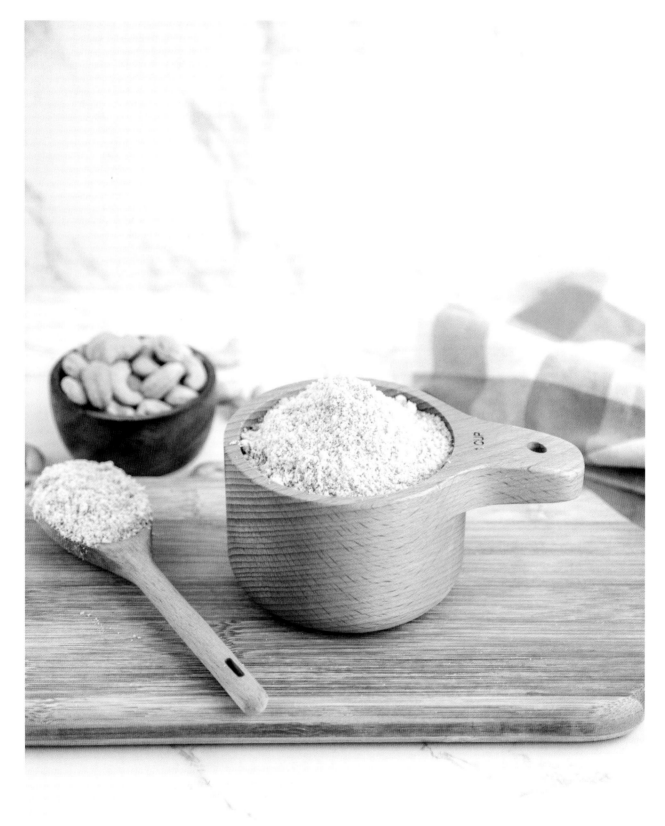

plant bacon

yield: 4 servings   prep time: 10 minutes   cook time: 10 to 25 minutes, depending on type

Crispy, smoky, and salty—this plant bacon is just as good as the real deal but without the saturated fat. Pick your base of mushrooms, coconut, or tempeh and get cooking! Use this as a crumbly topping on baked potatoes or casseroles, or place strips in a breakfast sandwich (page 140).

base:

1 tablespoon extra-virgin olive oil

2 tablespoons low-sodium soy sauce

½ teaspoon pure maple syrup

½ teaspoon liquid smoke

¼ teaspoon smoked paprika

¼ teaspoon ground black pepper

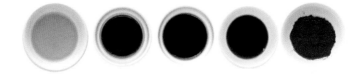

tempeh bacon:

1 (8-ounce) package tempeh, cut into ¼-inch-thick slices

1 tablespoon water

Heat the oil in a large skillet over medium heat. Add the tempeh and cook for 3 to 4 minutes on each side, until golden brown and crispy. Pour the water into the pan, then add the soy sauce, maple syrup, liquid smoke, paprika, and pepper. Let the tempeh brown for 2 to 3 minutes, then flip and cook for another 1 to 2 minutes, until browned on the other side. Store in a sealed container in the refrigerator for up to 5 days. Reheat in a skillet over medium heat until hot.

mushroom bacon:

4 ounces shiitake or portabella mushrooms, cut into ¼-inch-thick slices

Preheat the oven to 375°F and line a sheet pan with parchment paper. In a large bowl, combine the ingredients for the base. Add the mushrooms and toss to coat. Spread the mushrooms in a single layer on the prepared pan and bake for 15 minutes, flip, and bake for another 7 to 10 minutes, or until the mushrooms look dark and the edges are crisp. Let cool for 10 minutes. As the bacon cools, it will become crispier. Store in a sealed container in the refrigerator for up to 5 days. Reheat in a skillet over medium heat until hot.

coconut bacon:

2 cups unsweetened coconut chips

Preheat the oven to 325°F and line a sheet pan with parchment paper. In a large bowl, combine the ingredients for the base. Add the coconut and toss to coat. Spread the coconut chips in a single layer on the prepared pan. Bake for 5 minutes, toss, and bake for another 5 minutes, or until crispy and golden brown. Let cool for 10 minutes. As the bacon cools, it will become crispier. Store in a sealed container in the refrigerator for up to a week. Enjoy leftovers cold.

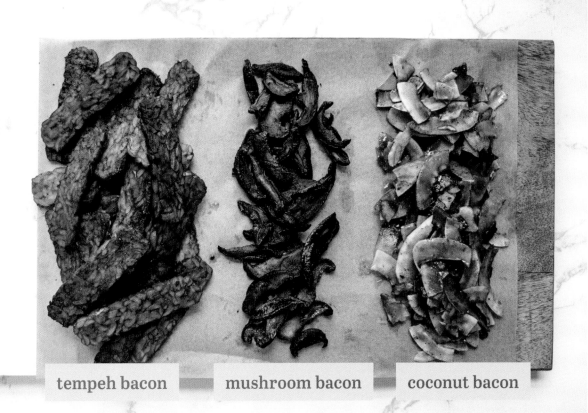

tempeh bacon   mushroom bacon   coconut bacon

simple tzatziki

yield: 1½ cups (¼ cup per serving)   prep time: 10 minutes

Re-create the yogurt cucumber sauce you love at Greek restaurants, at home! Rich and creamy with a lemony flavor and a hint of fresh dill, tzatziki can liven up any meal or savory snack. Besides using it as a dip for sliced veggies and pita, use it as a sandwich spread, salad topping, or condiment for grilled vegetables and lean proteins.

½ cup grated cucumber

2 tablespoons minced fresh dill fronds

2 cloves garlic, minced

1 cup plain Greek yogurt or plain nondairy yogurt (see notes)

1 tablespoon lemon juice

1 tablespoon extra-virgin olive oil, plus more for drizzling if desired

¼ teaspoon finely ground Himalayan pink salt

⅛ teaspoon ground black pepper

1. Place the cucumber in a clean kitchen towel and squeeze out the excess water.

2. Place all of the ingredients in a medium bowl and stir to combine. Finish with a drizzle of oil, if desired.

3. Store in a sealed container in the refrigerator for up to a week.

notes _____

For a super creamy sauce, I recommend using a higher-fat Greek yogurt (2% or higher).

If using nondairy yogurt, I recommend a plain almond milk yogurt.

If you don't have fresh dill, you can substitute another fresh herb, such as mint (most commonly used in tzatziki), parsley, or cilantro.

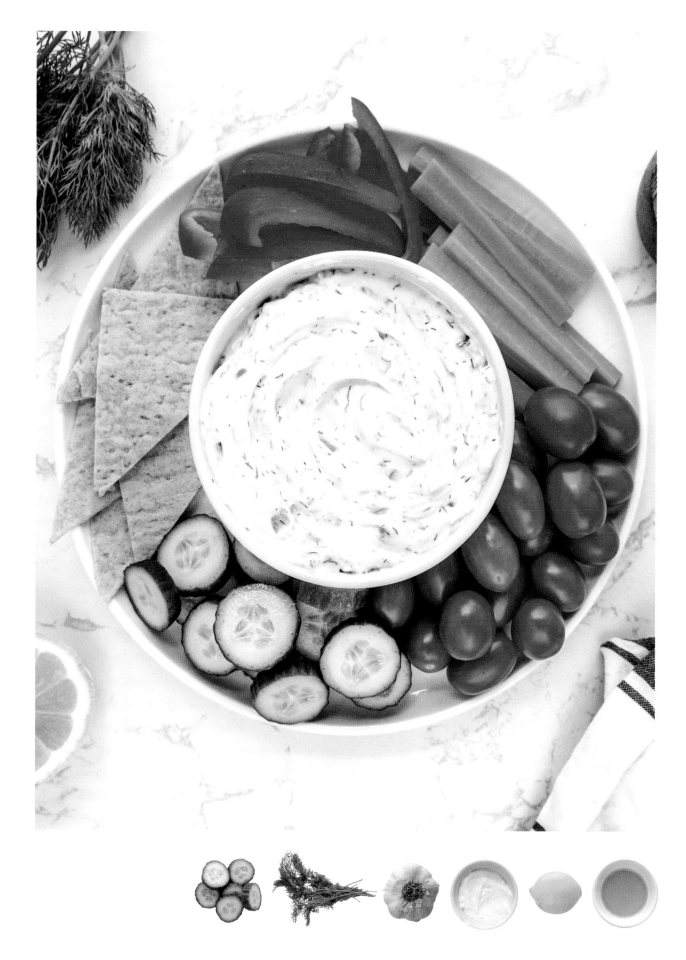

no-sugar all-purpose tomato sauce

yield: **2 cups (¼ cup per serving)**   prep time: **5 minutes**   cook time: **16 minutes**

If you've perused the tomato sauce aisle lately, you know it's hard to find a store-bought sauce without added sugar, a high sodium content, and hard-to-pronounce additives. The solution? Make your own! Keep this straightforward sauce on hand for easy pasta nights at home.

¼ cup extra-virgin olive oil

4 cloves garlic, minced

1 (28-ounce) can crushed tomatoes (unsalted and unflavored)

¼ cup water

1 teaspoon dried basil

½ teaspoon ground dried oregano

½ teaspoon finely ground Himalayan pink salt

¼ teaspoon ground black pepper

¼ teaspoon red pepper flakes (optional)

1. Pour the oil into a large saucepan over medium heat. When the oil is hot, add the garlic and sauté until lightly browned and fragrant, about 1 minute.

2. Add the crushed tomatoes, water, basil, oregano, salt, pepper, and red pepper flakes, if using.

3. Reduce the heat to a simmer and cook, stirring every few minutes, until thickened, about 15 minutes.

4. Serve immediately or store in a jar or other sealed container in the refrigerator for up to 2 weeks. Reheat in a small saucepan over medium heat.

note _____

Got fresh tomatoes on hand? Replace the canned crushed tomatoes with 3½ cups of diced fresh tomatoes. After completing Step 3, use an immersion blender to blend the sauce to your desired consistency.

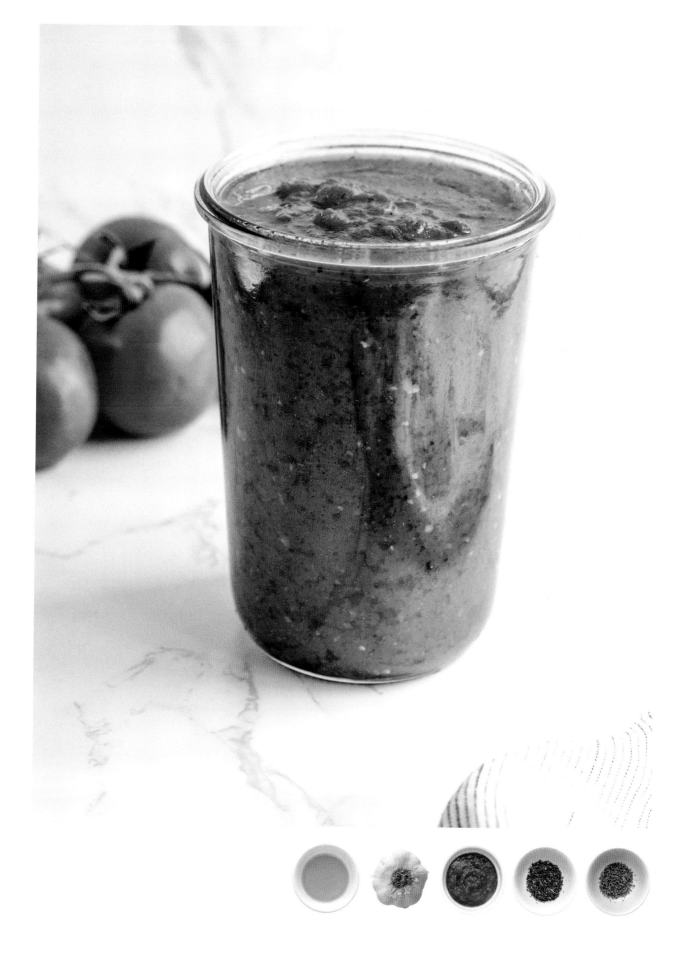

meaty mushroom grounds

yield: 2 cups (½ cup per serving)   prep time: 15 minutes
cook time: 15 to 35 minutes, depending on type

Mushrooms are like sponges—they soak up the flavors of the ingredients they are cooked with—while adding savory umami taste. Not to mention, replacing half the meat in your grounds with this versatile vegetable (botanically a fungi) lowers the fat, cholesterol, calories, and sodium while adding beneficial nutrients like potassium, B vitamins, and even vitamin D. This veggie is perfect for meat lovers looking to add more plants to their life and busy parents trying to sneak more veggies onto their kiddos' plates. Meet your new taco, spaghetti, burrito, and sloppy joe night staple—go 50/50 with meat and mushrooms or 100 percent with mushrooms alone. Either base can be flavored with the seasoning blend of your choice.

50/50 mushroom meat base:

8 ounces portabella mushrooms (2 large caps), stems removed

1 tablespoon extra-virgin olive oil

8 ounces lean ground beef

¼ teaspoon finely ground Himalayan pink salt

¼ teaspoon ground black pepper

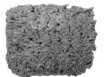

1. Put the mushroom caps in a food processor and pulse until finely chopped; the pieces should be similar in size to ground meat.

2. Pour the oil into a large skillet over medium heat. When the oil is hot, add the mushrooms and sauté until they begin to soften, about 2 minutes.

3. Add the beef and continue sautéing for another 7 to 10 minutes, stirring often to break the meat into small crumbles, until it is no longer pink and thoroughly combined with the mushrooms.

4. Drain any remaining liquid from the skillet. Stir in the salt, pepper, and seasonings for the flavor of your choice, if using, and cook for another minute, stirring often, until well combined and fragrant.

5. Enjoy immediately or store in a sealed container in the refrigerator for up to 2 days.

notes

Feel free to substitute other mushrooms, such as cremini or button. The most important thing is that they are processed to the same size as ground meat.

Any ground meat would work in place of ground beef, such as ground turkey, lamb, or chicken.

100% mushroom base:

8 ounces portabella mushrooms (2 large caps), stems removed

½ cup raw walnuts

½ cup shelled sunflower seeds

¼ teaspoon finely ground Himalayan pink salt

¼ teaspoon ground black pepper

1. Preheat the oven to 350°F. Line a sheet pan with parchment paper.

2. Place all of the ingredients, including the seasonings for the flavor of your choice, if using, in a food processor and pulse until finely chopped; the pieces should be similar in size to ground meat.

3. Spread the mixture into a thin layer on the prepared sheet pan and bake for 30 to 35 minutes, or until dried and crumbly.

4. Enjoy immediately or store in a sealed container in the refrigerator for up to 5 days.

flavor options

italian night:

1 teaspoon garlic powder

½ teaspoon dried basil

½ teaspoon ground dried oregano

¼ teaspoon finely ground Himalayan pink salt

⅛ teaspoon ground black pepper

mexican night:

1½ teaspoons chili powder

½ teaspoon ground cumin

¼ teaspoon ground dried oregano

¼ teaspoon garlic powder

¼ teaspoon finely ground Himalayan pink salt

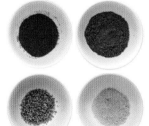

greek night:

1 teaspoon dried dill weed

1 teaspoon ground dried oregano

½ teaspoon garlic powder

¼ teaspoon finely ground Himalayan pink salt

⅛ teaspoon ground black pepper

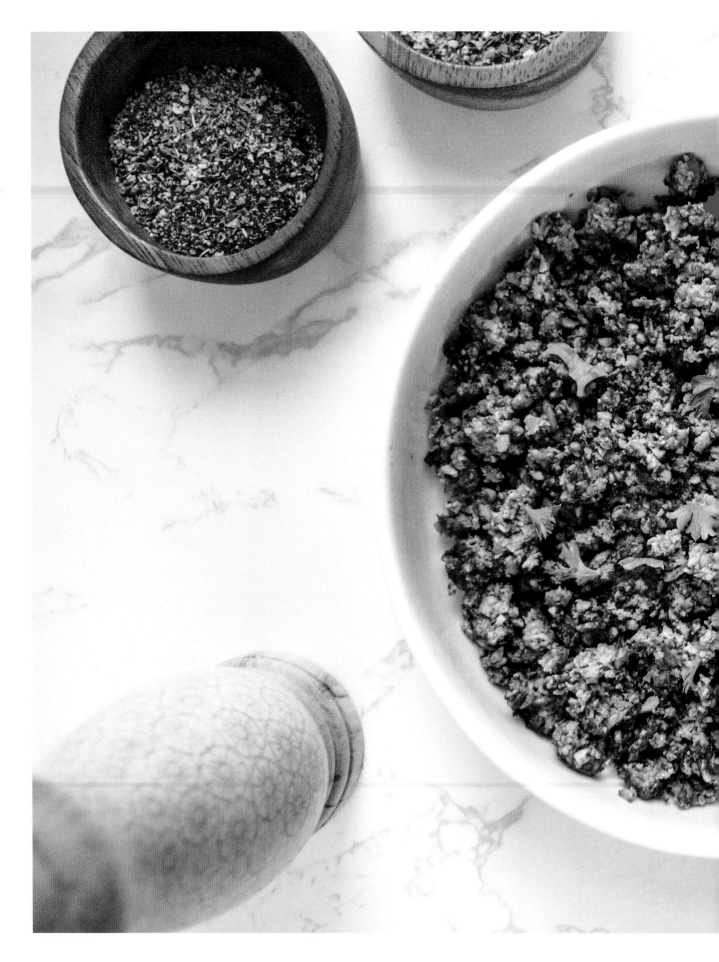

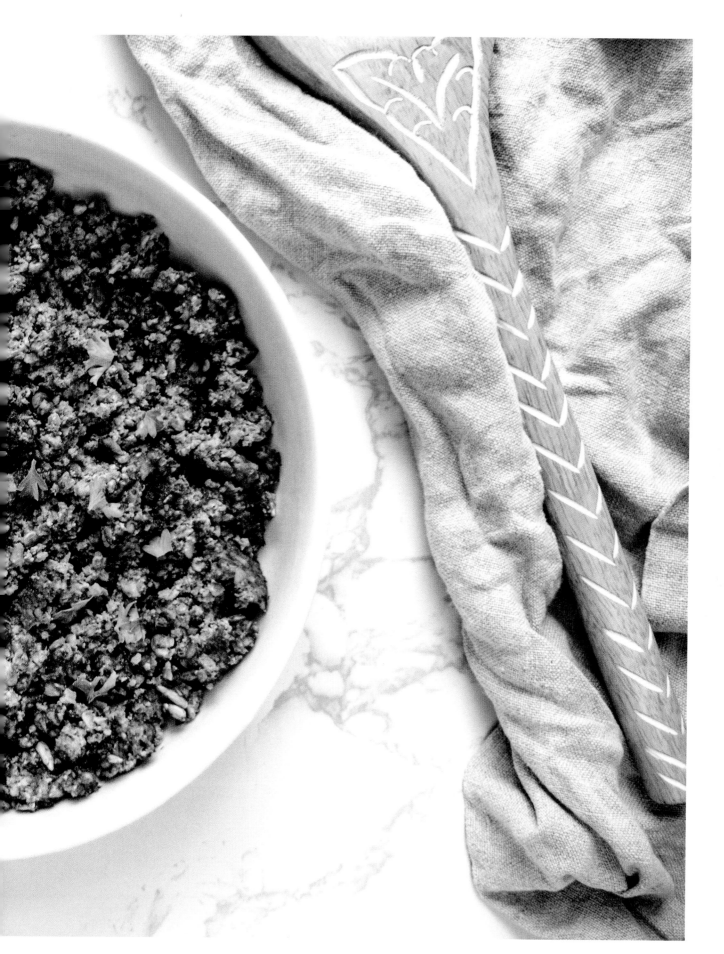

plants for breakfast

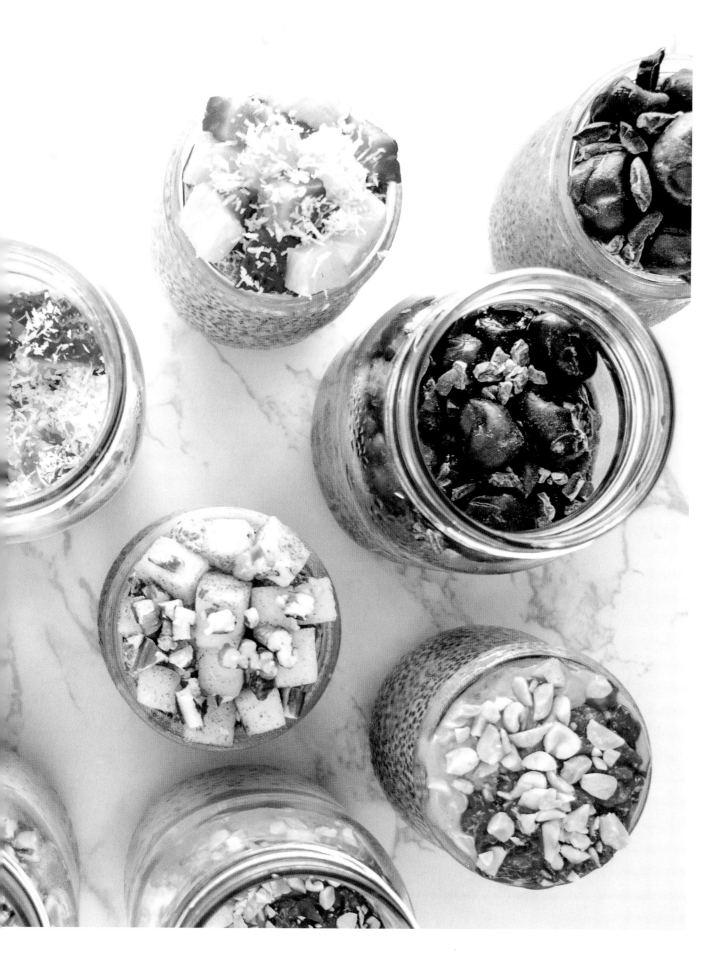

overnight breakfast

yield: 1 serving   prep time: 5 minutes, plus overnight to soak

Looking for a breakfast that "cooks" itself? Look no further than chia pudding and overnight oats. Both make a great base that can be flavored to suit your taste. In this recipe, I share six flavors that can be paired with either base (that makes 12 different breakfasts!). While oats soak up liquid overnight and soften to a consistency of warm cooked oats, chia seeds soak up to 10 times their weight in liquid to create a puddinglike consistency. Whether you are craving chewiness or creaminess in the a.m., you can't go wrong with either option.

overnight oats base:

½ cup rolled oats

½ cup unsweetened almond milk or coconut milk (see note)

¼ cup plain Greek yogurt or plain nondairy yogurt

2 teaspoons chia seeds

2 teaspoons pure maple syrup

¼ teaspoon pure vanilla extract

Put the base ingredients in a 16-ounce glass jar and mix until combined. If making the chocolate lover's flavor, mix in the cocoa powder. The remaining add-ins for this and the other flavors can be incorporated either with the base ingredients or added in the morning. Cover and refrigerate overnight to enjoy the next day.

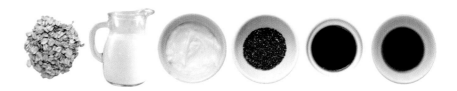

overnight chia pudding base:

3 tablespoons chia seeds

¾ cup unsweetened almond milk or coconut milk (see note)

2 teaspoons pure maple syrup

¼ teaspoon pure vanilla extract

Put the base ingredients in a small bowl and mix together using a fork. If making the chocolate lover's flavor, mix in the cocoa powder. The remaining add-ins for this and the other flavors can be incorporated either with the base ingredients or added in the morning. Let the mixture sit on the counter for 10 minutes to thicken and stir again to distribute the seeds. Cover and refrigerate overnight to enjoy the next day.

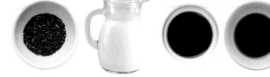

note _____

For the tropical flavor, use coconut milk in the base.

flavor options

chocolate lover's:

1 tablespoon unsweetened cocoa powder

¼ cup pitted or sliced cherries

1 teaspoon cacao nibs

Pinch of finely ground Himalayan pink salt

apple cinnamon:

½ medium apple, diced

¼ teaspoon ground cinnamon

2 tablespoons chopped raw pecans

grown-up pb&j:

½ cup mashed raspberries

1 tablespoon natural creamy peanut butter

1 tablespoon chopped roasted peanuts

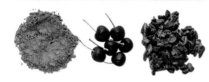

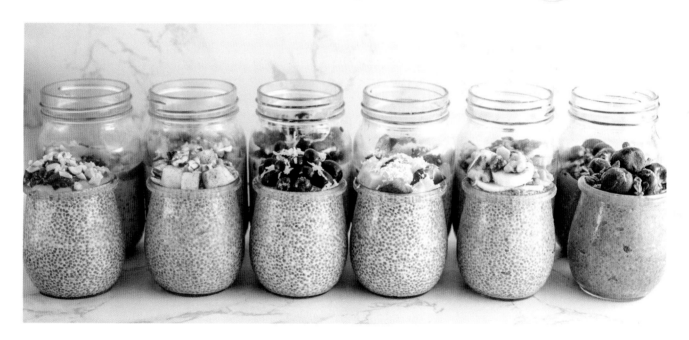

tropical *(see note)*:

¼ cup diced pineapple

¼ cup chopped strawberries

1 tablespoon unsweetened coconut flakes

banana bread:

½ medium banana, mashed

2 tablespoons chopped raw walnuts

¼ teaspoon ground cinnamon

blueberry lemon:

½ cup fresh blueberries

Grated zest of 1 lemon

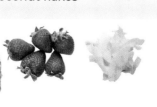 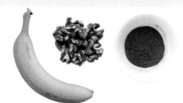 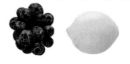

customizable make-ahead freezer breakfast sandwiches

yield: **12 sandwiches**   prep time: **15 minutes**   cook time: **15 minutes**

Skip the drive-through line on your way to work and pop one of these breakfast sandwiches in the microwave for two minutes while you fix your morning coffee. While these are made with a classic base of eggs, cheese, and toasted English muffins, they are customizable, so you can tailor the fillings to your preferences, from bacon to sliced avocado to fresh spinach. Prep these freezer sandwiches on Sunday and enjoy them all week long—your future self will thank you!

12 large eggs

¾ cup milk of choice

½ teaspoon finely ground Himalayan pink salt

¼ teaspoon ground black pepper

12 whole-grain English muffins, toasted

12 slices cheddar cheese or nondairy cheese of choice

12 slices bacon, cut in half crosswise and cooked, or Tempeh Bacon (page 126), cut in half crosswise

for serving (optional):

Fresh arugula or spinach

Sprouts

Sliced red onion

Sliced tomato

Sliced avocado

Hot sauce

1. Preheat the oven to 350°F and grease a sheet pan with cooking spray.

2. In a large bowl, whisk together the eggs, milk, salt, and pepper.

3. Pour the egg mixture into the prepared pan and bake until set, 12 to 15 minutes.

4. While the eggs are baking, toast the English muffins, then arrange them cut side up on a clean work surface.

5. Remove the eggs from the oven and allow to cool before cutting into 12 squares. Top the bottom half of an English muffin with an egg patty, a cheese slice, and 2 half pieces of cooked bacon. Top with the remaining muffin half. Repeat with the remaining English muffins, egg patties, cheese, and bacon.

6. Wrap each sandwich in foil and place in a freezer bag. Freeze for up to 3 months.

7. The sandwiches can be placed in the refrigerator to thaw overnight and then reheated, or reheated from frozen. To reheat a thawed sandwich:

   Oven or toaster oven method: Heat a foil-wrapped sandwich at 350°F for 15 to 20 minutes.

   Microwave method: Remove the sandwich from the foil and wrap it in a paper towel. Microwave for 1 minute, flip, and microwave for another 30 seconds, or until warmed through.

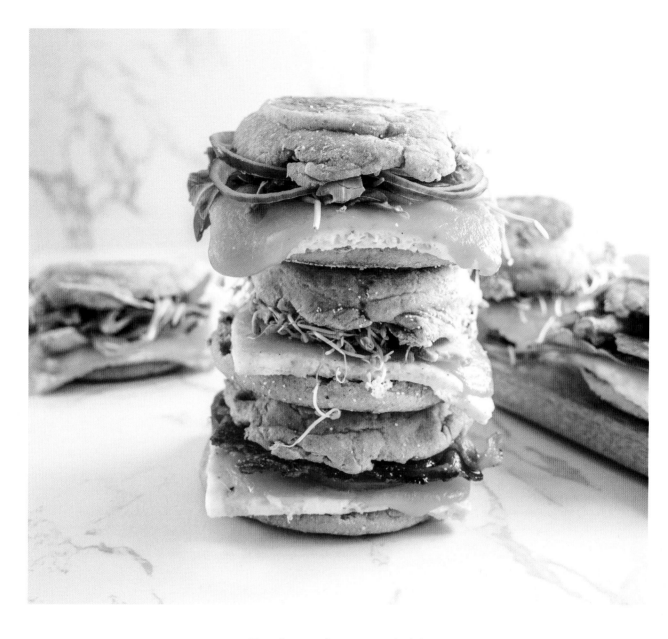

To reheat a frozen sandwich:

Oven or toaster oven method: Heat a foil-wrapped sandwich at 350°F for 30 minutes.

Microwave method: Remove the sandwich from the foil and wrap it in a paper towel. Microwave for 2 minutes, flip, and microwave for another minute, or until warmed through.

8. Add any additional desired fillings before consuming.

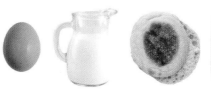

naturally sweetened banana oat pancakes

yield: **4 servings**   prep time: **5 minutes**   cook time: **15 minutes**

Sunday morning just got a whole lot easier (and more delicious!). These simple, naturally sweetened pancakes are made with everyday ingredients, and the batter is made in a blender. Unlike your standard boxed pancake mix, these have a base of oats, a whole grain packed with fiber to help keep you full until lunchtime.

2 large eggs

2 ripe medium-sized bananas

2 cups rolled oats

¼ cup unsweetened plant milk of choice

1 teaspoon pure vanilla extract

2 teaspoons baking powder

1 teaspoon ground cinnamon

Pinch of finely ground Himalayan pink salt

suggested toppings:

Pure maple syrup

Fresh fruit

Nuts

1. Place all of the ingredients in a high-powered blender or food processor and blend until smooth, 30 to 45 seconds. The batter will be thick.

2. Heat a large skillet over medium heat and grease the pan with cooking spray. Working in batches of 2 or 3 pancakes at a time, pour ¼ cup of batter for each pancake into the skillet. Use the back of a spoon to spread each pancake into a circle about 4 inches in diameter. Cook until little bubbles start to form on top and the edges start to turn golden brown, 1 to 3 minutes. Flip and cook until the other side is set, 20 to 40 seconds.

3. Serve with the toppings of your choice.

notes _____

To sweeten the batter further, add 1 to 3 tablespoons of pure maple syrup.

These pancakes can be frozen to eat at a later time. Simply allow them to cool completely, then place them in a freezer bag or other freezer-safe container and freeze for up to 3 months. To reheat, place frozen pancakes on a microwave-safe plate and microwave for 45 to 60 seconds, or until warm.

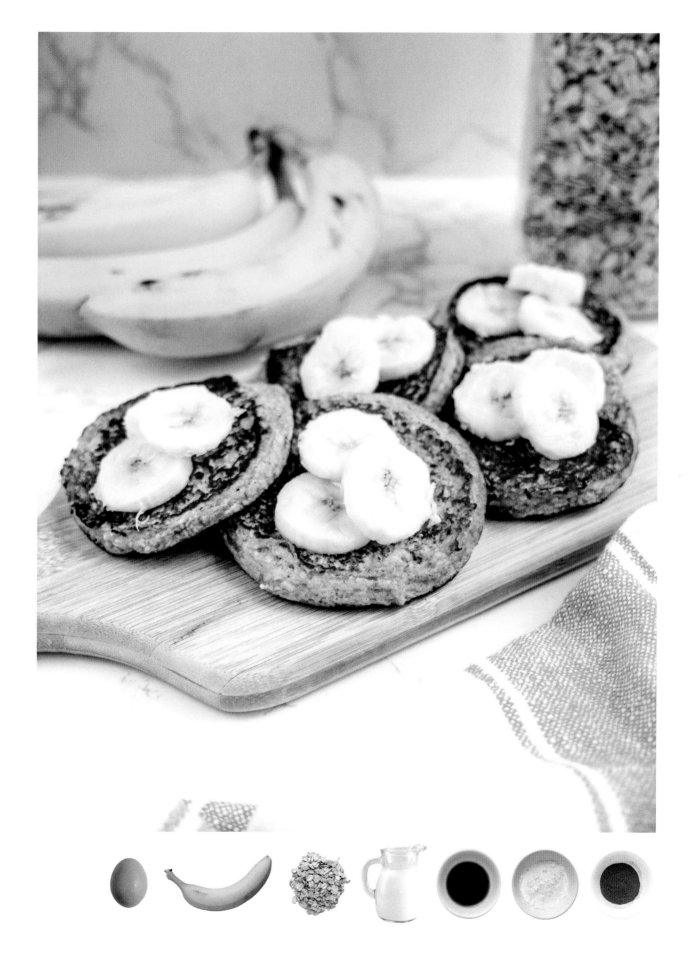

savory zucchini waffle minis

yield: **4 servings**   prep time: **10 minutes**   cook time: **40 minutes**

If you haven't tried savory waffles, you are missing out! Waffles get a bad rap in the nutrition department because they are often made with refined flour and sugar, making them more of a dessert than a nutritious start to the day. These waffles are not only packed with savory goodness, but they help you get in a serving of vegetables first thing in the a.m. Serve them with your favorite savory breakfast toppings, like eggs, smoked salmon, or sliced avocado, or enjoy them as is.

2 cups grated zucchini (about 2 medium zucchinis)

1 cup blanched almond flour

½ cup grated Parmesan cheese or plant-based parmesan, store-bought or homemade (page 124)

1 teaspoon baking powder

¼ teaspoon finely ground Himalayan pink salt

2 large eggs, beaten

1. Grease a nonstick waffle maker and preheat to medium-high heat.

2. Place the grated zucchini in a clean kitchen towel or piece of cheesecloth and squeeze out the liquid.

3. In a large bowl, whisk together the flour, cheese, baking powder, and salt. Add the zucchini and eggs and use a rubber spatula to mix until the batter is uniform.

4. Pour 3 to 4 tablespoons of the batter into the center of the preheated waffle maker and close the lid. Cook until golden brown and slightly crisp, 2 to 3 minutes. Remove the waffle and set aside. Repeat with the remaining batter to make a total of about 16 mini waffles.

5. Enjoy immediately. Store leftovers in a sealed container in the refrigerator, or place in a freezer bag or other freezer-safe container and freeze for up to 3 months. To reheat, pop the waffles in a toaster.

notes _____

You can also use this batter to make full-sized waffles.

For egg-free: Use 2 flax eggs. To make a flax egg, combine 1 tablespoon of flaxseed meal with 3 tablespoons of water in a small bowl and set aside to thicken for 5 minutes.

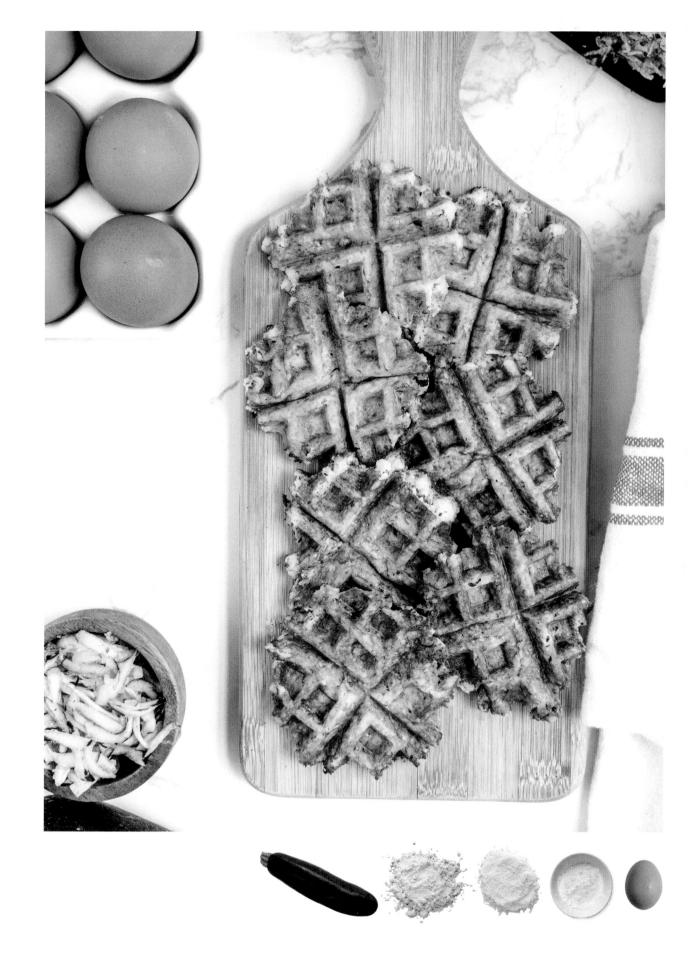

all-day energy smoothie

6 WAYS

yield: **1 serving**   prep time: **5 minutes**

A smoothie is an easy way to pack a boatload of nutrition into your day in one convenient beverage. Unlike your typical smoothie shop options, which are typically fruit-focused and often contain added sugar, these are formulated with a range of whole-food ingredients, including vegetables and plant proteins, to provide lasting energy. Though I give you six delicious flavor combinations, you can use my dietitian-approved smoothie-building formula below to build an all-day energy smoothie using whatever ingredients you have in your fridge and pantry.

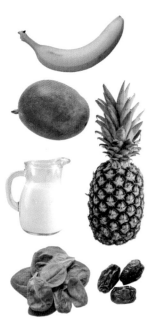

Place all of the ingredients for the smoothie flavor of your choice in a blender, pouring in the liquid last, and blend until smooth. Add more liquid or ice as needed to achieve the desired consistency.

Turn the page for FLAVOR OPTIONS.

build an all-day energy smoothie

Here is your ultimate guide to getting as much nutrition into your busy day, all in one meal. Follow this formula to a build a smoothie that actually fills you up and leaves you with lasting energy.

MILD-TASTING VEGGIES (1–2 servings)

Handful of raw leafy green vegetables (spinach, kale, etc.)

¼–½ cup frozen riced cauliflower or zucchini

¼–½ cup pure pumpkin puree

¼–½ cup chopped celery, peeled and chopped cucumbers, or peeled and shredded carrots

FRUIT (1–2 servings)

1 medium banana, sliced and frozen

1 cup frozen berries or mango or pineapple chunks

1–2 soft pitted medjool dates

1 large orange or 1 medium grapefruit, peeled and segmented

Juice of ½ lemon or lime

PROTEIN

1 scoop plant-based protein powder

¼–⅓ cup plain Greek yogurt

2–3 ounces soft or silken tofu

FIBER-RICH FATS

1 tablespoon natural creamy nut butter

1–2 tablespoons raw nuts, such as almonds, walnuts, and/or cashews

1–2 tablespoons raw seeds, such as chia, flax, and/or sunflower

⅓ medium avocado (rich in good fats, but botanically a fruit)

NUTRITIOUS MIX-INS for flavor and texture

Unsweetened cocoa powder

Spices, such as cardamom, cinnamon, ginger, pumpkin pie spice, or turmeric powder

Extracts, such as vanilla, peppermint, almond, or maple

Nutrient-rich powders, such as matcha, spirulina, or wheatgrass

¼ cup rolled oats

Handful of fresh herbs, such as cilantro or parsley

LIQUID (½–1 cup)

Water

Unsweetened plant milk, regular milk, or kefir

detox green smoothie:

1 cup frozen pineapple chunks

½ Granny Smith apple, chopped

⅓ cup peeled and sliced cucumbers

1 cup baby spinach

1 scoop unflavored or vanilla plant-based protein powder

Juice of ½ lime

Small handful of fresh cilantro leaves

1 cup water

¼ teaspoon ginger powder

berry blast smoothie:

1 cup frozen mixed berries (any type)

1 medium banana, sliced and frozen

½ cup frozen riced cauliflower

¼ cup plain Greek yogurt

1 tablespoon chia seeds

1 cup unsweetened plant milk of choice

pumpkin pie smoothie:

⅓ cup pure pumpkin puree

½ medium banana, sliced and frozen

1 soft pitted medjool date

1 tablespoon natural creamy almond butter

¼ teaspoon pumpkin pie spice

1 cup unsweetened plant milk of choice

peanut butter cup smoothie:

1 medium banana, sliced and frozen

¼ cup rolled oats

¼ cup frozen riced cauliflower

1 soft pitted medjool date

1 tablespoon natural creamy peanut butter

1 teaspoon unsweetened cocoa powder

1 scoop chocolate plant-based protein powder

1 cup unsweetened plant milk of choice

immunity smoothie:

1 medium carrot, peeled and shredded

1 cup frozen mango chunks

1 medium orange, peeled and segmented

¼ cup plain Greek yogurt

⅛ teaspoon ginger powder

⅛ teaspoon turmeric powder

1 cup water

the everyday green smoothie:

½ medium banana, sliced and frozen

½ cup frozen mango chunks

½ cup frozen pineapple chunks

1 cup baby spinach

1 scoop vanilla plant-based protein powder

1 cup unsweetened plant milk of choice

customizable lower-sugar granola

yield: 9 servings (½ cup per serving)   prep time: 10 minutes, plus 45 minutes to cool
cook time: 20 minutes

Yogurt bowls and smoothies are simply incomplete without a sprinkling of crunchy granola. Forgo the store-bought variety and make your own low-sugar option customized with the nuts and seeds of your choice for a boost of plant protein and good-for-you fats.

3 cups rolled oats

1 cup raw or dry-roasted nuts, such as pecans, sliced almonds, or walnuts, or pepitas

¼ cup seeds, such as chia seeds, hemp seeds, shelled sunflower seeds, or flaxseeds

1 teaspoon finely ground Himalayan pink salt

1 teaspoon ground cinnamon

¼ cup extra-virgin olive oil

⅓ cup pure maple syrup

1 teaspoon pure vanilla extract

1. Preheat the oven to 350°F. Line a sheet pan with parchment paper.

2. In a large bowl, combine the oats, nuts, seeds, salt, and cinnamon.

3. In a small bowl, combine the oil, maple syrup, and vanilla. Pour the wet mixture over the oat mixture and combine using a rubber spatula.

4. Transfer the granola to the prepared pan and spread in an even layer. Bake for 15 to 20 minutes, stirring halfway through the baking time, until golden brown.

5. Let the granola cool completely, about 45 minutes. It will get crunchier as it cools. Store in a sealed container in the refrigerator for up to 2 weeks.

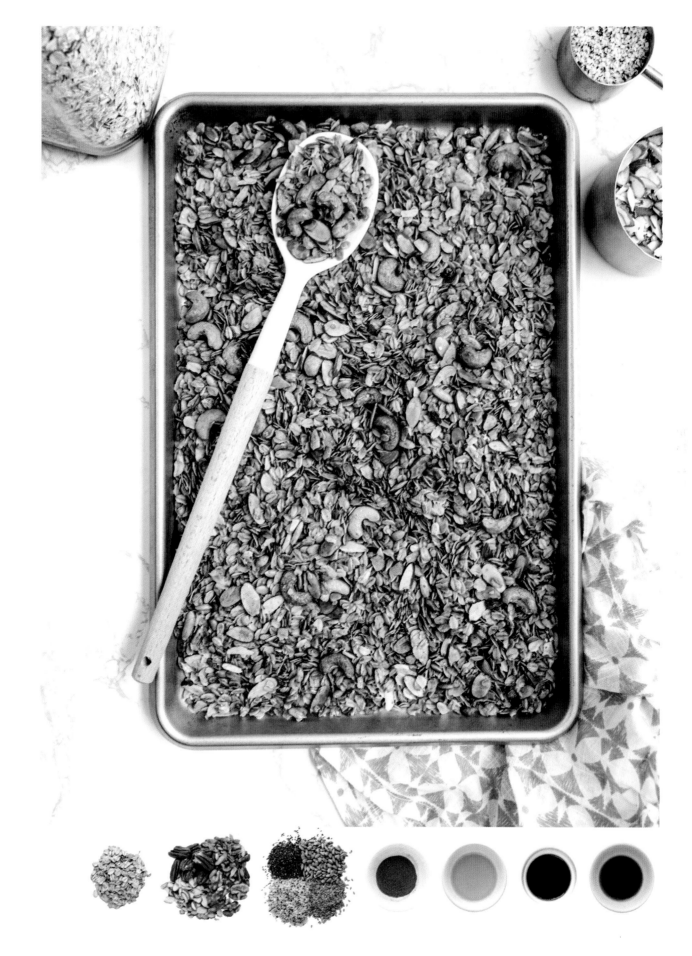

sweet potato toast, savory or sweet

yield: **4 toasts (2 servings)**   prep time: **5 minutes**   cook time: **18 minutes**

Not your typical toast! If you are confused by the overwhelming number of choices in the bread aisle, grab a sweet potato from the produce section for sweet potato "toast," a naturally gluten-free, lower-calorie, nutrient-dense alternative. This fiber-rich veggie can serve as a vehicle for your favorite sweet or savory toppings while adding a boost of beta-carotene antioxidants to your day, which are important for skin and immune health.

toast:

1 large sweet potato (about 8 ounces), scrubbed

sweet toppings:

Unsweetened nut butter of choice, banana, crushed walnuts, and cinnamon

Tahini and diced apples sautéed with cinnamon

Ricotta, fresh figs, raw manuka honey, and crushed pistachios

Natural creamy almond butter, mashed raspberries, and sliced almonds

Coconut butter, toasted unsweetened coconut flakes, and bee pollen

savory toppings:

Mashed avocado, lemon juice, and everything bagel seasoning

Cream cheese, smoked salmon, red onion, and capers

Pesto, fried egg, and red pepper flakes

Hummus, store-bought or homemade (page 120), sliced cucumbers, and fresh dill

Fresh mozzarella, sliced tomato, and fresh basil

1. Preheat the oven to 425°F. Line a sheet pan with parchment paper or grease it with cooking spray.

2. Slice off the ends of the sweet potato, then cut lengthwise into four ¼-inch-thick planks, discarding the ends. Arrange the planks in a single layer on the prepared pan, spray with cooking spray, and bake until fork-tender, 15 to 18 minutes, flipping halfway through.

3. Transfer the sweet potato slices to a wire rack to cool before topping.

4. Store leftover sweet potato slices in a sealed container in the refrigerator for up to a week or in the freezer for up to 3 months. To reheat, warm refrigerated slices on a pan in a toaster oven until crisp, about 2 minutes, or frozen slices for 4 to 5 minutes.

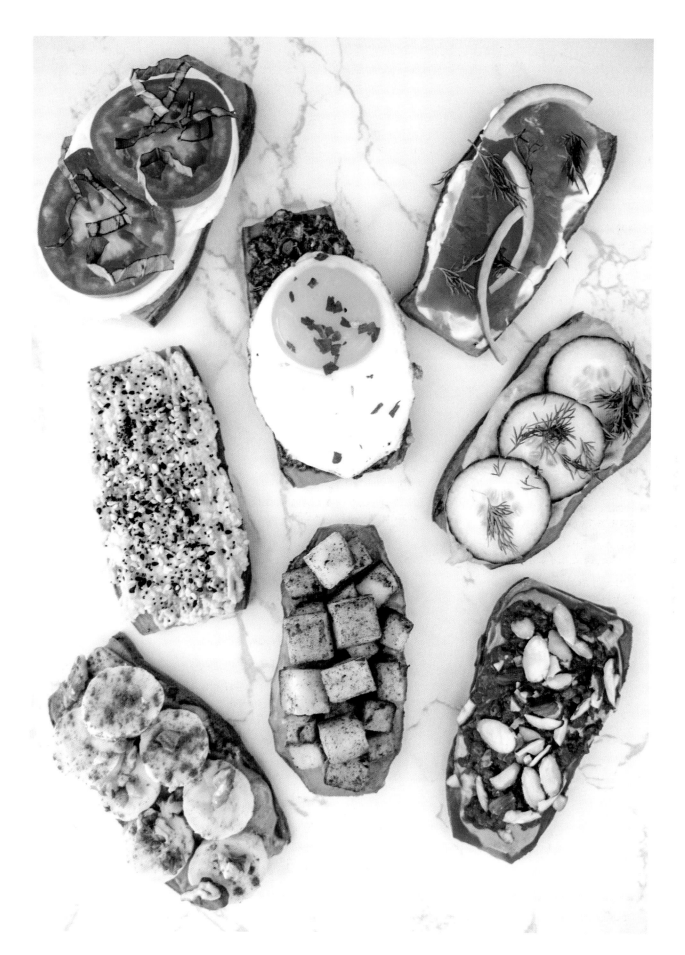

very veggie shakshuka

yield: **2 servings**   prep time: **10 minutes**   cook time: **28 minutes**

Weekend or weekday, shakshuka is an easy breakfast for any day of the week. Thought to have originated in North Africa and the Middle East, this simple recipe of eggs poached in a sauce of simmered tomatoes, onions, and spices is nourishing and satisfying and pairs perfectly with whole-grain toast. The simple yet bold flavors are a match for mild-tasting vegetables like mushrooms and spinach, making them a great plant-powered addition to this traditional dish.

1 tablespoon extra-virgin olive oil

½ medium yellow onion, chopped

1 cup sliced portabella mushrooms

4 cloves garlic, minced

2 cups fresh spinach

1 (28-ounce) can crushed tomatoes

1 teaspoon ground cumin

1 teaspoon paprika

¼ teaspoon finely ground Himalayan pink salt

⅛ teaspoon ground black pepper

4 large eggs

suggested toppings:

Crumbled feta cheese

Chopped fresh flat-leaf parsley

1. Preheat the oven to 375°F.

2. Heat the oil in a 10-inch oven-safe skillet over medium-high heat. Add the onion and mushrooms and cook until soft, about 5 minutes. Add the garlic and spinach and cook, stirring often, until the garlic is fragrant and the spinach is wilted, about 3 minutes.

3. Pour the tomatoes into the skillet and stir in the cumin, paprika, salt, and pepper. Simmer until the mixture has thickened, about 10 minutes.

4. Make four small wells in the sauce using the back of a spoon and gently crack an egg into each well. Season the eggs with salt.

5. Transfer the skillet to the oven and bake until the eggs are just set, 7 to 10 minutes. If desired, sprinkle feta and/or parsley on top before serving.

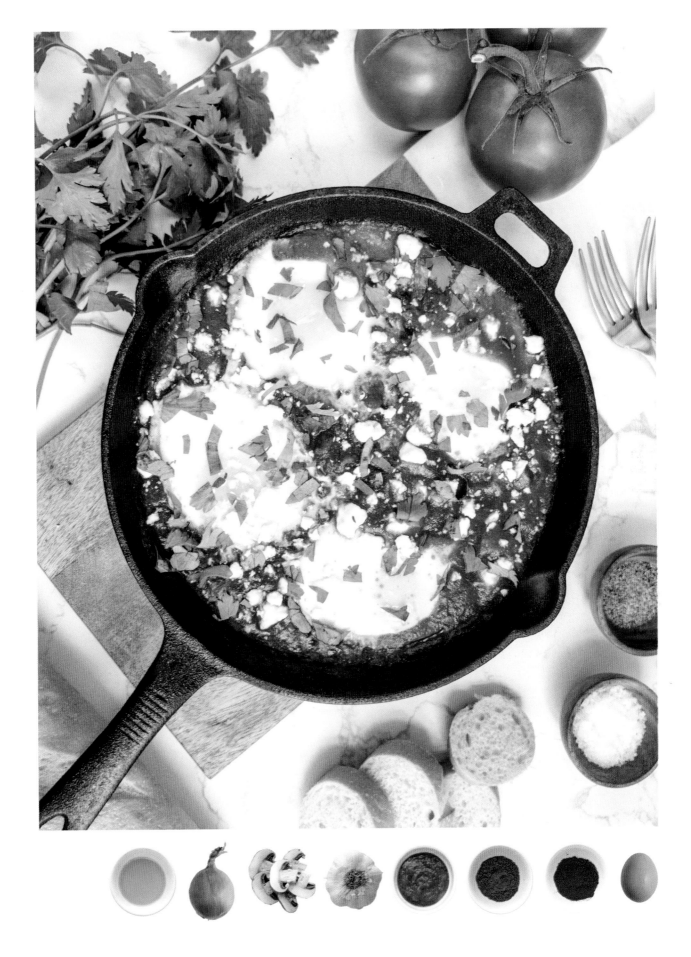

basic breakfast burritos

yield: **4 burritos (1 per serving)**   prep time: **15 minutes**   cook time: **33 minutes**

Kick-start your morning with a breakfast that has everything you need—energizing carbohydrates, satiating protein, and good-for-you fats. The best part? These freezer-friendly burritos can be made ahead of time to reheat and eat for weeks to come for breakfast (or any time of the day).

2 tablespoons avocado oil, divided

2 medium Yukon Gold potatoes (about 12 ounces), diced

¼ teaspoon finely ground Himalayan pink salt, divided

⅛ teaspoon ground black pepper

4 large eggs

¼ cup unsweetened nut milk of choice

2 cups fresh spinach

4 (10-inch) whole-grain tortillas, warmed

4 slices regular bacon, cooked, or Tempeh Bacon (page 126)

½ medium avocado, thinly sliced

½ cup pico de gallo, store-bought or homemade (page 116), or ½ cup salsa

note _____

For the burritos you plan to freeze, I recommend making them without avocado and adding the avocado fresh right before enjoying.

1. Preheat the oven to 425°F.

2. In a large bowl, toss together 1 tablespoon of the oil, the potatoes, ⅛ teaspoon of the salt, and the pepper. Arrange the potatoes on a sheet pan in a single layer. Roast until tender on the inside and slightly crisp on the outside, 20 to 30 minutes, tossing halfway through.

3. When the potatoes are nearly done, prepare the eggs: In a large bowl, whisk together the eggs, milk, and remaining ⅛ teaspoon of salt. Heat the remaining tablespoon of oil in a medium nonstick skillet over medium heat, then cook the eggs until set, stirring occasionally with a rubber spatula to scramble them. Set aside.

4. When the potatoes are done, remove them from the oven and stir in the spinach. The hot potatoes will help wilt the spinach. Return the pan to the oven and bake until the spinach is completely wilted, another 2 to 3 minutes.

5. To assemble the burritos, place a tortilla on a square piece of foil. Spoon one-quarter of the potato and spinach mixture into the center and top with one-quarter of the eggs, a slice of bacon, one-quarter of the avocado (see note), and 2 tablespoons of pico de gallo, leaving space around the edges. Fold the sides of the tortilla, including the foil, over the filling, then roll from the bottom up. Repeat with the remaining ingredients to make 4 burritos.

6. Serve immediately or store in a sealed container in the freezer to enjoy later. To reheat frozen burritos, remove the foil and microwave on high for 2 to 3 minutes, or place in a 350°F oven for 12 to 15 minutes, until warmed through.

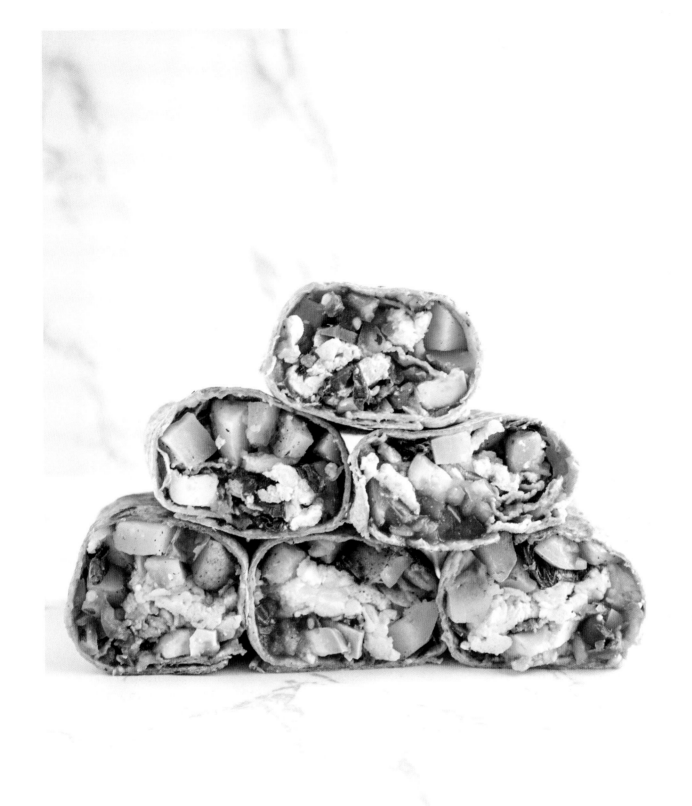
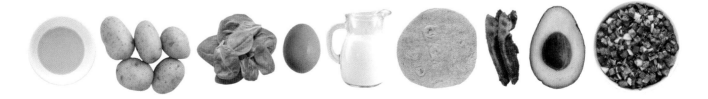

customizable blender oat cups

6 WAYS

yield: 6 oat cups (1 per serving)   prep time: 15 minutes   cook time: 18 minutes

These subtly sweet, gluten-free oat cups are a delicious way to start your day with a dose of whole-grain goodness. Though the base is infinitely customizable, I've given you a start with six flavors that run the gamut of the seasons, from Blueberry Almond to Pumpkin Spice.

base:

1 tablespoon flaxseed meal

3 tablespoons water

2½ cups rolled oats

1 teaspoon ground cinnamon

2 teaspoons baking powder

⅛ teaspoon finely ground Himalayan pink salt

¼ cup plus 2 tablespoons unsweetened applesauce

¼ cup pure maple syrup

¼ cup coconut oil

¼ cup unsweetened plant milk of choice

1 teaspoon pure vanilla extract

1. Preheat the oven to 350°F. Grease 6 wells of a standard-size 12-well muffin pan with cooking spray or line them with paper cups.

2. Make a flax egg by combining the flaxseed meal and water in a small bowl and allow to sit for 5 minutes.

3. Place the oats, cinnamon, baking powder, and salt in a food processor and process until combined and the oats are broken down into a flour.

4. Add the flax egg, applesauce, maple syrup, oil, milk, and vanilla to the food processor and process until the batter is smooth. Carefully remove the blade from the food processor bowl, add the ingredients for the flavor of your choice, and fold in by hand using a rubber spatula.

5. Divide the batter evenly among the prepared wells of the muffin pan, filling each about three-quarters full. Bake until a toothpick comes out clean when inserted into the center of an oat cup, 15 to 18 minutes. Let cool in the pan for 5 minutes, then transfer to a cooling rack. Serve warm.

6. Store in a sealed container in the refrigerator for up to a week.

notes _____

Customize these oat cups using your own combination of ingredients: 2 teaspoons of spice, ¼ cup of nuts or seeds, and 1 cup of fresh fruit or ½ to 1 cup of grated or pureed vegetables like carrot or sweet potato.

For no-added-sugar oat cups, omit the maple syrup and replace the applesauce with 2 large ripe bananas, mashed.

Turn the page for FLAVOR OPTIONS.

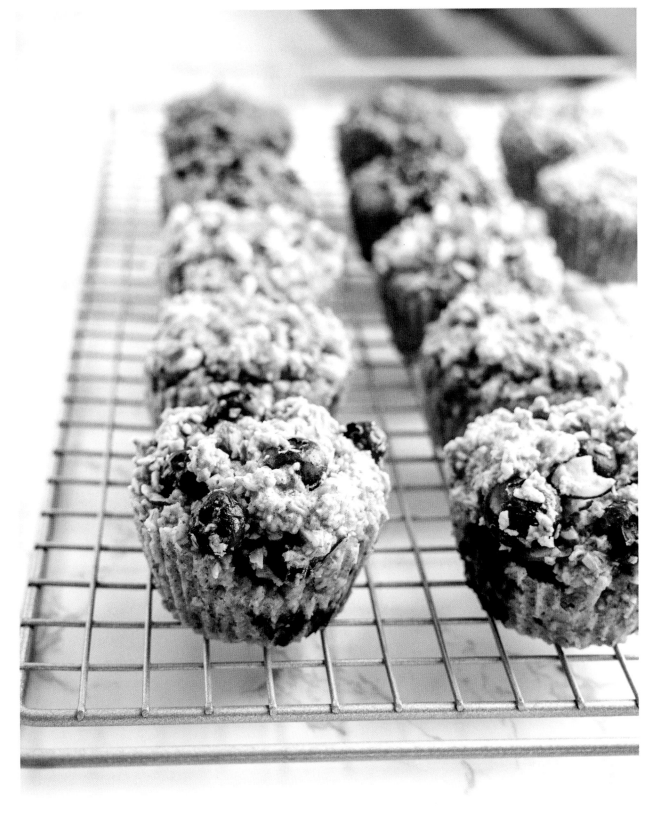

flavor options

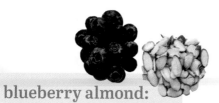

blueberry almond:

1 cup fresh or frozen blueberries

¼ cup sliced raw almonds

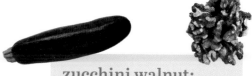

zucchini walnut:

1 cup grated zucchini

½ cup chopped raw walnuts

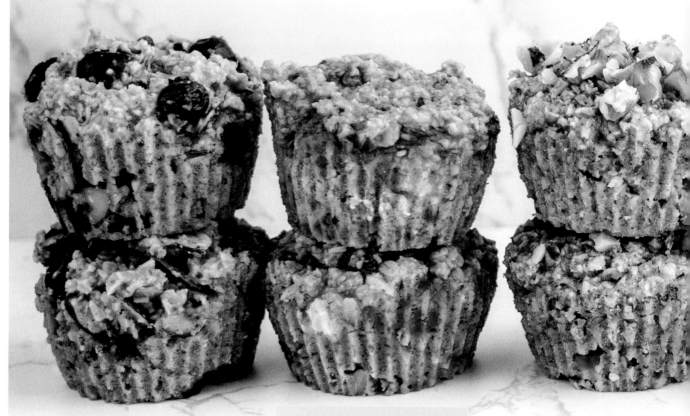

raspberry cream cheese:

1 cup mashed fresh or frozen raspberries

¼ cup cream cheese, softened

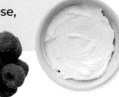

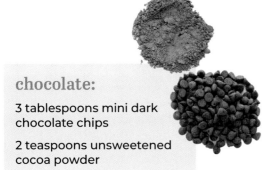

chocolate:

3 tablespoons mini dark chocolate chips

2 teaspoons unsweetened cocoa powder

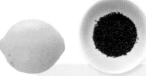

lemon poppy seed:

Grated zest and juice of ½ lemon

1 tablespoon poppy seeds

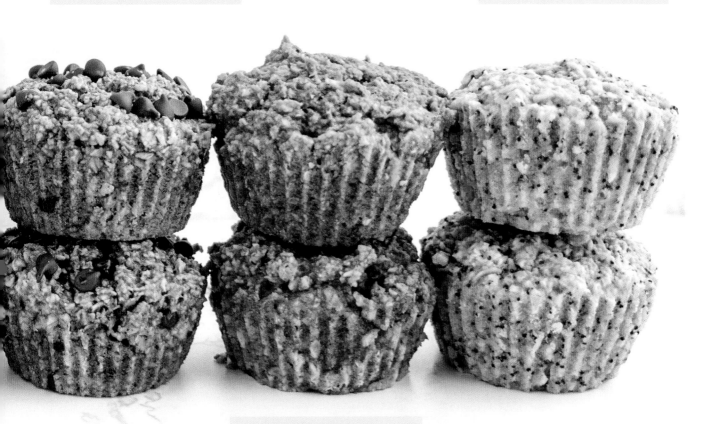

pumpkin spice:

½ cup pure pumpkin puree

2 teaspoons pumpkin pie spice

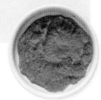

note

In the mood for a lemony oat cup but don't have poppy seeds? Replace them with chia seeds.

almond flour bagels

yield: **6 bagels (1 per serving)**   prep time: **15 minutes**   cook time: **20 minutes**

This recipe is based on a bagel-making hack that uses just two ingredients: self-rising flour and Greek yogurt—no yeast or boiling required. Except this recipe adds a gluten-free twist, using a combination of almond flour and tapioca flour as the base. Along with improving the texture, the yogurt gives the bagels a sourdough-like flavor, reminiscent of yeasted bagels. These protein-packed bagels will keep you full all morning long—especially when topped with mashed avocado and a fried egg or Tempeh Bacon (page 126) to build a complete meal.

1 cup blanched almond flour

¾ cup tapioca flour

1 tablespoon baking powder

½ teaspoon finely ground Himalayan pink salt

1 large egg, separated

1 cup plain nonfat Greek yogurt

suggested toppings:

Everything bagel seasoning

Poppy seeds

Sesame seeds

notes _____

For dairy-free: Swap the yogurt for 1 cup of blended silken tofu.

For egg-free: Replace the egg with 3 tablespoons of aquafaba (the liquid left over from cooked/canned chickpeas). Use the entire amount in the dough only, omitting the egg yolk wash.

1. Preheat the oven to 400°F. Line a baking sheet with parchment paper.

2. In a large bowl, whisk together the almond flour, tapioca flour, baking powder, and salt.

3. Place the egg white in a medium bowl; place the yolk in a small bowl, beat it with a fork, and set aside. Add the yogurt to the egg white and whisk until combined.

4. Pour the yogurt–egg white mixture into the bowl with the dry ingredients and combine using a rubber spatula until a sticky dough forms.

5. Divide the dough into 6 equal portions. Shape each portion into a ball, flatten it slightly, and use your thumb to make a hole in the center.

6. Place the bagels on the prepared pan. Brush the egg yolk on top of the bagels, then sprinkle them with the desired toppings.

7. Bake until the tops are golden, about 20 minutes. Allow to cool before slicing. Store leftover bagels in a sealed container in the refrigerator for up to 2 days or freeze for longer storage. To reheat, slice and toast the bagels before serving.

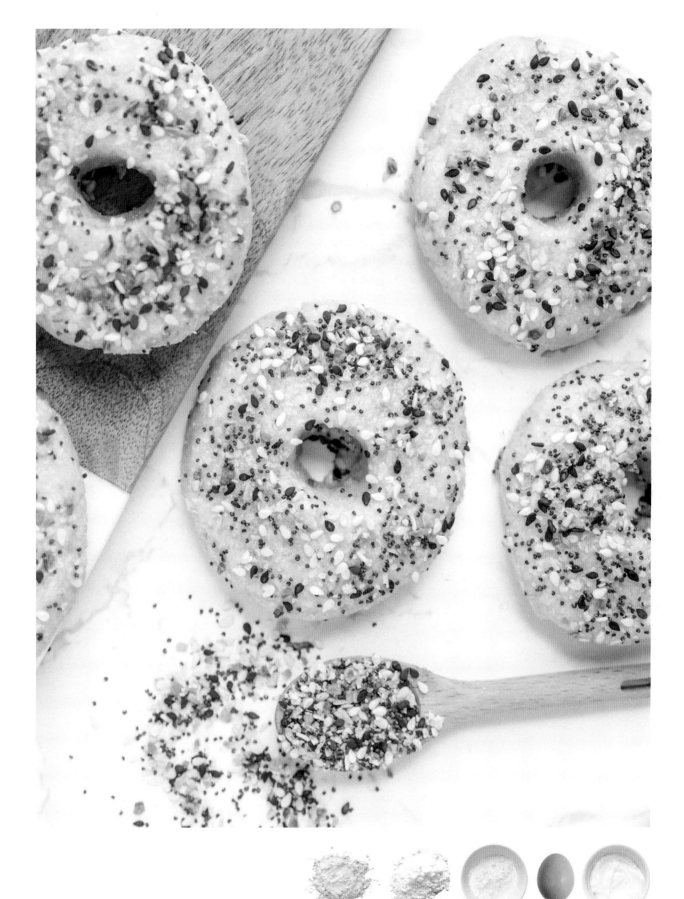

morning glory baked oatmeal

yield: **4 servings**   prep time: **10 minutes**   cook time: **30 minutes**

This baked oatmeal puts a cakelike spin on the iconic Morning Glory muffins. The array of textures and flavors from chewy whole-grain oats, shredded coconut, and grated carrots and apple will have you looking forward to breakfast.

2 cups rolled oats

¼ cup unsweetened shredded coconut

2 teaspoons ground cinnamon

1 teaspoon baking powder

Pinch of finely ground Himalayan pink salt

1 cup unsweetened plant milk of choice

⅓ cup pure maple syrup

¼ cup unsweetened applesauce

1 medium apple (any type), grated

⅔ cup peeled and grated carrots

¼ cup raisins

⅓ cup chopped raw walnuts (optional)

1. Preheat the oven to 375°F and grease an 8-inch square baking dish with cooking spray.

2. In a large bowl, whisk together the oats, coconut, cinnamon, baking powder, and salt.

3. In a medium bowl, mix together the milk, maple syrup, and applesauce. Pour into the bowl with the dry ingredients and stir in the apple, carrots, raisins, and walnuts, if using.

4. Transfer the batter to the prepared baking dish. Bake until a toothpick comes out clean when inserted into the center, 25 to 30 minutes. Let cool slightly before slicing into 4 portions. Serve warm.

5. Store leftovers in a sealed container in the refrigerator for up to 5 days. To reheat, microwave for 1 minute or bake covered in foil for 20 minutes at 300°F.

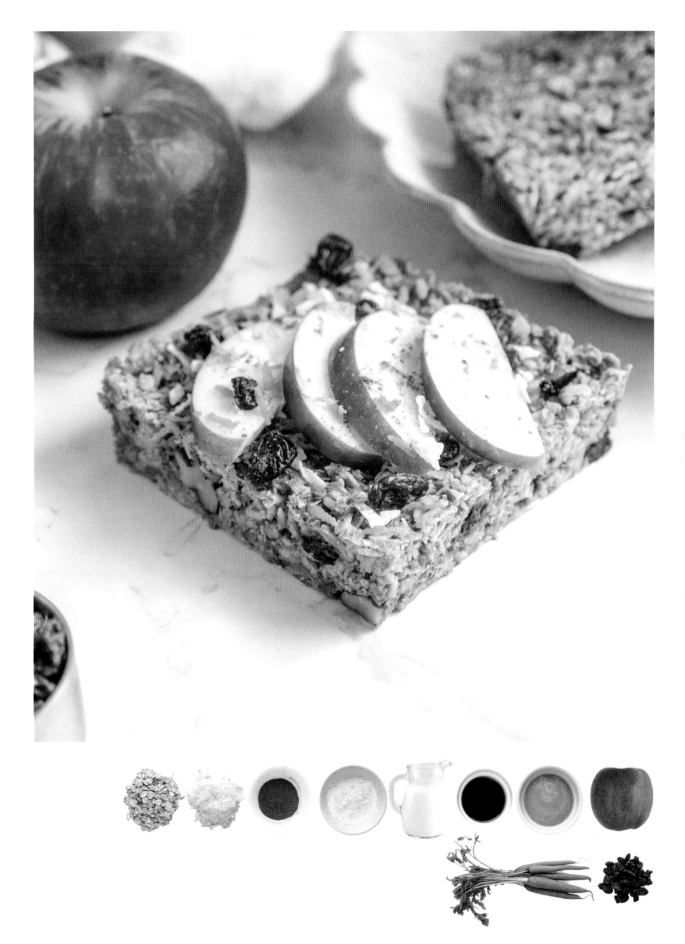

avo toast

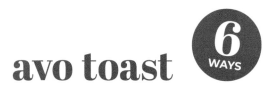

6 WAYS

yield: **2 servings**   prep time: **10 minutes**

Botanically a fruit, avocados are "nature's butter." This mild-tasting toast spread provides a dose of good-for-you unsaturated fat and pairs seamlessly with toppers like fresh salad greens, eggs, and Tempeh Bacon bits (page 126) while effortlessly boosting the absorption of important vitamins A, D, E, and K.

base:

1 medium ripe avocado

1 teaspoon lemon juice

1 teaspoon extra-virgin olive oil

⅛ teaspoon finely ground Himalayan pink salt

2 slices whole-grain sprouted bread, toasted

additional toppings (optional):

Chopped fresh herbs, such as dill or cilantro

Salad greens

Sautéed mushrooms or asparagus

Sliced jalapeño, red onion, or green onion

Sprouts

Cheese, such as crumbled feta

Chickpea Poppers (page 230)

Egg, cooked as desired

Smoked salmon

Tempeh Bacon bits (page 126) or regular bacon bits

Everything bagel seasoning

Red pepper flakes

Balsamic vinegar

Drizzle of extra-virgin olive oil

Drizzle of pesto, store-bought or homemade (page 114)

Hot sauce

1. To make the base, take the avocado and carefully slice it open by running a knife all around the exterior, cutting through to the pit in the center. Twist the two halves to open. Remove the pit and scoop the flesh into a small bowl. Add the lemon juice, oil, and salt and mash using a potato masher or fork until mostly smooth.

2. Use a butter knife or fork to evenly spread the avocado mixture on the pieces of toasted bread.

3. *For the savory umami, Caprese, plant BLT, chili mango, and brain booster flavors:* Top the toast with the ingredients listed.

For the cucumber ribbon flavor: Cut off the ends of the cucumber and slice into long ribbons using a vegetable peeler. Place the cucumber ribbons on the toast. In a small bowl, whisk together the vinegar, oil, soy sauce, sesame seeds, and red pepper flakes, if using. Drizzle the mixture on top of the toast.

Turn the page for FLAVOR OPTIONS.

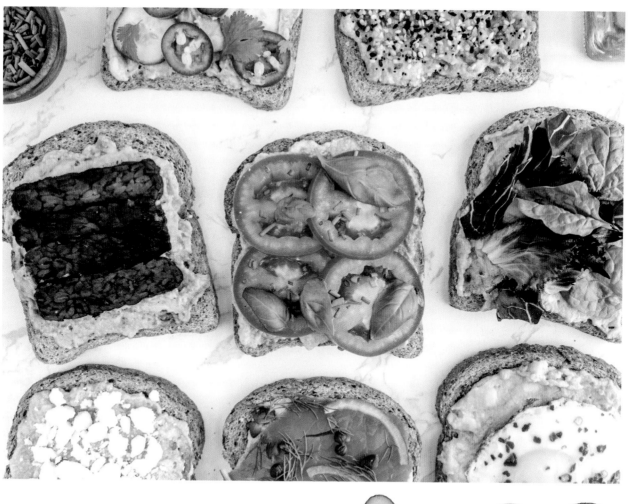

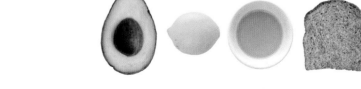

🌱 tips

Choosing the perfect avocado:
Dark-colored avocados tend to be riper and will yield to firm but gentle pressure in the palm of your hand.

Storing avocados:
Store avocados in the fridge if you plan to eat them within 2 weeks, depending on their level of ripeness when you purchase them.
Store avocados at room temperature if you plan to eat them within 1 to 3 days, depending on their level of ripeness when you purchase them.

Ripening avocados fast:
Store avocados in a brown paper bag with an apple or banana for 2 to 3 days to speed up the ripening process. The naturally occurring plant hormone ethylene found in these fruits can help trigger ripening. The brown bag helps trap the gas and speed up the process.

flavor options

savory umami:

2 small sheets roasted seaweed, crumbled

½ teaspoon sesame seeds

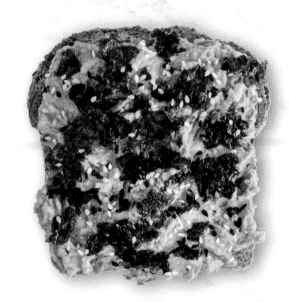

chili mango:

½ mango, thinly sliced

2 tablespoons chopped fresh mint leaves

1 teaspoon lime juice

Chili powder, to taste

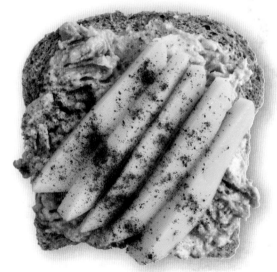

plant BLT:

1 cup loosely packed arugula

1 cup cherry tomatoes, halved

2 slices Tempeh Bacon (page 126), crumbled, ⅓ cup Mushroom or Coconut Bacon (page 127), or 2 slices regular bacon, cooked and crumbled

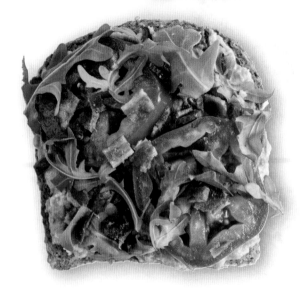

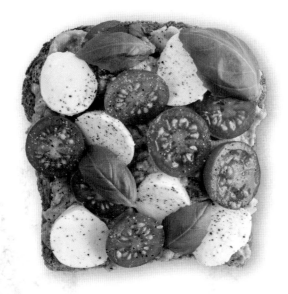

caprese:

1 Roma tomato, sliced into rounds

2 ounces fresh mozzarella pearls

Chopped fresh basil leaves

Balsamic glaze, for drizzling (optional)

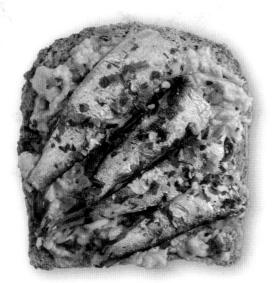

brain booster:

1 (3¾-ounce) can sardines in water, drained

1 tablespoon lemon juice

¼ cup loosely packed flat-leaf parsley leaves

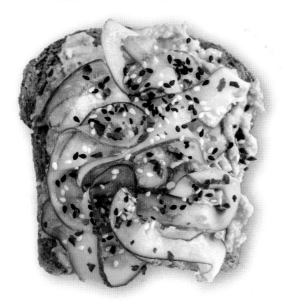

cucumber ribbon:

1 small Persian cucumber, peeled

1 teaspoon unseasoned rice vinegar

1 teaspoon toasted sesame oil

½ teaspoon low-sodium soy sauce

½ teaspoon toasted sesame seeds

Red pepper flakes, for topping (optional)

hash brown breakfast casserole

yield: **6 servings**   prep time: **10 minutes**   cook time: **35 minutes**

Breakfast comes together in a flash with frozen shredded hash browns, eggs, and chopped vegetables. This casserole has a perfectly crunchy top and a creamy soft interior; you'll want to (and can) enjoy it for breakfast more days than one. For a plant-based take, use crumbled tofu in place of the eggs (see the note below) and omit the cheese.

1 (1-pound) bag frozen shredded hash browns (about 3 cups)

1 cup fresh spinach, chopped

1 medium red bell pepper, diced

¼ medium yellow onion, diced

⅓ cup shredded cheddar cheese

6 large eggs

⅓ cup unsweetened plant milk of choice

¼ teaspoon finely ground Himalayan pink salt

⅛ teaspoon ground black pepper

Sliced green onions, for topping (optional)

1. Preheat the oven to 400°F. Grease a 9 by 13-inch baking dish with cooking spray.

2. Put the hash browns, spinach, bell pepper, onion, and cheese in the prepared baking dish and stir to combine.

3. In a large bowl, whisk together the eggs, milk, salt, and pepper. Pour the mixture into the prepared baking dish to evenly coat the hash brown mixture.

4. Bake until the eggs are set and the potatoes are cooked, 30 to 35 minutes. Top with sliced green onions, if desired.

5. Store leftovers in a sealed container in the refrigerator for up to 3 days.

note _____

For egg-free: Use a 14-ounce block of extra-firm tofu, crumbled, in place of the eggs.

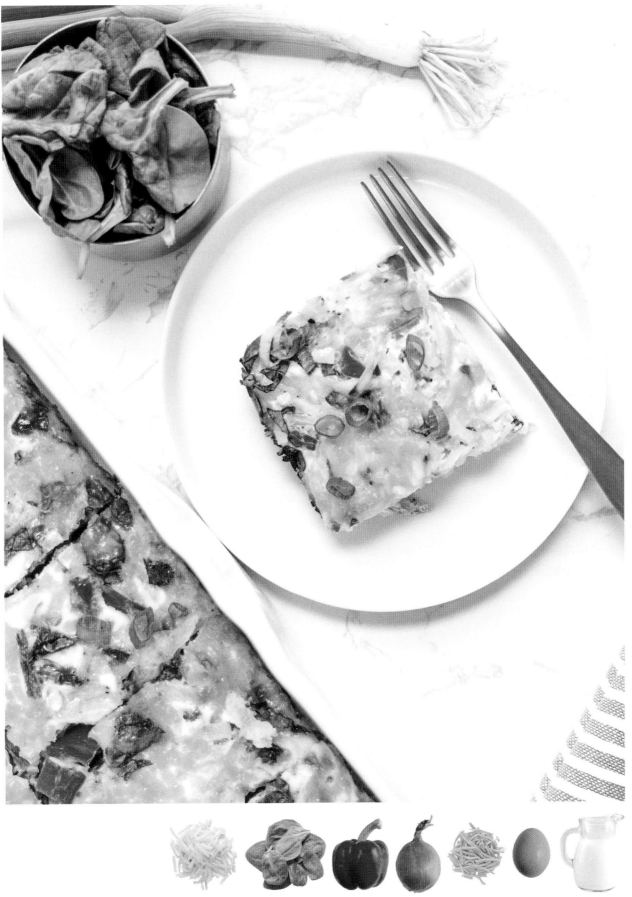

oatmeal breakfast cakes

yield: 2 cakes (1 per serving)   prep time: 5 minutes   cook time: 35 minutes

Is it breakfast or is it dessert? How about both! This breakfast cake is made with a base of fiber-rich whole-grain oats and sweetened exclusively with banana (unless you opt to add dark chocolate chips). Be sure to use a natural peanut butter (made with one ingredient—peanuts) as opposed to a sweetened or salted variety. If you are an oatmeal lover looking to switch up your morning meal, try this fun take.

⅔ cup rolled oats

1 large ripe banana

1 large egg

2 tablespoons natural creamy peanut butter

1 teaspoon pure vanilla extract

¼ teaspoon baking powder

Pinch of finely ground Himalayan pink salt

¼ cup mini dark chocolate chips (optional)

1. Preheat the oven to 350°F. Grease two 8-ounce oven-safe ramekins.

2. Blend all of the ingredients except the chocolate chips in a food processor or blender until smooth. Stir in the chocolate chips by hand, if using.

3. Divide the batter between the prepared ramekins. Bake for 30 to 35 minutes, or until a toothpick inserted in the center comes out clean.

4. Enjoy immediately.

notes

Feel free to use any creamy nut butter, such as cashew or almond, in place of the peanut butter. Just make sure it's unsweetened and unsalted. If you use salted nut butter, omit the pinch of salt from this recipe.

To make this cake more of a dessert, you can add 2 to 3 teaspoons of pure maple syrup to the batter in Step 2.

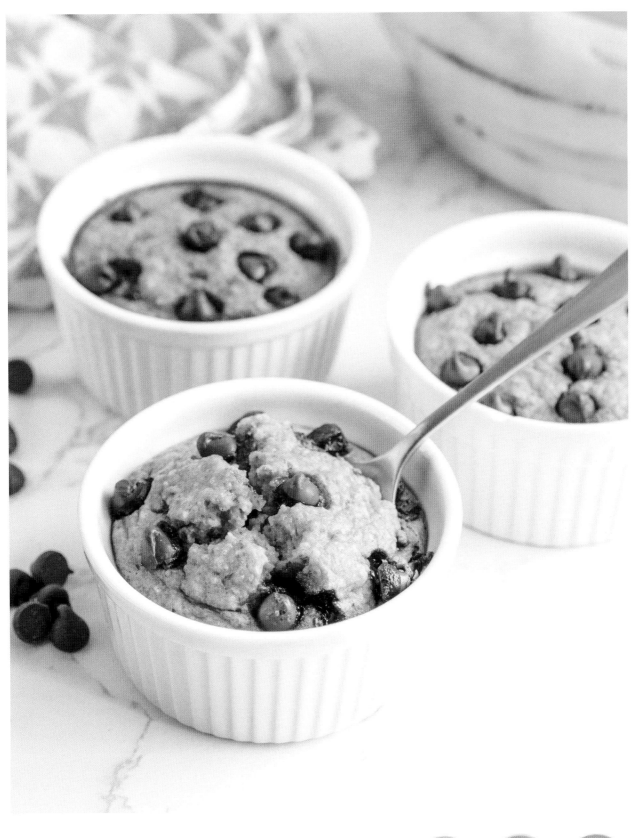

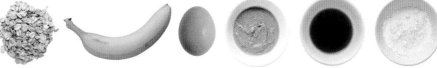

CHAPTER 8:

salads and soups

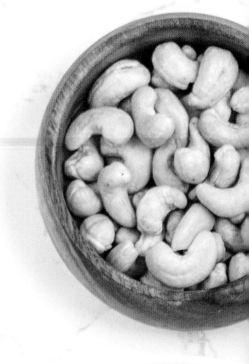

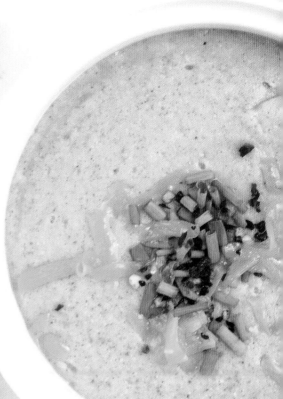

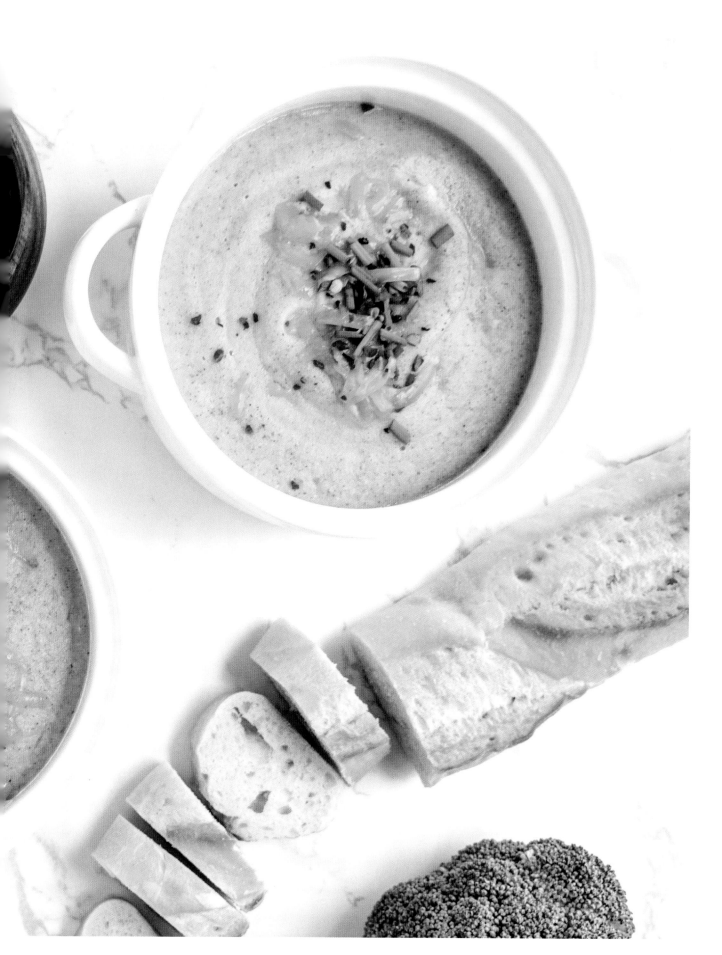

salad jar

yield: **1 serving**   prep time: **10 minutes**   cook time: **8 minutes (for tempeh taco version)**

Building a layered salad jar that stays fresh and perfectly crisp is an art but, once mastered, can transform lunch. The idea is simple: start with a flavorful dressing and layer with food groups—protein, vegetables, fruit, whole grains, good fats, and leafy greens. These six versions are my favorite combinations, but you can use the formula on page 179 to create your own customized jars with just about any mix of ingredients you have on hand. *Tip:* If using fruit that browns when exposed to air, such as apple, pear, or avocado, add it the day you plan to eat the salad.

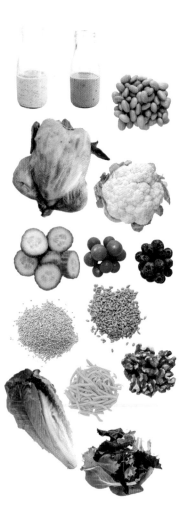

To make all of the jars except the tempeh taco, layer the ingredients in a 24-ounce lidded jar in the order listed and store in the refrigerator for up to 3 days. Pour out onto a plate when ready to eat.

To make the tempeh taco jar, warm the oil in a medium skillet over medium-high heat. Add the tempeh and taco seasoning and sauté until crispy on the outside, about 5 minutes. Remove from the pan and set aside. Add the corn to the skillet and cook until charred, about 3 minutes. Remove the pan from the heat and set aside. Layer the ingredients in a jar starting with the dressing followed by the tempeh, corn, bell peppers, tomatoes, rice, cheese, and romaine.

antioxidant salad jar:

2 tablespoons balsamic vinaigrette, store-bought or homemade (page 110)

3 ounces shredded rotisserie chicken

½ cup diced red onions

½ cup chopped cucumbers

¼ cup chopped strawberries

¼ cup blueberries

½ cup cooked quinoa

2 tablespoons chopped raw walnuts

1 handful spinach

california cobb salad jar:

2 tablespoons green goddess dressing, store-bought or homemade (page 111)

1 hard-boiled egg, chopped

1 slice bacon, cooked and crumbled, or ¼ cup crumbled Tempeh Bacon (page 126)

½ cup chopped cucumbers

½ cup halved cherry tomatoes

½ medium avocado, diced

2 tablespoons blue cheese crumbles (optional)

1 handful chopped romaine lettuce

mediterranean medley salad jar:

2 tablespoons balsamic vinaigrette, store-bought or homemade (page 110)

½ cup cooked chickpeas

⅓ cup chopped Persian cucumbers

⅓ cup diced red onions

⅓ cup chopped bell peppers (any color)

½ cup halved cherry tomatoes

½ cup cooked farro

¼ cup pitted kalamata olives

2 tablespoons crumbled feta cheese

1 handful arugula

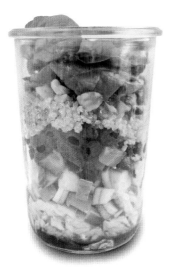
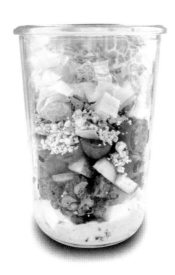
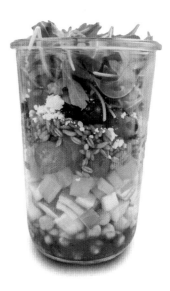

steakhouse salad jar:

2 tablespoons balsamic vinaigrette, store-bought or homemade (page 110)

3 ounces cooked and sliced lean steak, or 2 large portabella mushroom caps, diced and sautéed until softened

½ cup cooked barley

½ cup thinly sliced red onions

½ cup chopped cucumbers

½ cup halved cherry tomatoes

2 tablespoons blue cheese crumbles

1 handful mixed greens

thai peanut salad jar:

2 tablespoons peanut dressing, store-bought or homemade (page 110)

3 ounces firm tofu, cubed, or ½ cup steamed shelled edamame

½ cup shredded red cabbage

½ cup shredded carrots

½ cup mandarin orange segments

½ cup cooked brown rice

2 tablespoons roasted peanuts, chopped

1 handful arugula

tempeh taco salad jar:

2 teaspoons avocado oil

3 ounces tempeh, crumbled

½ teaspoon taco seasoning

½ cup frozen corn

2 tablespoons ranch dressing, store-bought or homemade (page 111)

½ cup diced green bell peppers

½ cup halved cherry tomatoes

½ cup cooked brown rice

2 tablespoons shredded cheddar cheese

1 handful chopped romaine lettuce

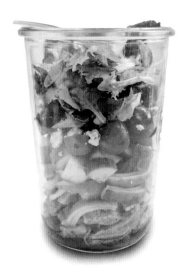
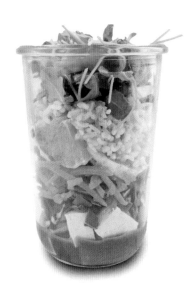
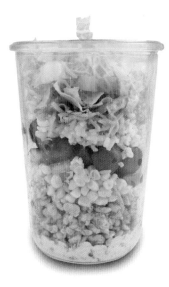

salad jar formula (from bottom to top in a 24-ounce jar):

DRESSING
(1–3 tablespoons)

Balsamic
Green goddess
Peanut
Ranch

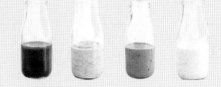

+

PROTEIN
(3–4 ounces or ½ cup cooked)

Beans
Tofu
Egg
Chicken
Steamed shelled edamame

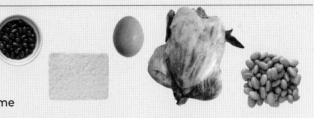

+

DENSE, FIRM, CRISP VEGGIES
(1 cup)

Bell peppers
Carrots
Cucumbers
Cooked or raw broccoli or cauliflower florets

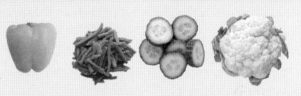

+

SOFT, DELICATE VEGGIES/ FRUIT
(½ cup)

Avocado
Tomatoes
Berries
Oranges
Apple
Pear

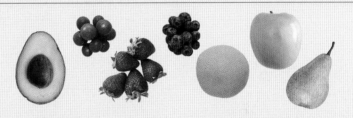

+

WHOLE GRAINS/ GRAIN SWAPS
(½ cup cooked)

Rice
Pasta
Quinoa
Farro
Riced cauliflower

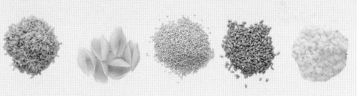

+

FATS
(1–2 tablespoons)

Nuts
Seeds
Cheese
Olives

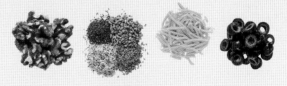

+

LEAFY GREENS
(1 handful)

Arugula
Romaine
Spinach
Mixed greens

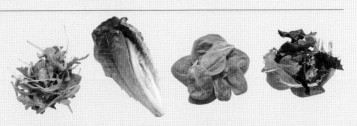

creamy cream-less butternut squash soup

yield: **4 servings**   prep time: **15 minutes**   cook time: **30 minutes**

Fill your kitchen with the cozy scent of fresh rosemary and simmering vegetables, and fill your belly with this nourishing, creamless butternut squash soup. It is made with a base of squash, carrots, and potatoes, which gives it creaminess without the cream. Serve this silky-smooth soup piping hot with crusty bread.

1 tablespoon extra-virgin olive oil

½ small yellow onion, chopped

4 cloves garlic, minced

1 medium butternut squash (about 2 pounds), peeled, seeded, and cubed

1 large russet potato (about 8 ounces), scrubbed and chopped

1 large carrot (about 3 ounces), peeled and chopped

3 cups low-sodium vegetable broth

1 tablespoon minced fresh rosemary

⅛ teaspoon ground nutmeg

1 teaspoon finely ground Himalayan pink salt

⅛ teaspoon ground black pepper

suggested toppings:

Roasted pepitas

Sour cream

1. Heat the oil in a large pot over medium heat. Add the onion and cook, stirring frequently, until softened, 4 to 5 minutes. Stir in the garlic and sauté until fragrant, about 30 seconds.

2. Add the squash, potato, carrot, broth, rosemary, nutmeg, salt, and pepper. Bring to a boil, then reduce the heat to medium-low and simmer until the vegetables are tender, 15 to 20 minutes.

3. Using an immersion blender, blend the soup until smooth. Alternatively, let the soup cool for at least 10 minutes and then, working in batches, pour the soup into a regular blender and blend until thick and silky.

4. Serve topped with a sprinkle of pepitas and/or a dollop of sour cream, if desired.

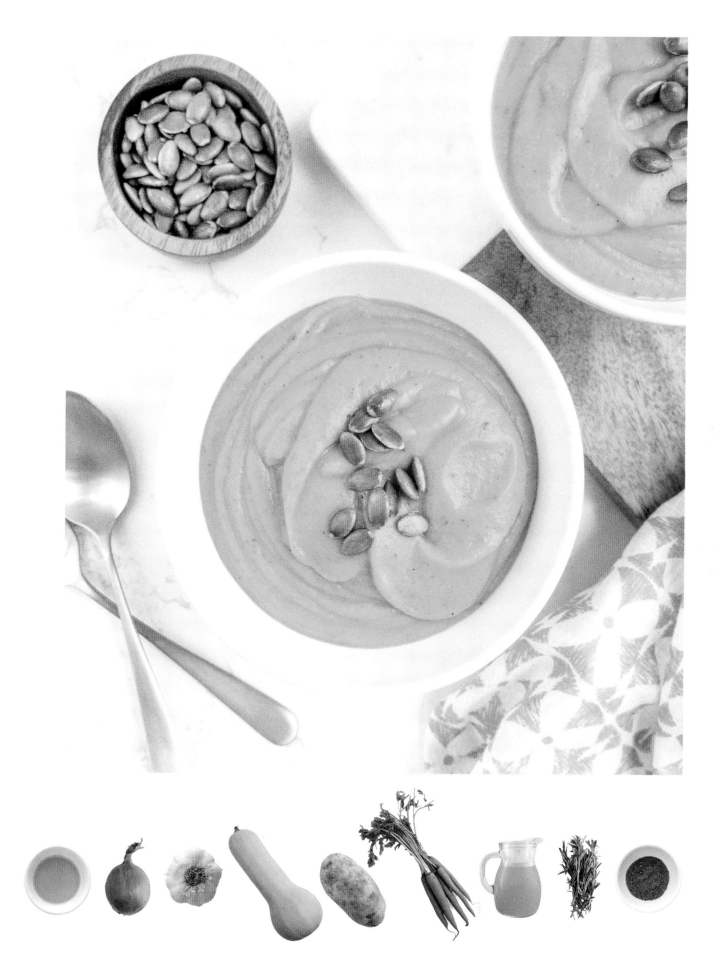

lettuce-less greek salad

yield: **4 servings**   prep time: **20 minutes**   cook time: **20 to 30 minutes**

Authentic Greek salads skip the lettuce and get right to the good stuff! This lettuce-less salad can be served as a hearty side dish or a complete meal. Crispy chickpeas serve as the plant protein source but can be swapped with shredded rotisserie chicken for additional staying power.

salad:

1 (15-ounce) can no-salt-added chickpeas, drained and rinsed well, or 1½ cups cooked chickpeas (see page 44)

2 tablespoons extra-virgin olive oil

¼ teaspoon finely ground Himalayan pink salt

1 large English cucumber (about 10 ounces), halved lengthwise and sliced into thin half-moons

2 cups cherry tomatoes, halved

1 cup pitted kalamata olives, halved

½ medium red onion, thinly sliced

⅓ cup crumbled feta cheese

dressing:

¼ cup extra-virgin olive oil

Juice of 1 lemon

1 teaspoon finely ground Himalayan pink salt

1 teaspoon ground black pepper

¼ cup fresh dill fronds, chopped

1. Preheat the oven to 425°F and line a sheet pan with parchment paper.

2. Spread the chickpeas in a single layer on the prepared pan and toss with the oil and salt. Roast until golden brown and crisp, 20 to 30 minutes. Set aside.

3. In a medium bowl, whisk together the dressing ingredients.

4. Put the cucumber, tomatoes, olives, red onion, feta, and roasted chickpeas in a large bowl. Pour the dressing over the top and toss the ingredients to combine.

5. Serve immediately. Store leftovers, covered, in the refrigerator and eat within a day.

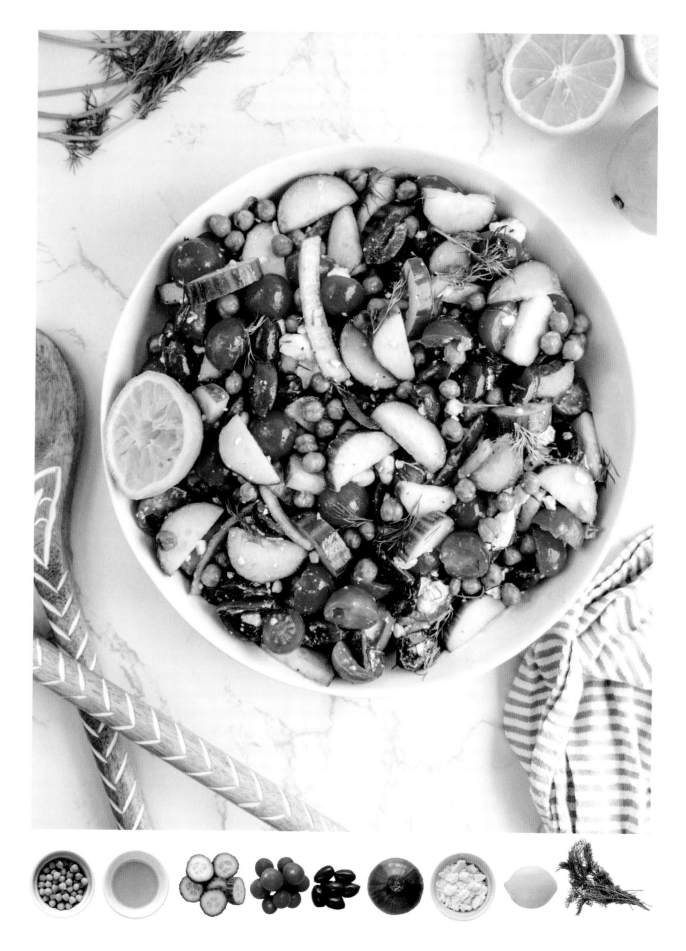

everyday quinoa salad

yield: **4 servings**   prep time: **15 minutes**   cook time: **15 minutes**

A staple quinoa salad is an essential when you are eating mostly plant-based. Quinoa, while classified as a whole grain, is actually an edible seed that comes in various colors, including black, red, yellow, and white. It is also considered a complete protein—plus, it packs more protein by weight than grains like rice or farro, with 8 grams per cup of cooked quinoa. While this dish can serve as a complete meal, you can also enjoy it as a hearty complement to lean proteins.

1 cup quinoa (any color)

2 cups water

1 (15-ounce) can no-salt-added chickpeas, drained and rinsed well, or 1½ cups cooked chickpeas (see page 44)

1 cup chopped English cucumbers

1 medium red bell pepper, chopped

½ cup diced red onions

1 cup chopped fresh flat-leaf parsley

quick lemon dressing:

2 tablespoons extra-virgin olive oil

Juice of ½ lemon

2 cloves garlic, minced

Finely ground Himalayan pink salt and ground black pepper

1. Rinse and drain the quinoa in a fine-mesh strainer. Combine the quinoa and water in a 2-quart saucepan and bring to a boil over medium-high heat. Lower the heat to a simmer, cover the pan, and cook until the liquid is absorbed, about 15 minutes. Set aside to cool.

2. To make the dressing, whisk together the oil, lemon juice, and garlic in a small bowl. Season to taste with salt and pepper.

3. Transfer the cooled quinoa to a large bowl and add the chickpeas, cucumbers, bell pepper, onions, and parsley. Pour the dressing on top and toss to combine. For the best flavor, chill for 1 to 2 hours before serving to allow the flavors to mingle.

4. Store leftovers in a sealed container in the refrigerator for up to 5 days.

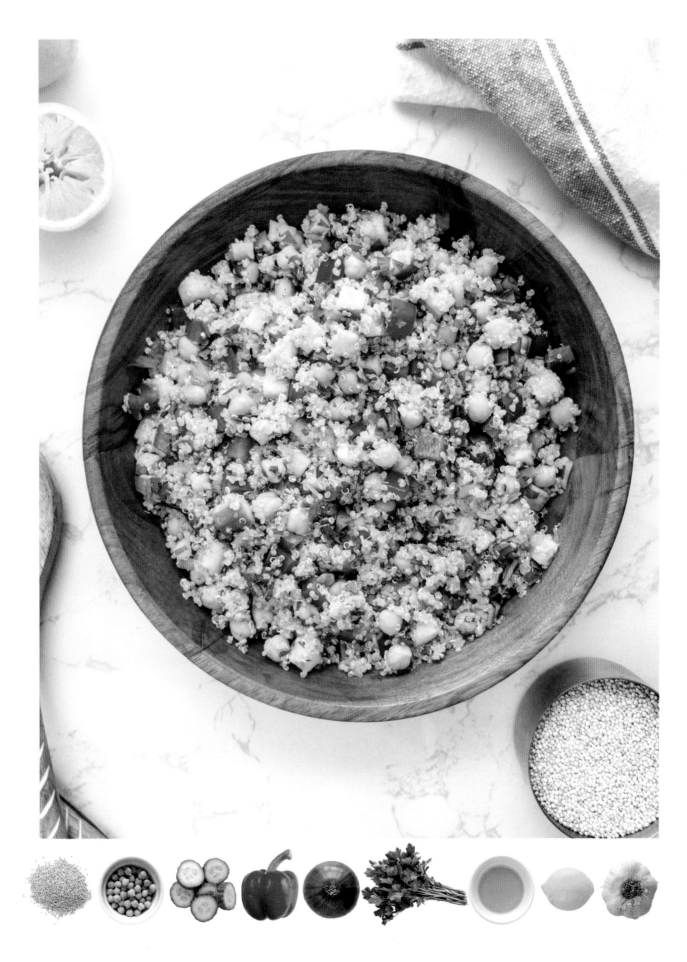

tex-mex chopped salad

yield: **2 servings**   prep time: **10 minutes**   cook time: **15 minutes**

There is no shortness of crunch in this chopped salad made with crisp romaine, charred corn, and toasted tortilla strips brought together with a creamy two-ingredient taco ranch dressing. Packed with texture and bold flavors, this salad is a lunchtime dream!

1 (10-inch) whole-grain tortilla, cut into 1-inch strips

Finely ground Himalayan pink salt

1 tablespoon avocado oil

8 ounces boneless, skinless chicken breasts, cut into 1-inch pieces, or 8 ounces tempeh, crumbled

Ground black pepper

1 cup frozen corn

5 cups chopped romaine lettuce

2 Roma tomatoes, diced

1 cup cooked black beans

¼ cup chopped fresh cilantro

Lime wedges, for serving (optional)

dressing:

¼ cup ranch dressing, store-bought or homemade (page 111)

½ teaspoon taco seasoning

1. Preheat the oven to 350°F. Line a sheet pan with parchment paper.

2. Place the tortilla strips on the prepared pan in a single layer, spray with cooking spray, and season with salt. Bake for 3 to 5 minutes, or until crisp.

3. To make the dressing, whisk together the ranch dressing and taco seasoning in a small bowl. Set aside.

4. Pour the oil into a large skillet over medium-high heat.

If using chicken, place the chicken in the pan and sauté until no longer pink, 5 to 6 minutes. Season with salt and pepper to taste. Remove the chicken to a plate and set aside.

If using tempeh, place the crumbled tempeh in the pan and sauté until slightly crisp, about 5 minutes. Season with salt and pepper to taste. Remove the tempeh to a plate and set aside.

5. Place the corn in the skillet and cook until slightly charred, about 3 minutes. Remove from the pan.

6. In a large bowl, toss together the chicken or tempeh, corn, romaine, tomatoes, beans, cilantro, and dressing. Divide between two plates, top with the tortilla strips, and serve with lime wedges, if desired.

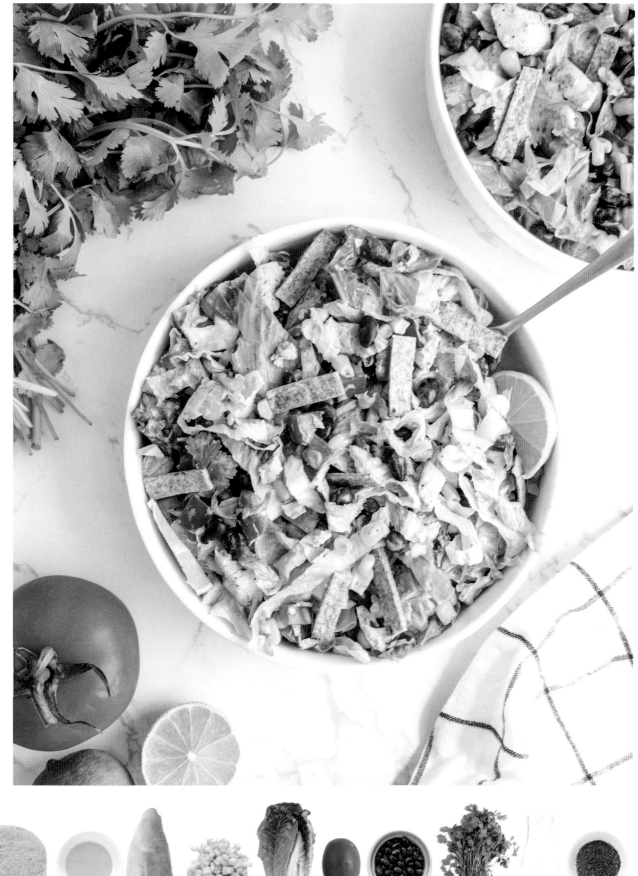
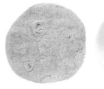 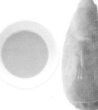 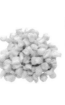 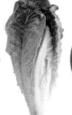 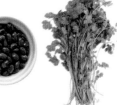

veggie chili

yield: 6 servings   prep time: 10 minutes   cook time: 35 minutes

Nothing says cozy like a bowl of warm, hearty chili. This simple version is packed with veggie goodness—you won't even miss the meat (but you can swap out a can of beans for some meat for additional staying power; see the note below). You can "beef" it up with even more plant-based goodness by adding another cup of chopped vegetables, such as carrots, celery, and/or sweet potato. Or choose the classic mirepoix (2 parts diced onions to 1 part each diced carrots and celery)—just omit the onion from the ingredient list.

1 tablespoon extra-virgin olive oil

1 medium yellow onion, diced

1½ cups frozen corn

2 medium green bell peppers, diced

2 cloves garlic, minced

1 (14.5-ounce) can diced fire-roasted tomatoes (with juices)

1 (15-ounce) can no-salt-added kidney beans, drained and rinsed well, or 1½ cups cooked kidney beans (see page 44)

1 (15-ounce) can no-salt-added pinto beans, drained and rinsed well, or 1½ cups cooked pinto beans (see page 44)

1 tablespoon chili powder

1 tablespoon ground cumin

3 cups water

Finely ground Himalayan pink salt and ground black pepper

suggested toppings:

Sour cream

Diced red onions

Sliced jalapeño

Chopped fresh cilantro

1. Heat the oil in a large pot over medium-high heat. Add the onion, corn, and bell peppers. Cook, stirring frequently, until tender, about 5 minutes. Add the garlic and sauté until fragrant, about 30 seconds.

2. Stir in the tomatoes, beans, chili powder, cumin, and water. Stir to combine, bring to a boil, then reduce to a simmer and cook, covered, for 30 minutes, or until thickened. Season to taste with salt and pepper.

3. Serve immediately, topped as desired. Store leftovers in a sealed container in the refrigerator for up to 5 days.

notes

For a heartier dish, replace 1 can of beans with 1 pound of lean ground beef or turkey. Begin by browning the meat and draining the excess fat, then add the onion, corn, and bell peppers and proceed with the rest of the recipe.

For extra flavor, you can replace the water with vegetable broth.

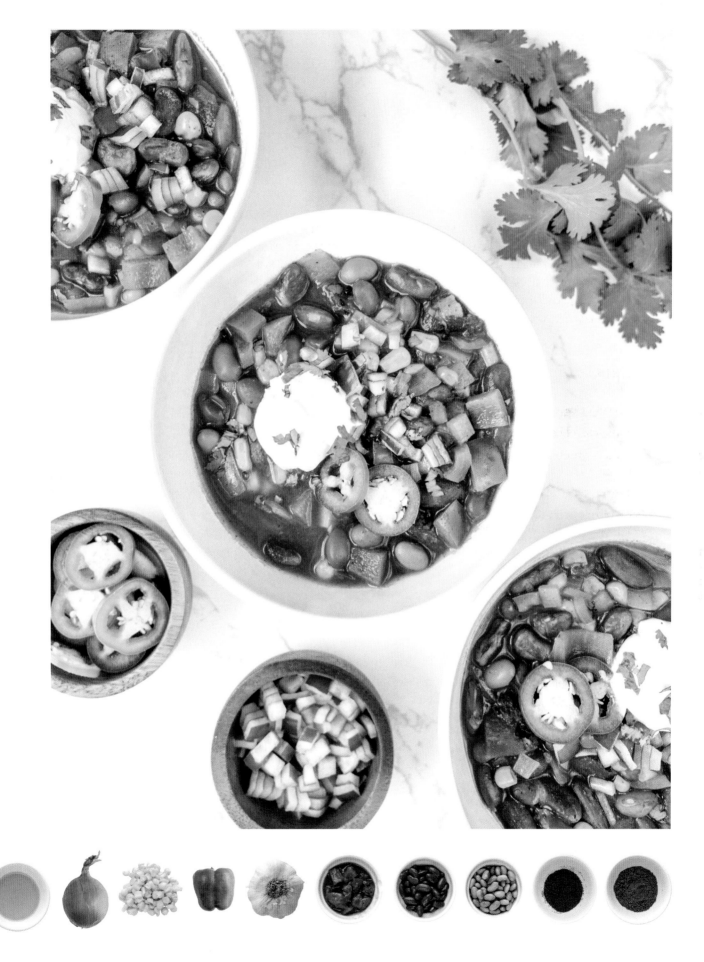

avocado chicken salad

yield: **2 servings**   prep time: **15 minutes**   cook time: **12 minutes**

This super satisfying salad is packed with a trifecta of nutrients that keep you fuller longer—protein, fiber, and good fats. To save time in the kitchen, use shredded rotisserie chicken from the grocery store. Enjoy this salad as is, scooped up with whole-grain crackers or endive leaves, in a sandwich, or stuffed into a whole-grain pita or butter lettuce cups.

8 ounces boneless, skinless chicken breasts

1 tablespoon avocado oil

1 cup frozen corn

1 large avocado, pitted, peeled, and diced

¼ cup diced red onions

¼ cup chopped fresh cilantro

1 clove garlic, minced

1 tablespoon lime juice

½ teaspoon finely ground Himalayan pink salt

¼ teaspoon ground black pepper

1. To poach the chicken, place it in a medium saucepan, fill with an inch of water, and bring to a boil. Reduce the heat to a simmer and cover the pan with a lid. Simmer until the chicken reaches an internal temperature of 165°F and is opaque through the middle, 10 to 12 minutes.

2. Meanwhile, char the corn: Warm the oil in a small skillet over medium-high heat. Cook the corn until slightly charred, about 4 minutes. Transfer to a large bowl.

3. When the chicken is done, remove it from the cooking water and place it on a clean work surface. Shred the chicken using two forks.

4. Place the chicken in the bowl with the corn. Add the avocado, red onions, cilantro, garlic, lime juice, salt, and pepper and stir to combine. Enjoy immediately.

note _____

For meat-free: You can use a 15-ounce can of no-salt-added chickpeas, drained, rinsed well, and mashed, in place of the chicken, similar to my Chickpea Tuna-Less Salad (page 260).

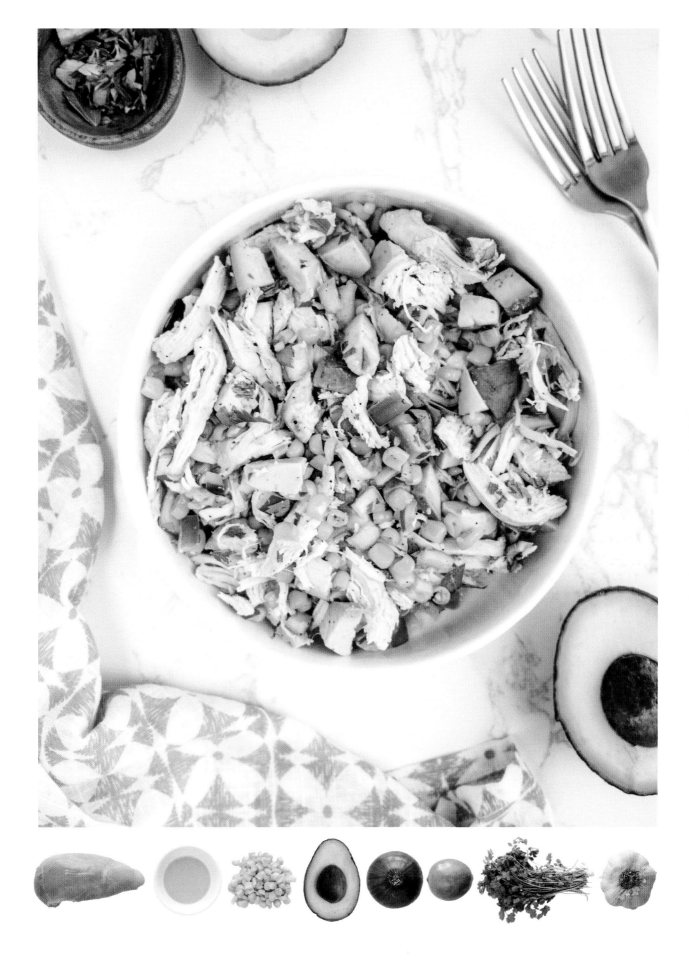

cauliflower rice tabbouleh

yield: **4 servings**   prep time: **15 minutes, plus 30 minutes to chill**   cook time: **5 minutes**

Try this lightened-up, vegetable-packed spin on traditional Middle Eastern tabbouleh that replaces bulgur with riced cauliflower while still packing the same fresh lemon-herb flavor. Enjoy it as a side dish or pair it with a protein to build a complete meal.

1 tablespoon extra-virgin olive oil

1 medium head cauliflower (about 1½ pounds), cored, cut into florets, and riced, or 4 cups prericed cauliflower

½ teaspoon finely ground Himalayan pink salt

1 bunch fresh flat-leaf parsley, thick stems removed

4 green onions, chopped

¼ cup fresh mint leaves

½ large English cucumber, diced

2 Roma tomatoes, seeded and diced

dressing:

2 tablespoons extra-virgin olive oil

Juice of ½ lemon

1 clove garlic, minced

1 teaspoon finely ground Himalayan pink salt

½ teaspoon ground black pepper

1. Heat the oil in a large skillet over medium-high heat. Add the riced cauliflower, season with the salt, and cook, stirring often, until tender and slightly crisp, 4 to 5 minutes. Transfer to a large bowl and place in the refrigerator to cool.

2. Put the parsley, green onions, and mint in a food processor and pulse until finely minced, about 10 seconds. Transfer the mixture to the bowl with the cauliflower and add the cucumber and tomatoes.

3. In a small bowl, whisk together the dressing ingredients. Pour the dressing over the salad and stir to combine.

4. Chill the tabbouleh for at least 30 minutes to let the flavors mingle. Store leftovers in a sealed container for up to 4 days.

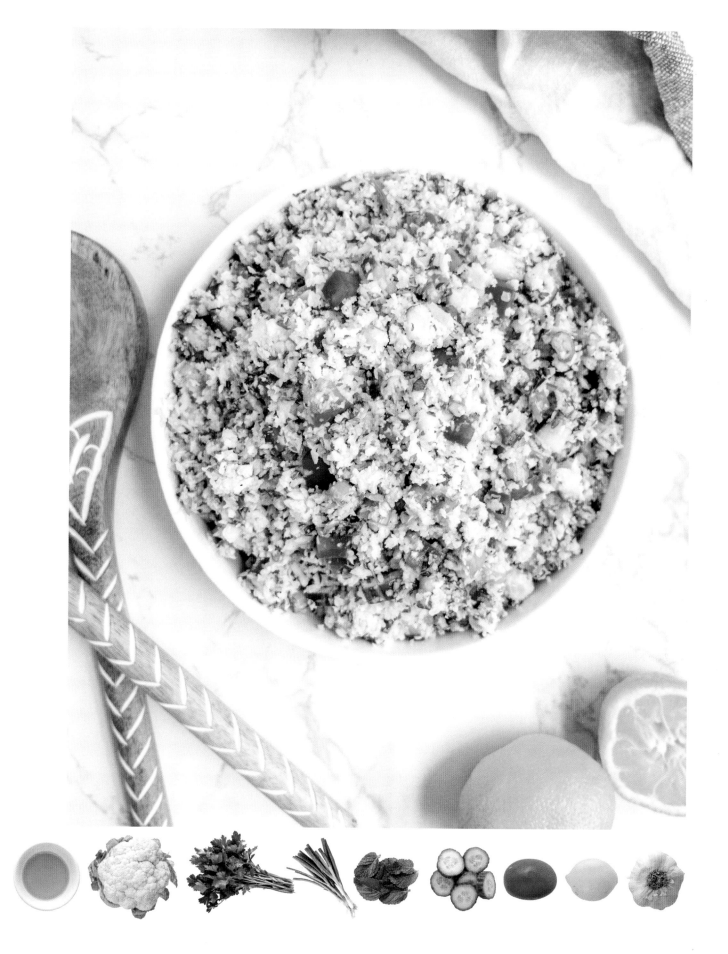

greenest green goddess salad

yield: **4 servings**   prep time: **15 minutes**

Looking for a unique way to eat your greens? Crunchy meets creamy in this seriously addicting chopped salad. It's made with a base of five flavorful green vegetables and coated in a creamy plant-based dressing made with even more greens (parsley, basil, dill, and avocado). It doesn't get any greener (or tastier!) than this.

1 small head green cabbage (about 1 pound), shredded

4 small Persian cucumbers, finely diced

1 bunch green onions, sliced

⅓ cup sliced fresh chives

1 cup green goddess dressing, store-bought or homemade (page 111)

Place all of the ingredients in a large bowl and toss to combine. Store leftovers in a sealed container in the refrigerator for up to 2 days.

note _____

A mandoline or food processor works well for shredding the cabbage.

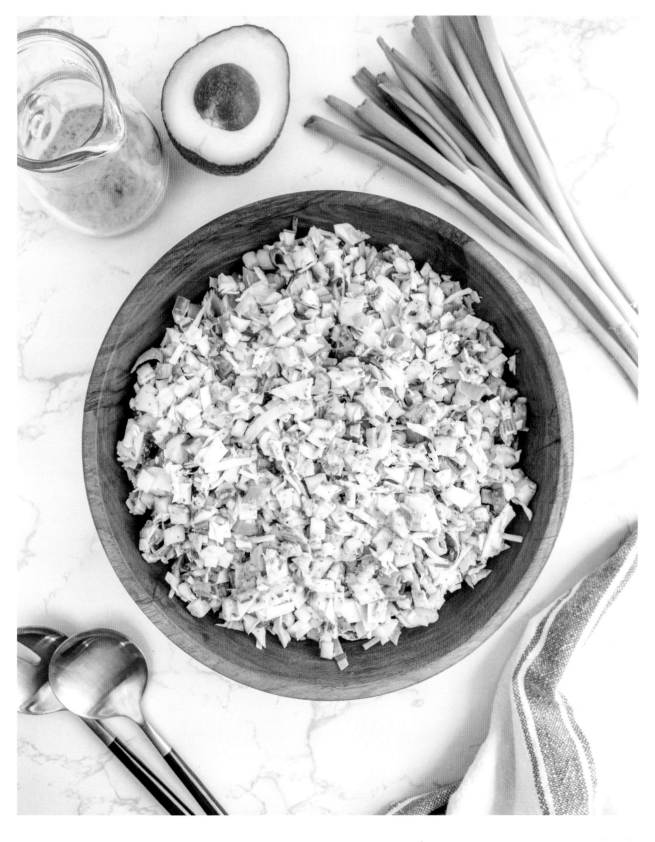

   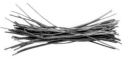

creamy broccoli cauliflower soup

yield: 4 servings   prep time: 10 minutes, plus 20 minutes to soak cashews   cook time: 40 minutes

Broccoli and cauliflower come together in this creamy, decadent-tasting soup. The secret ingredients? Cashews and potatoes, which give the soup a silky-smooth texture without the addition of cream or butter.

⅓ cup raw cashews

1 tablespoon extra-virgin olive oil

1 small yellow onion, chopped

3 cloves garlic, minced

1 large head broccoli (about 1 pound), cut into small florets

1 small head cauliflower (about 12 ounces), cut into small florets

1 large russet potato (about 8 ounces), scrubbed and chopped

1 teaspoon finely ground Himalayan pink salt

½ teaspoon ground black pepper

4 cups reduced-sodium vegetable broth

suggested toppings:

Shredded cheddar cheese

Chopped fresh chives

Red pepper flakes

1. Put the cashews in a medium bowl and cover with water. Soak for at least 20 minutes or up to an hour to soften, then drain.

2. Heat the oil in a large pot over medium heat. Add the onion and cook until softened, 3 to 4 minutes. Stir in the garlic and sauté until fragrant, about 30 seconds.

3. Add the broccoli, cauliflower, potato, salt, and pepper to the pot with the onion and garlic. Pour in the broth and bring to a boil. Reduce to a simmer, cover, and cook until the vegetables are tender, 25 to 30 minutes.

4. Let the soup cool for 10 minutes, then, working in batches, pour it into a blender with the cashews and puree until smooth. Serve topped with cheese, chives, and red pepper flakes, if desired.

5. Store leftovers in a sealed container in the refrigerator for up to 4 days or in the freezer for up to 3 months.

note _____

For a soup that is both creamy and chunky, blend only some of the soup and leave the remaining vegetables whole.

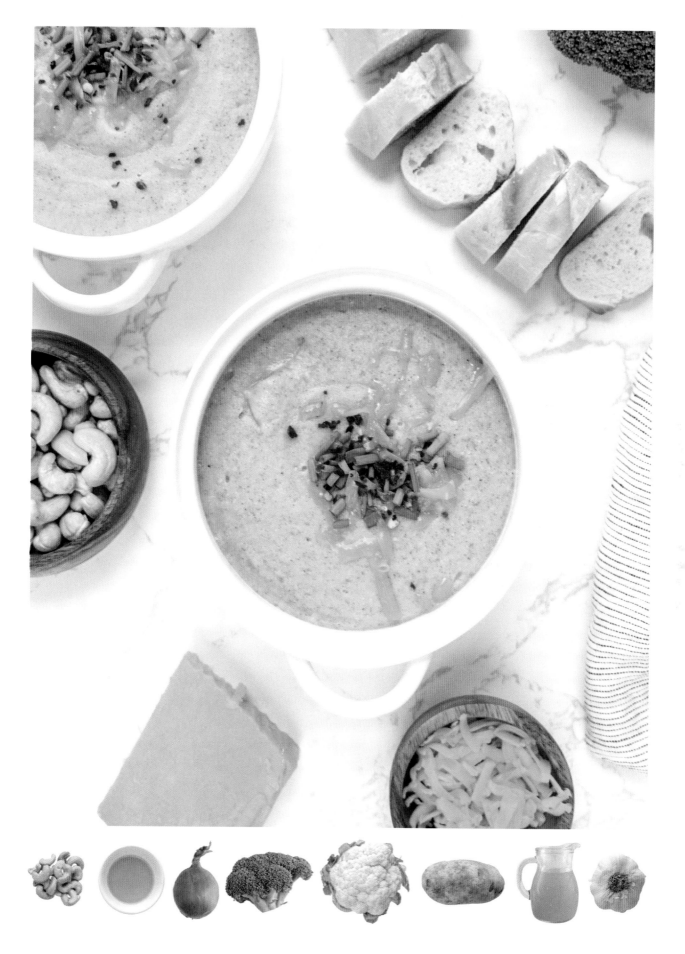

kale romaine caesar salad with chickpea croutons

yield: **4 servings**   prep time: **10 minutes**

Kale meets romaine in this nutritionally elevated Caesar salad that you won't find on a standard restaurant menu. Mixing up your leafy greens helps you get a range of vitamins, minerals, and phytonutrients. Instead of traditional bread croutons, add some plant protein–packed crunch with roasted chickpeas.

1 large bunch kale, stemmed and coarsely chopped (about 4 cups)

⅓ cup Caesar dressing, store-bought or homemade (page 111)

1 head romaine lettuce, chopped (about 4 cups)

2 tablespoons grated Parmesan cheese or plant-based parmesan, store-bought or homemade (page 124)

Finely ground Himalayan pink salt to taste

Ground black pepper to taste

1½ cups Garlic Herb Chickpea Poppers (page 230) or store-bought roasted chickpeas

1. Place the kale in a large bowl and pour the dressing on top. Using your hands, massage the kale with the dressing until slightly softened, about 1 minute.

2. Add the romaine, Parmesan, salt, pepper, and chickpeas and toss to combine. Serve immediately.

notes _____

I don't recommend storing leftover salad; the lettuce will get soggy after a day.

If you aren't a fan of kale, feel free to replace it with arugula, spinach, or more romaine.

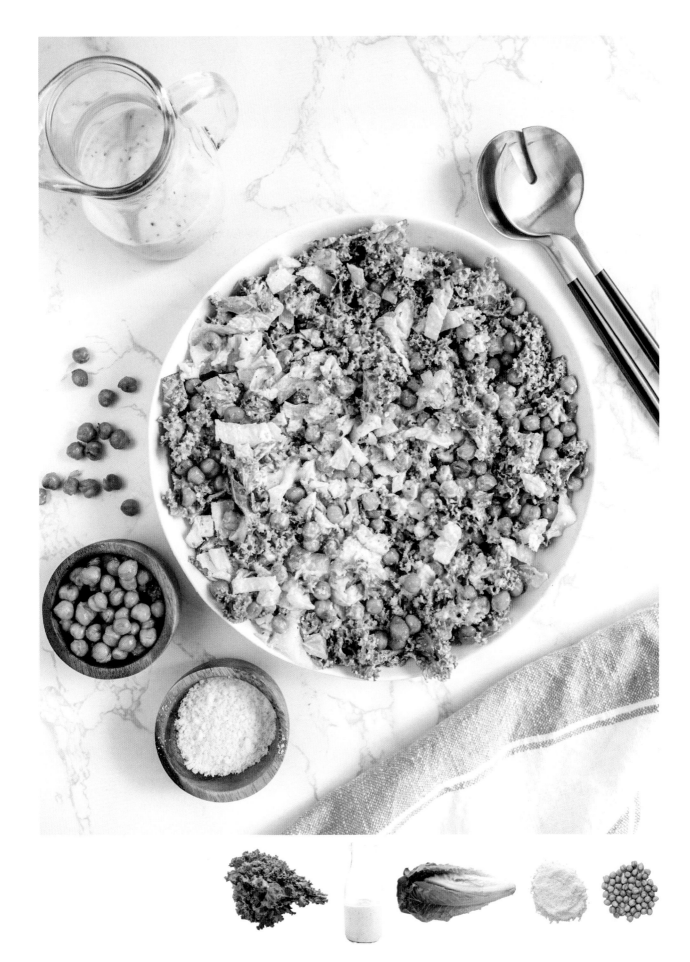

romaine "wedge" salad

yield: **2 servings**   prep time: **10 minutes**

Traditional wedge salads leave much to be desired nutritionally, as they are typically made with nutrient-poor leafy greens (iceberg lettuce) and blanketed with ingredients that are high in saturated fat. This recipe elevates the nutrition while delivering the crunch factor by using romaine as the base, which offers key nutrients, including vitamin C, vitamin K, and folate, and plant-based tempeh bacon and a low-fat, protein-rich Greek yogurt ranch dressing as toppings.

1 large head romaine lettuce or romaine heart, or 2 heads baby romaine ("Little Gems")

¼ cup ranch dressing, store-bought or homemade (page 111)

1 cup diced tomatoes

1 medium avocado, diced

2 slices Tempeh Bacon (page 126), crumbled, or regular bacon, cooked and crumbled

¼ cup blue cheese crumbles

2 teaspoons chopped fresh chives

Finely ground Himalayan pink salt and ground black pepper

1. Wash the romaine and trim the end(s). If using a large head or heart, cut it in half lengthwise.

2. Place each romaine wedge on a serving plate and spoon the dressing over them. Sprinkle the tomatoes, avocado, bacon, cheese, and chives on top of the wedges before serving. Season with salt and pepper to taste.

note _____

For dairy-free: Omit the blue cheese and use a dairy-free ranch dressing.

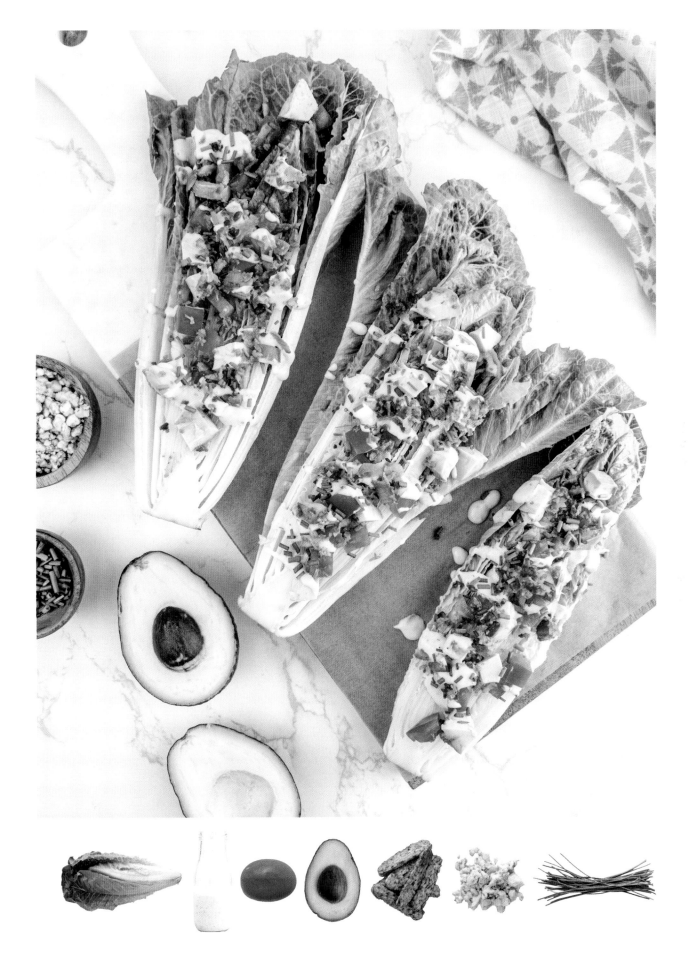

tuscan-style artichoke salad

yield: **4 servings**   prep time: **10 minutes**   cook time: **30 minutes**

Artichokes, a source of gut-loving prebiotic fiber, take center stage in a simple-to-make salad perfect for a picnic, barbecue, potluck, or weeknight dinner. Made with Tuscan-inspired ingredients and dressed in a red wine vinaigrette, this salad is full of vibrant colors and fresh flavor.

1 medium red bell pepper, halved, seeds and membranes removed

1 cup green beans, ends trimmed

1 (12-ounce) jar marinated artichokes, drained and halved

1 cup cooked chickpeas

½ cup sliced sun-dried tomatoes packed in oil

½ medium red onion, thinly sliced

½ cup pitted kalamata olives

¼ cup fresh basil leaves, for topping

dressing:

3 tablespoons extra-virgin olive oil

2 tablespoons red wine vinegar

2 tablespoons minced fresh basil

¼ teaspoon finely ground Himalayan pink salt

⅛ teaspoon ground black pepper

1. Preheat the oven to 450°F. Line a sheet pan with parchment paper.

2. Place the bell pepper halves on the prepared pan, cut side down. Roast until the skin of the pepper is black and the flesh is tender, 25 to 30 minutes. Allow to cool before removing and discarding the skin with your hands. Chop the pepper and transfer to a large bowl.

3. Bring a medium pot of salted water to a boil over high heat. Add the green beans and cook until tender, about 2 minutes. Drain the beans and add them to the bowl with the roasted red pepper.

4. Add the artichokes, chickpeas, sun-dried tomatoes, onion, and olives to the bowl and toss to combine.

5. In a small bowl, whisk together the ingredients for the dressing. Pour over the salad and toss to combine. Top with the basil leaves.

note

To save time, you can use ½ cup of chopped jarred roasted red peppers and skip Steps 1 and 2.

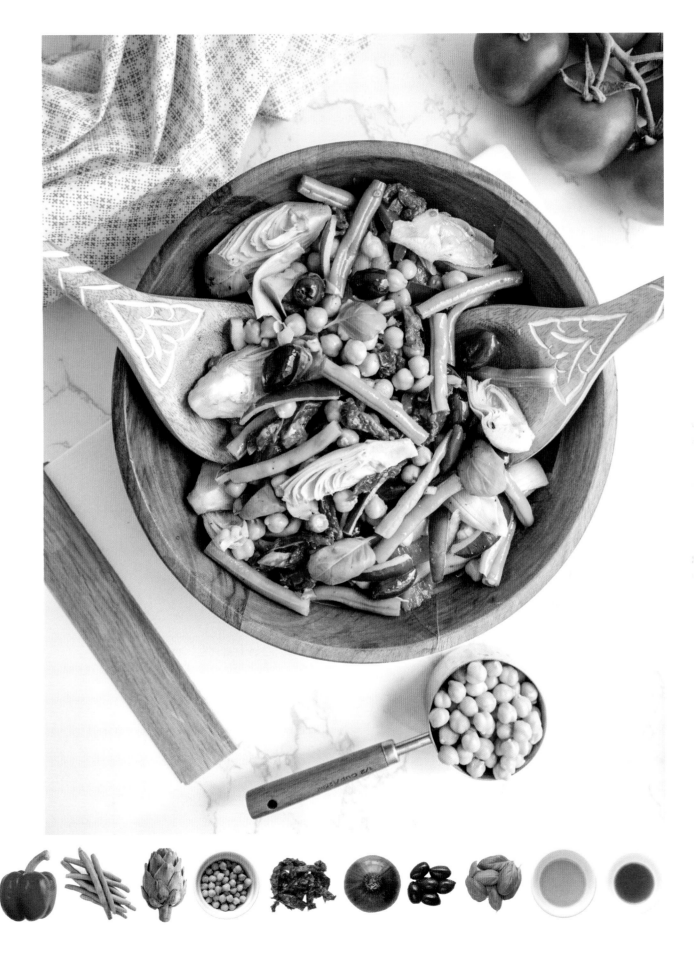

easy taco soup

yield: **4 servings**   prep time: **15 minutes**   cook time: **30 minutes**

The only thing easier than taco night is taco soup night. Simplify taco Tuesday with this hearty one-pot meal. This super satisfying soup is packed with protein, thanks to ground beef and two types of beans, plus it boasts a fair dose of vegetables, of course. While toppings are optional, I can't go without diced avocado and crushed tortilla chips.

1 tablespoon avocado oil

1 pound lean ground beef

½ medium yellow onion, diced

1 (15-ounce) can no-salt-added black beans, drained and rinsed well, or 1½ cups cooked black beans (see page 44)

1 (15-ounce) can no-salt-added pinto beans, drained and rinsed well, or 1½ cups cooked pinto beans (see page 44)

1 (14.5-ounce) can diced fire-roasted tomatoes

1½ cups frozen or fresh corn

½ cup tomato sauce, store-bought or homemade (page 130)

2 tablespoons taco seasoning

2 cups low-sodium beef broth

1 teaspoon finely ground Himalayan pink salt

½ teaspoon ground black pepper

suggested toppings:

Shredded cheese

Sour cream

Diced avocado

Chopped fresh cilantro

Sliced jalapeño

Sliced green onions

Crushed tortilla chips

1. Heat the oil in a large pot. Brown the beef and onion in the oil, using a wooden spoon to break up the clumps of meat. Drain and return to the pot.

2. Add the black beans, pinto beans, tomatoes, corn, tomato sauce, taco seasoning, broth, salt, and pepper to the pot. Bring to a boil, then reduce to a simmer and cook for 10 to 15 minutes to let the flavors blend and thicken the soup to the desired consistency.

3. Serve with the toppings of your choice. Store leftovers in a sealed container in the refrigerator for up to 3 days.

note _____

For meat-free: Replace the beef broth with vegetable broth and the ground beef with another can of beans, such as kidney beans.

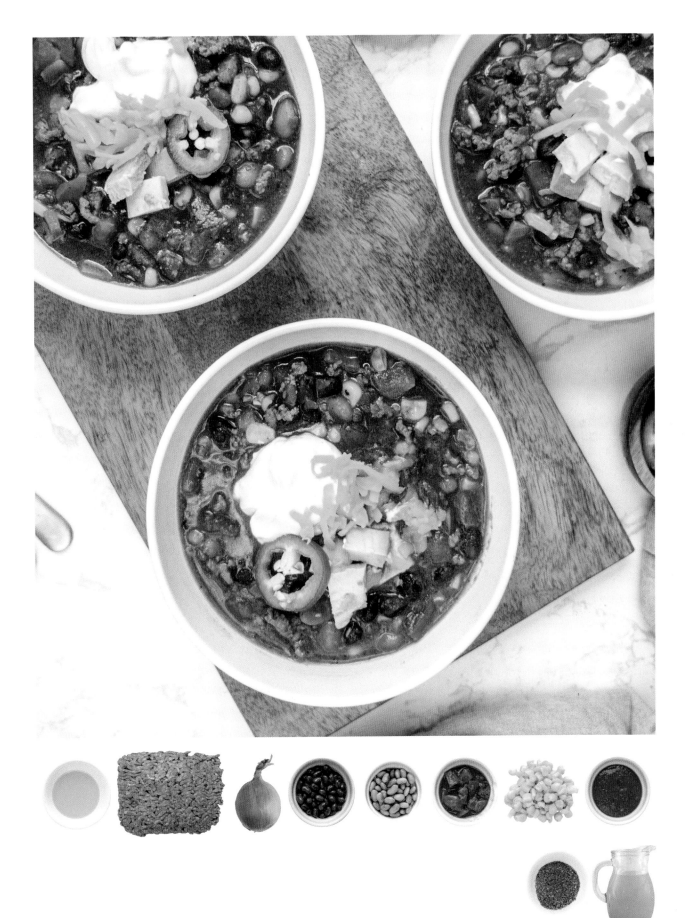

crunchy broccoli cauliflower salad

yield: **4 servings**   prep time: 10 minutes, plus 30 minutes to chill

Make over your crunchy broccoli salad with a dose of cauliflower. While this salad is traditionally prepared with a mayonnaise-based dressing, this version uses a creamy tahini Caesar dressing. You can go with the traditional choice of bacon or up the plant ratio by using tempeh or coconut bacon instead. For a touch of sweetness, I suggest adding diced apple.

½ cup shelled sunflower seeds

½ large head broccoli (about 8 ounces), cut into bite-sized florets

½ small head cauliflower (about 8 ounces), cut into bite-sized florets

½ small red onion, diced

1 medium apple, diced (optional)

3 slices bacon, cooked and crumbled, 3 slices Tempeh Bacon (page 126), crumbled, or ⅓ cup Coconut Bacon (page 127)

⅓ cup shredded sharp cheddar cheese (optional)

⅓ cup Plant-Based Caesar Dressing (page 111), store-bought Caesar dressing, or ranch dressing, store-bought or homemade (page 111)

1. Preheat the oven to 350°F.

2. Spread the sunflower seeds on a sheet pan in a single layer. Toast until lightly browned, about 10 minutes.

3. Place the broccoli, cauliflower, onion, apple (if using), bacon, cheese (if using), and toasted sunflower seeds in a large bowl. Pour the dressing on top and toss to coat. Place in the refrigerator for at least 30 minutes to allow the flavors to combine.

4. Store leftovers in a sealed container in the refrigerator for up to 3 days.

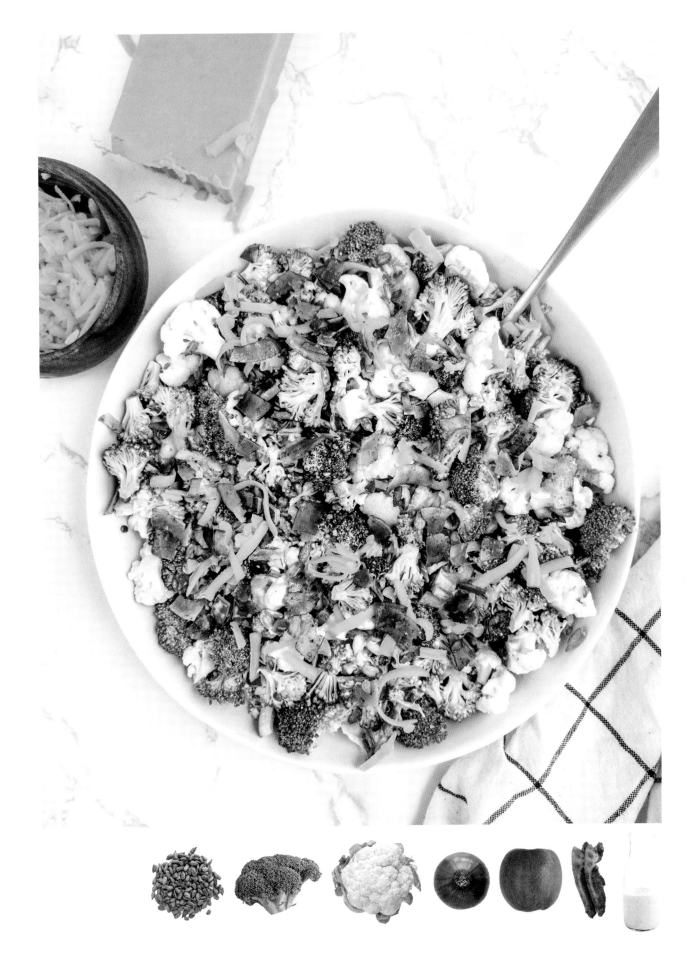

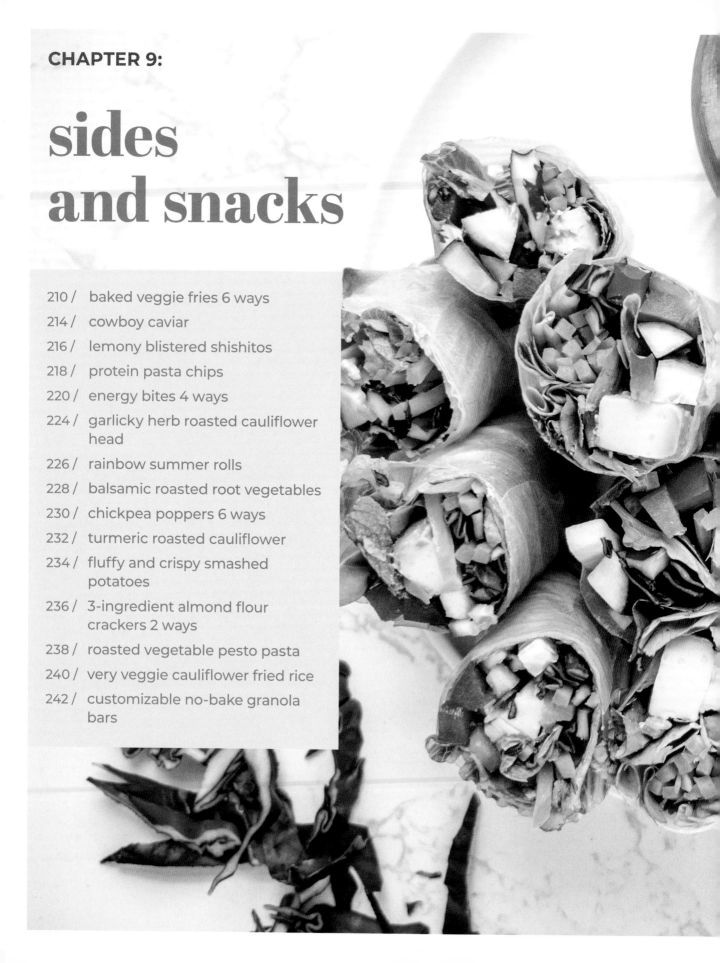

CHAPTER 9:

sides and snacks

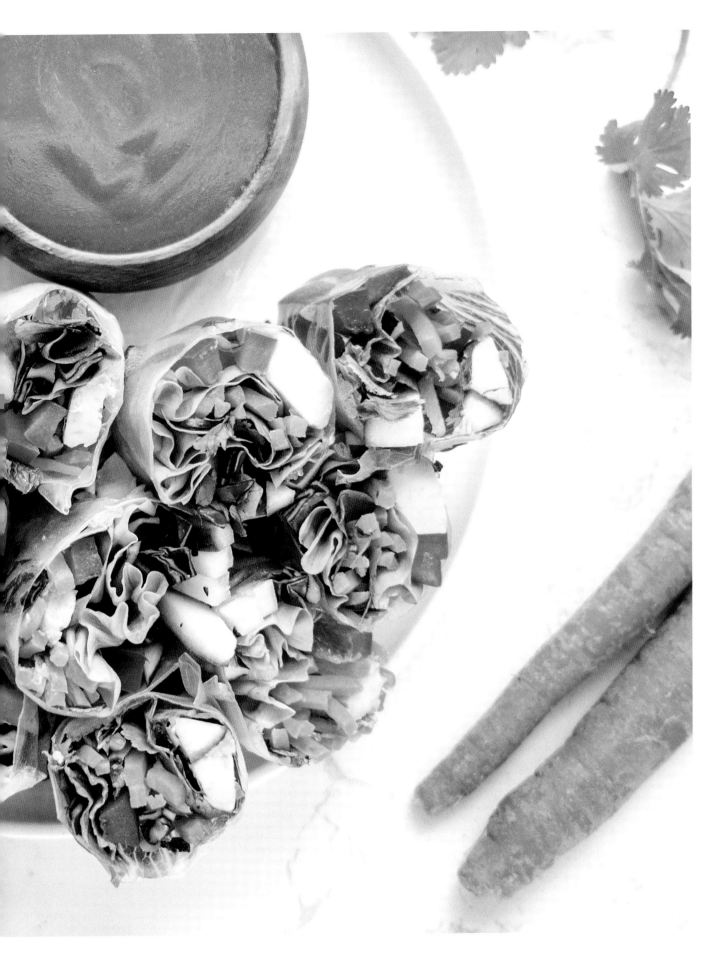

baked veggie fries

yield: 2 servings   prep time: 15 minutes, plus 30 minutes to soak russet potato fries
cook time: 25 to 35 minutes, depending on type

French fries can be made from more than potatoes. While not much beats the classic taste of potato fries (so recipes are included!), there are so many great veggies that hold up in the oven to deliver that similar salty satisfaction. French fries get a bad rap because of the oil they are cooked in and the method of preparation (frying). These are baked and made with a good-for-you oil and flavorful seasonings, which are all you really need to transform humble veggies into your next addicting, can't-just-eat-one side dish or snack.

sweet potato fries:

1 tablespoon extra-virgin olive oil

½ teaspoon finely ground Himalayan pink salt

⅛ teaspoon ground black pepper

2 large sweet potatoes (about 1 pound), scrubbed and sliced into ¼-inch-wide sticks

Preheat the oven to 425°F and line a sheet pan with parchment paper. In a large bowl, whisk together the oil, salt, and pepper. Place the potatoes in the bowl and toss to coat. Arrange the fries in a single layer on the prepared pan. Bake for 15 minutes, flip, and bake for another 15 to 20 minutes, until slightly crisp on the outside and fluffy on the inside.

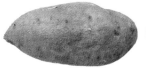

rosemary parsnip fries:

1 tablespoon extra-virgin olive oil

½ teaspoon finely ground Himalayan pink salt

⅛ teaspoon ground black pepper

1 tablespoon chopped fresh rosemary

5 medium parsnips (about 1 pound), peeled and cut into ½-inch-wide sticks

Preheat the oven to 425°F and line a sheet pan with parchment paper. In a large bowl, whisk together the oil, salt, pepper, and rosemary. Place the parsnip sticks in the bowl and toss to coat. Arrange the fries in a single layer on the prepared pan. Bake for 10 minutes, flip, and bake for another 10 to 15 minutes, until slightly crisp on the outside and tender on the inside.

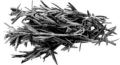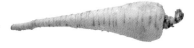

smoky jicama fries:

1 tablespoon extra-virgin olive oil

½ teaspoon finely ground Himalayan pink salt

½ teaspoon smoked paprika

1 medium jicama (about 1 pound), peeled and cut into ½-inch-wide sticks

Preheat the oven to 425°F and line a sheet pan with parchment paper. In a large bowl, whisk together the oil, salt, and paprika. Place the jicama sticks in the bowl and toss to coat. Arrange the fries in a single layer on the prepared pan. Bake for 10 minutes, flip, and bake for another 10 to 15 minutes, until slightly crisp on the outside and tender on the inside.

carrot fries:

1 tablespoon extra-virgin olive oil

½ teaspoon finely ground Himalayan pink salt

1 tablespoon chopped fresh flat-leaf parsley

6 medium carrots (about 1 pound), peeled and cut into ½-inch-wide sticks

Preheat the oven to 425°F and line a sheet pan with parchment paper. In a large bowl, whisk together the oil, salt, pepper, and parsley. Place the carrot sticks in the bowl and toss to coat. Arrange the fries in a single layer on the prepared pan. Bake for 10 minutes, flip, and bake for another 10 to 15 minutes, until slightly crisp on the outside and tender on the inside.

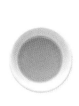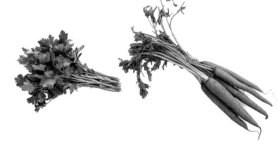

garlic potato wedges:

3 large russet potatoes (about 1 pound), scrubbed and cut into 1-inch-wide wedges

1 tablespoon extra-virgin olive oil

2 cloves garlic, minced

½ teaspoon finely ground Himalayan pink salt

½ teaspoon onion powder

⅛ teaspoon ground black pepper

Place the potato wedges in a large bowl and cover with water. Soak for 30 minutes. Preheat the oven to 425°F and line a sheet pan with parchment paper. In a small bowl, whisk together the oil, garlic, salt, onion powder, and pepper. Drain the potatoes, dry them and the bowl thoroughly, and place back in the bowl. Pour the oil mixture over the wedges and toss to coat. Arrange the wedges in a single layer on the prepared pan. Bake for 15 minutes, flip, and bake for another 15 to 20 minutes, until slightly crisp on the outside and fluffy on the inside.

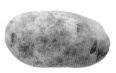

beet fries:

1 tablespoon extra-virgin olive oil

½ teaspoon finely ground Himalayan pink salt

2 tablespoons grated Parmesan cheese or plant-based parmesan, store-bought or homemade (page 124)

1 pound beets (about 2 large beets), peeled and sliced into ½-inch-wide sticks

Preheat the oven to 425°F and line a sheet pan with parchment paper. In a large bowl, whisk together the oil, salt, and Parmesan. Place the beet sticks in the bowl and toss to coat. Arrange the fries in a single layer on the prepared pan. Bake for 10 minutes, flip, and bake for another 10 to 15 minutes, until slightly crisp on the outside and tender on the inside.

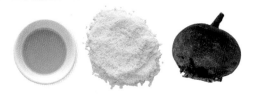

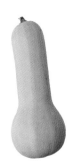

notes

Make sure the fries are cut uniformly for even cooking.

Soaking the russet potato wedges before baking helps remove the excess starch, which yields crispier fries.

It doesn't stop here! You can also transform butternut squash, celeriac, green beans, plantains, rutabaga, and more into your next fry obsession.

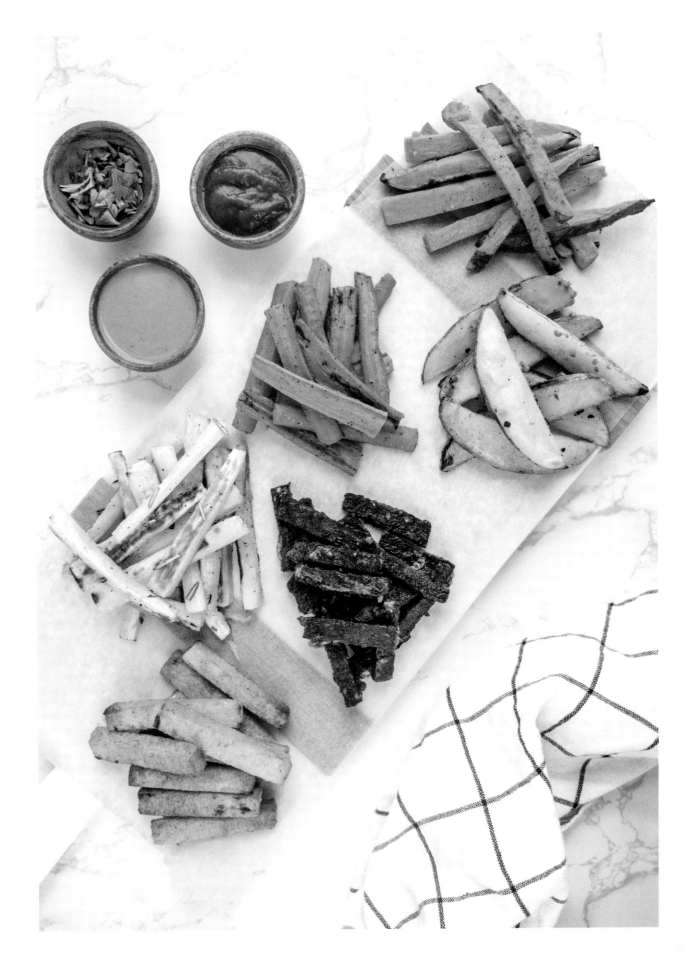

cowboy caviar

yield: 16 servings (½ cup per serving)   prep time: 15 minutes

A summer potluck menu is incomplete without a bowl of cowboy caviar (also known as Texas caviar). This salad of black beans, black-eyed peas, diced vegetables, and a vinaigrette-style dressing is best enjoyed as a dip for tortilla chips (or even endive leaves) but can also be served as a side salad or topping for lean proteins off the grill.

1 (15-ounce) can no-salt-added black beans, drained and rinsed well, or 1½ cups cooked black beans (see page 44)

1 (15-ounce) can no-salt-added black-eyed peas, drained and rinsed well, or 1½ cups cooked black-eyed peas (see page 44)

2 Roma tomatoes, diced

2 medium bell peppers (any color), diced

1½ cups frozen corn, defrosted

½ medium red onion, diced

⅓ cup finely chopped fresh cilantro

dressing:

¼ cup extra-virgin olive oil

Juice of ½ lime

½ teaspoon finely ground Himalayan pink salt

¼ teaspoon ground black pepper

1. In a large bowl, combine the black beans, black-eyed peas, tomatoes, bell peppers, corn, red onion, and cilantro. Stir using a rubber spatula until the ingredients are well combined.

2. To make the dressing, whisk together the oil, lime juice, salt, and pepper in a small bowl.

3. Pour the dressing over the other ingredients and stir well.

4. Store leftovers in the refrigerator, covered, for up to 5 days.

note

Other tasty add-ins include diced avocado and finely diced jalapeño for some heat.

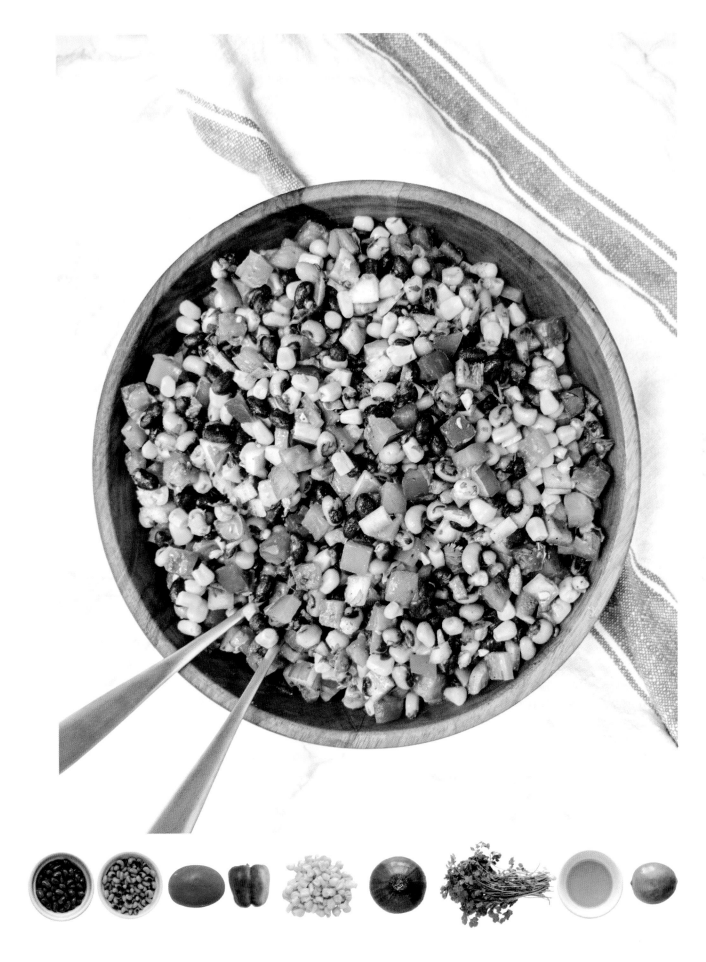

lemony blistered shishitos

yield: **2 servings**   prep time: **5 minutes**   cook time: **4 minutes**

They aren't sweet like bell peppers and they aren't spicy like jalapeños—they're shishitos! Blistered shishito peppers are like potato chips—you can't just eat one. But you should know that eating shishito peppers is like a game of Russian roulette; one out of ten will pack a spicy punch due to its level of capsaicin. However, even the hottest ones are quite mild.

6 ounces shishito peppers (about 3 heaping cups), rinsed and patted dry

2 tablespoons avocado oil, divided

Juice of ½ lemon

Sea salt flakes, for topping

1. Put the peppers in a large bowl and toss with 1 tablespoon of the oil.

2. Pour the remaining tablespoon of oil into a large skillet over medium-high heat. When the oil is hot, add the peppers in one even layer. Work in batches if needed to avoid overcrowding in the skillet.

3. Let the peppers cook undisturbed for 1 to 2 minutes, until charred. Stir and continue cooking for another 1 to 2 minutes, until charred and blistered all over.

4. Squeeze the lemon juice over the peppers and sprinkle sea salt flakes on top. Use tongs to toss once and transfer to a serving plate.

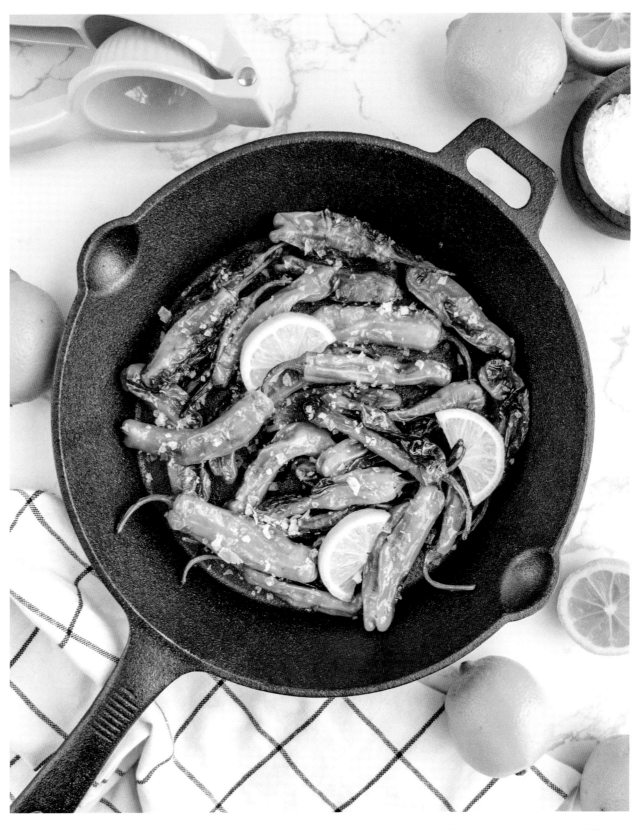

protein pasta chips

yield: **4 servings**   prep time: **10 minutes**   cook time: **40 minutes**

Craving some savory crunch? Try protein pasta chips made with a base of short chickpea pasta that's been cooked, coated in oil and seasonings, and crisped in the oven. While you can use any pasta in this recipe, I recommend chickpea because it has more protein, fiber, and naturally occurring micronutrients than regular pasta.

8 ounces short chickpea or red lentil pasta, such as rigatoni, farfalle, penne, or shells

1 tablespoon extra-virgin olive oil

3 tablespoons grated Parmesan cheese or plant-based parmesan, store-bought or homemade (page 124)

1 teaspoon dried oregano leaves

½ teaspoon garlic powder

½ teaspoon finely ground Himalayan pink salt

⅛ teaspoon ground black pepper

Tomato sauce, store-bought or homemade (page 130), warmed, for serving (optional)

1. Preheat the oven to 400°F. Line a sheet pan with parchment paper.

2. Bring a large pot of salted water to a boil. Cook the pasta according to the package instructions until al dente. Drain, rinse under cold water to stop the cooking, and return to the pot. Toss the pasta over low heat for 30 seconds to evaporate any remaining water. Remove from the heat and toss with the oil, Parmesan, oregano, garlic powder, salt, and pepper.

3. Spread the pasta in a single layer on the prepared sheet pan. Bake for 30 to 35 minutes, tossing halfway through, until crisp.

4. Serve with tomato sauce for dipping, if desired.

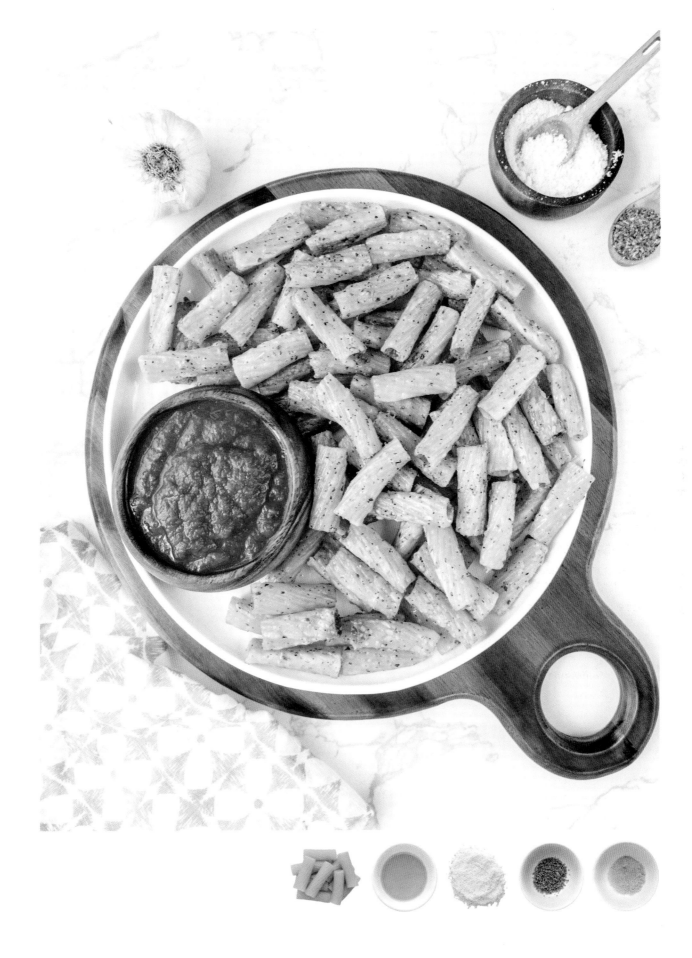

energy bites 4 WAYS

yield: 12 bites (1 per serving)   prep time: 15 minutes, plus 20 minutes to soak dates and 10 minutes to chill bites

The perfect on-the-go snack. These bites are balanced with energizing carbohydrates, filling fiber, and satiating plant protein to help fuel your afternoon and bridge the gap between meals.

brownie bites:

2 cups soft pitted medjool dates (about 12 large dates)

1 cup raw almonds

1 cup raw cashews

2 tablespoons unsweetened cocoa powder

½ teaspoon pure vanilla extract

Pinch of finely ground Himalayan pink salt

¼ cup mini dark chocolate chips

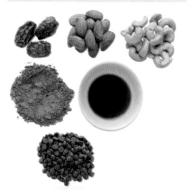

chocolate peanut butter cup bites:

2 cups soft pitted medjool dates (about 12 large dates)

2 cups raw peanuts

2 tablespoons natural creamy peanut butter

½ teaspoon pure vanilla extract

Pinch of finely ground Himalayan pink salt

¼ cup mini dark chocolate chips

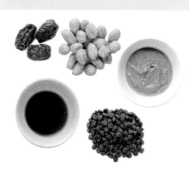

blueberry lemon bites:

1 cup soft pitted medjool dates (about 6 large dates)

1 cup raw almonds

1 cup raw cashews

1 cup unsweetened dried blueberries

1 teaspoon lemon juice

½ teaspoon pure vanilla extract

Pinch of finely ground Himalayan pink salt

Grated zest of 1 lemon

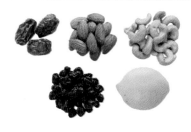

pineapple coconut bites:

1 cup soft pitted medjool dates (about 6 large dates)

1 cup raw pistachios

1 cup raw walnuts

1 cup chopped unsweetened dried pineapple rings

¼ cup unsweetened shredded coconut, plus more for rolling

½ teaspoon pure vanilla extract

Pinch of finely ground Himalayan pink salt

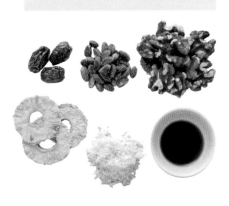

note

You can use any variety of raw nuts, such as pecans, pistachios, or walnuts.

1. Line a sheet pan with parchment paper.

2. Place the dates in a large bowl and cover with water. Set aside to soak and soften for 20 minutes, then drain.

3. *To make the brownie bites,* place the almonds and cashews in a food processor and process until crumbly, about 20 seconds. Add the drained dates and the remaining ingredients, except the chocolate chips, and blend until a slightly sticky dough forms. If the dough is too dry, add water 1 teaspoon at a time. Fold in the chocolate chips by hand using a rubber spatula.

4. *To make the chocolate peanut butter bites,* place the peanuts in a food processor and process until crumbly, about 20 seconds. Add the drained dates and the remaining ingredients except the chocolate chips and blend until a slightly sticky dough forms. If the dough is too dry, add water 1 teaspoon at a time. Fold in the chocolate chips by hand using a rubber spatula.

5. *To make the blueberry lemon bites,* place the almonds and cashews in a food processor and process until crumbly, about 20 seconds. Add the drained dates and the remaining ingredients except the lemon zest and blend until a slightly sticky dough forms. If the dough is too dry, add water 1 teaspoon at a time. Fold in the lemon zest by hand using a rubber spatula.

6. *To make the pineapple coconut bites,* place the pistachios and walnuts in a food processor and process until crumbly, about 20 seconds. Add the drained dates and the remaining ingredients and blend until a slightly sticky dough forms. If the dough is too dry, add water 1 teaspoon at a time.

7. Scrape the mixture into a bowl. Using your hands, roll about 2 tablespoons at a time into 1-inch balls. If making the pineapple coconut bites, roll the balls in shredded coconut. Place the bites on the prepared pan and refrigerate for 10 minutes to harden.

8. Store in a sealed container in the refrigerator for up to a week.

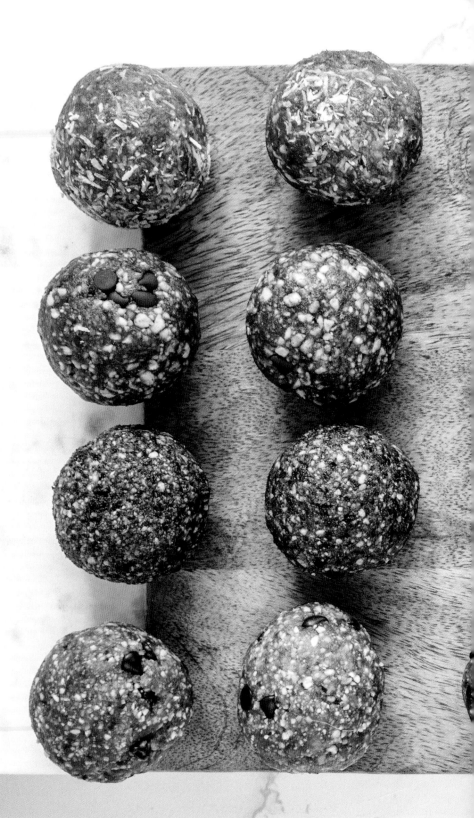

pineapple
coconut bites

brownie bites

blueberry
lemon bites

chocolate
peanut butter
cup bites

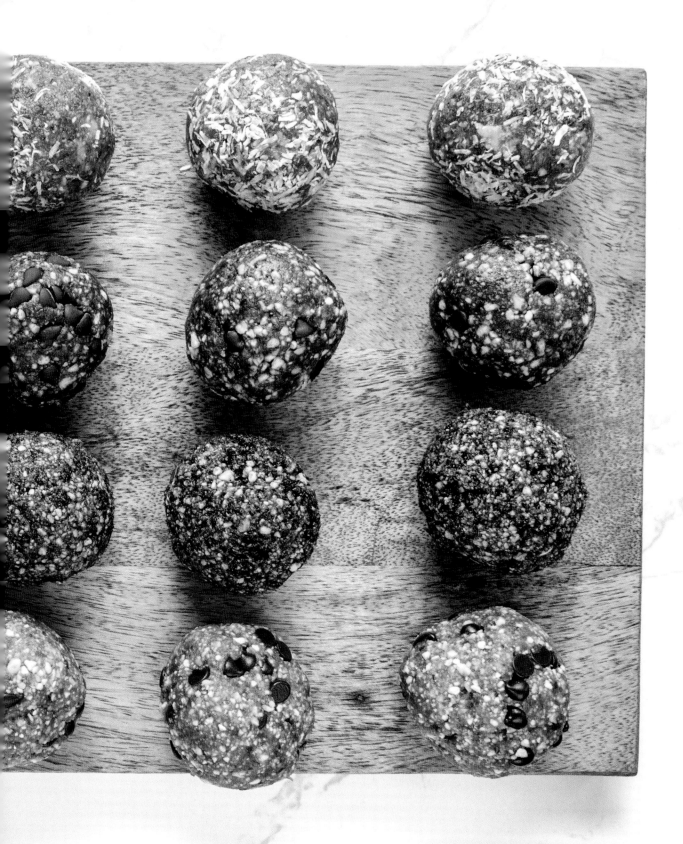

garlicky herb roasted cauliflower head

yield: **4 servings**   prep time: **10 minutes**   cook time: **50 minutes**

Save time chopping and cook up the entire cauliflower head instead. This mild-tasting cruciferous vegetable soaks up the flavors you cook it with—in this case, savory garlic, flavorful Parmesan, and aromatic herbs. The outside of the head gets perfectly crispy while the inside stays soft and tender.

1 large head cauliflower (about 2 pounds)

3 tablespoons extra-virgin olive oil

3 cloves garlic, minced

2 tablespoons grated Parmesan cheese or plant-based parmesan, store-bought or homemade (page 124), divided

1 teaspoon dried basil

1 teaspoon dried parsley

¼ teaspoon finely ground Himalayan pink salt

⅛ teaspoon ground black pepper

Chopped fresh flat-leaf parsley, for topping

1. Preheat the oven to 400°F.

2. Trim and discard the leaves from the head of cauliflower, then cut off enough of the base of the stalk to allow the head to lie flat but remain intact.

3. In a small bowl, whisk together the oil, garlic, 1 tablespoon of the cheese, the dried herbs, salt, and pepper.

4. Place the cauliflower on a sheet pan and brush with three-quarters of the herbed oil.

5. Cover the pan tightly with foil and bake for 30 minutes. Remove the foil and bake for another 10 to 15 minutes, or until tender and slightly crisp.

6. Remove the cauliflower from the oven, brush the remaining herbed oil on top, and sprinkle with the remaining tablespoon of cheese. Set the oven to broil and broil the cauliflower until the cheese begins to turn golden brown, 3 to 5 minutes. Top with fresh parsley before serving.

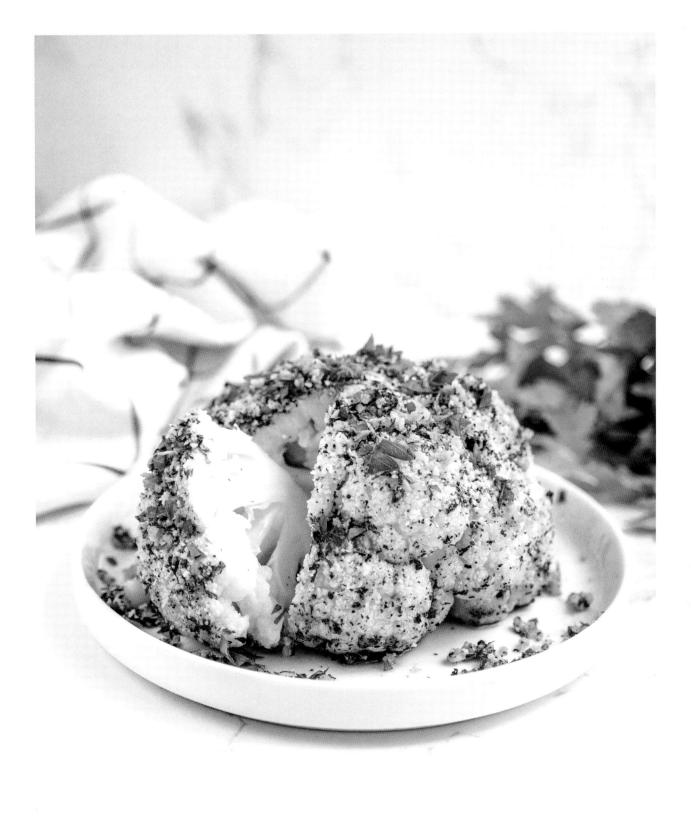

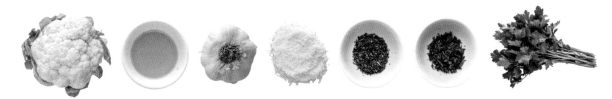

rainbow summer rolls

yield: **8 rolls**   prep time: **20 minutes**

Summer rolls may be something you only expect on a restaurant menu, but they are surprisingly easy to make at home once you get ahold of some rice paper. Made with fresh and flavorful herbs (basil, mint, and cilantro) along with crunchy, colorful vegetables, these rolls are a bright and refreshing light bite.

8 (10-inch) rice paper wrappers

8 butter lettuce leaves, stems removed

1 cup fresh basil leaves

1 cup fresh cilantro leaves

½ cup fresh mint leaves

1½ cups shredded or julienned carrots

1 cup shredded red cabbage

1 medium red bell pepper, thinly sliced

½ English cucumber, cut into matchsticks

1 large avocado, thinly sliced

Peanut sauce, store-bought, or homemade Peanut Dressing/ Dip (page 110), for serving (optional)

1. Working one at a time, place a rice paper wrapper in a large bowl of water for 10 to 15 seconds, then transfer to a clean work surface. Place one-eighth of the lettuce, basil, cilantro, and mint in the center of the wrapper. Top with one-eighth of the carrots, cabbage, bell pepper, cucumber, and avocado. Bring the bottom edge of the wrapper tightly over the filling, then fold in the sides and continue rolling from bottom to top.

2. Repeat with the remaining rice paper wrappers and filling ingredients.

3. Serve with peanut sauce for dipping, if desired. Store leftover rolls in a sealed container in the refrigerator for up to 2 days.

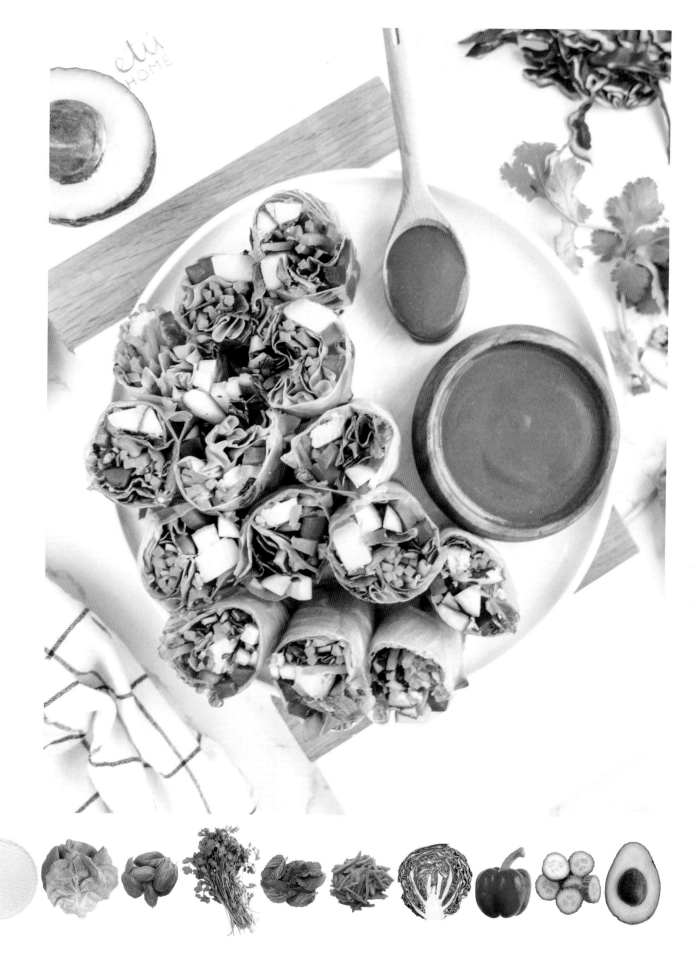

balsamic roasted root vegetables

yield: **4 servings**   prep time: **15 minutes**   cook time: **50 minutes**

Nothing says fall fare like roasted root vegetables—but this effortless side dish is great right through winter and into spring. Among all the types of veggies, the root variety is higher in carbohydrates and starch so can be treated more like a grain than a green on your plate. Tender and caramelized, with an earthy touch of thyme, this dish is one that you'll want to make any time you have hearty produce on hand.

marinade:

3 tablespoons extra-virgin olive oil

2 tablespoons balsamic vinegar

1 tablespoon ground dried thyme

1 teaspoon finely ground Himalayan pink salt

¼ teaspoon ground black pepper

1 pound baby potatoes, cut into quarters

8 ounces carrots, peeled and cut into 1-inch pieces

8 ounces parsnips, peeled and cut into 1-inch pieces

2 medium beets, peeled and cut into 1-inch pieces

1 large red onion, peeled and cut into 1-inch wedges

1. Preheat the oven to 425°F.

2. In a small bowl, whisk together the marinade ingredients.

3. Put the root vegetables in a large bowl. Pour the marinade on top and toss to coat.

4. Pour the vegetable mixture onto a sheet pan and spread out in a single layer. Roast until tender and slightly crisp, 45 to 50 minutes, tossing halfway through.

notes

You can use any root vegetable you like in this dish, such as celeriac, rutabaga, sweet potatoes, and turnips. The key is to cut them to similar sizes so they cook evenly.

If you use red beets, the other vegetables may take on a bit of red color. If you'd like to avoid that, use golden beets instead.

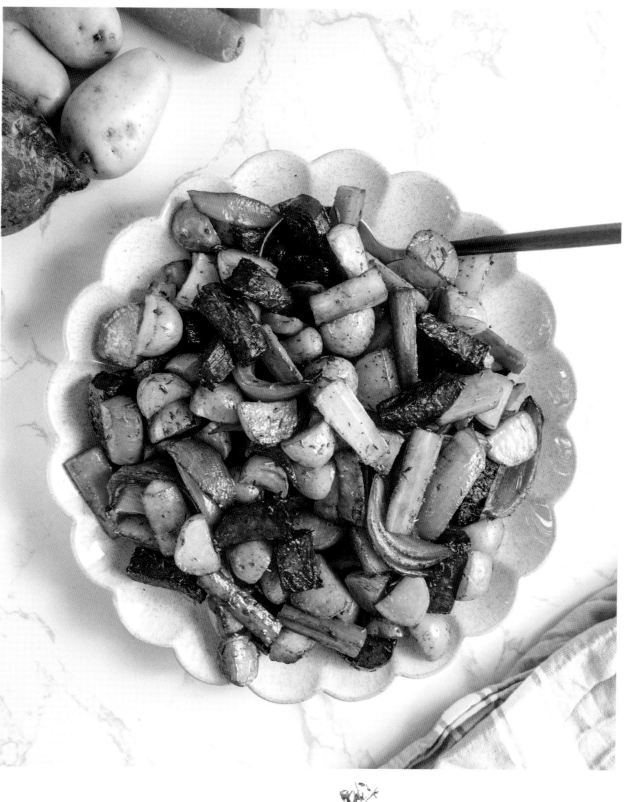

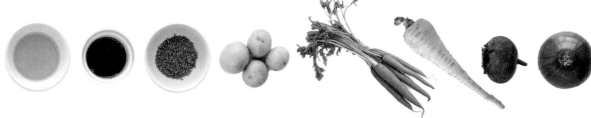

chickpea poppers

6 WAYS

yield: 1½ cups (¼ cup per serving)   prep time: **5 minutes**   cook time: **30 minutes**

Transform the can of chickpeas sitting in your pantry into your next addicting sweet or savory snack—roasted chickpea poppers. In addition to snacking on them by the handful, you can use this protein-packed plant-based recipe as a crouton swap atop a salad or soup or in a sandwich or wrap.

base:

1 (15-ounce) can no-salt-added chickpeas, drained and rinsed well, or 1½ cups cooked chickpeas (see page 44)

1 tablespoon extra-virgin olive oil

¼ teaspoon finely ground Himalayan pink salt

1. Preheat the oven to 425°F. Grease a sheet pan with cooking spray or line it with parchment paper.

2. Place the chickpeas in a clean kitchen towel and gently pat dry. Remove and discard any loose skins. Drying the chickpeas helps ensure they get crispy in the oven.

3. Transfer the chickpeas to the prepared pan and spread out in a single layer. Toss with the oil and salt. If making the Sweet Honey or BBQ flavor, add those ingredients now.

4. Bake until golden and crisp, 25 to 30 minutes, stirring halfway through.

5. Remove the chickpeas from the oven. If making the spiced, "cheezy," garlic herb, or everything bagel flavor, toss the still-warm chickpeas with the ingredients for your choice of flavor.

6. Store leftovers in a jar or other sealed container in the refrigerator and enjoy within 5 days.

note _____

Chickpea poppers are best the day they are made and will lose their crispiness over time. To recrisp them, reheat in a 250°F oven for 10 to 15 minutes.

flavor options

spiced:

1 teaspoon chili powder

½ teaspoon ground cumin

½ teaspoon cayenne pepper

"cheezy":

2 tablespoons grated Parmesan cheese or plant-based parmesan, store-bought or homemade (page 124)

sweet honey:

1 tablespoon raw manuka honey

1 teaspoon ground cinnamon

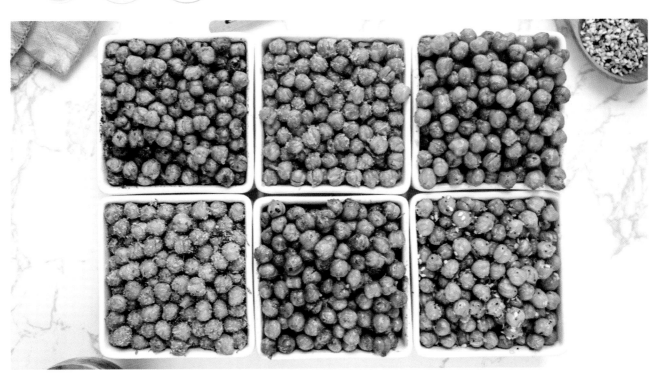

garlic herb:

1 teaspoon garlic powder

½ teaspoon onion powder

1 teaspoon dried dill weed

1 teaspoon dried parsley

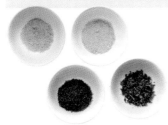

BBQ:

1 tablespoon pure maple syrup

½ teaspoon paprika

½ teaspoon chili powder

½ teaspoon garlic powder

¼ teaspoon ground black pepper

everything bagel:

1 tablespoon everything bagel seasoning

turmeric roasted cauliflower

yield: **4 servings**   prep time: **15 minutes**   cook time: **30 minutes**

In this earthy, savory side dish, the bright yellow super spice turmeric takes center stage. Slightly peppery with a subtle ginger taste, this native-to–Southeast Asia spice has been used culinarily for thousands of years as well as in Ayurvedic medicine. Promising research has highlighted the significant anti-inflammatory properties of curcumin, the main active component of turmeric.

2 tablespoons extra-virgin olive oil

1 tablespoon minced garlic

1 teaspoon finely ground Himalayan pink salt

1 teaspoon turmeric powder

½ teaspoon ground cumin

½ teaspoon paprika

½ teaspoon ground black pepper

1 large head cauliflower (about 2 pounds), cored and cut into 1-inch florets (3 to 4 cups florets)

Juice of ½ lemon

3 tablespoons chopped fresh cilantro, for topping

1. Preheat the oven to 450°F. Line a sheet pan with parchment paper or grease it with cooking spray.

2. In a small bowl, whisk together the oil, garlic, salt, and spices.

3. Place the cauliflower florets in a large bowl, drizzle with the oil mixture, and toss to coat.

4. Spread the cauliflower in a single layer on the prepared pan and bake until tender and crisp, 25 to 30 minutes, tossing halfway through cooking. Top with the lemon juice and cilantro before serving.

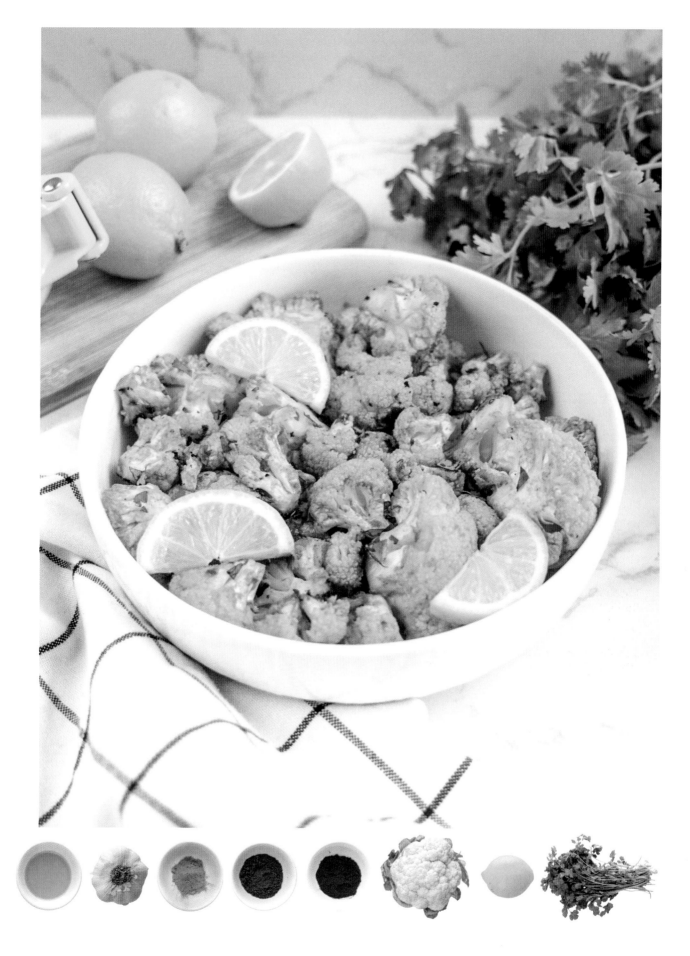

fluffy and crispy smashed potatoes

yield: **4 servings**   prep time: **10 minutes**   cook time: **55 minutes**

Meet your new favorite way to prepare potatoes! These smashed potatoes are as crispy on the outside as they are fluffy on the inside. They are made with just a handful of ingredients, but you can top them with whatever your heart desires, like Parmesan cheese, Plant-Based Parm (page 124), red pepper flakes, or whatever chopped fresh herbs you have on hand. Dill or chives would be a great alternative to parsley.

1 pound small yellow potatoes, scrubbed

1 tablespoon extra-virgin olive oil

½ teaspoon finely ground Himalayan pink salt

⅛ teaspoon ground black pepper

2 tablespoons finely chopped fresh flat-leaf parsley, for topping

Sea salt flakes, for topping (optional)

1. Place the potatoes in a large pot and cover them with water by about 1 inch. Bring to a boil over medium-high heat. Cook until the potatoes are soft and easy to pierce, 15 to 20 minutes.

2. While the potatoes are cooking, preheat the oven to 425°F and grease two sheet pans with cooking spray.

3. Drain the potatoes in a large colander and let them cool and dry for 5 minutes.

4. Evenly distribute the potatoes over the prepared pans, make a small slit in the top of each potato using a knife, and then use a potato masher or fork to gently smash each potato so it is about ¼ inch thick.

5. In a small bowl, combine the oil, salt, and pepper. Use a pastry brush to brush the oil mixture over the potatoes.

6. Bake the potatoes for 30 to 35 minutes, or until golden and crisp. Sprinkle the parsley and sea salt flakes, if using, on top and serve hot.

🌱 note _____

The thinner you smash the potatoes, the crispier they will be!

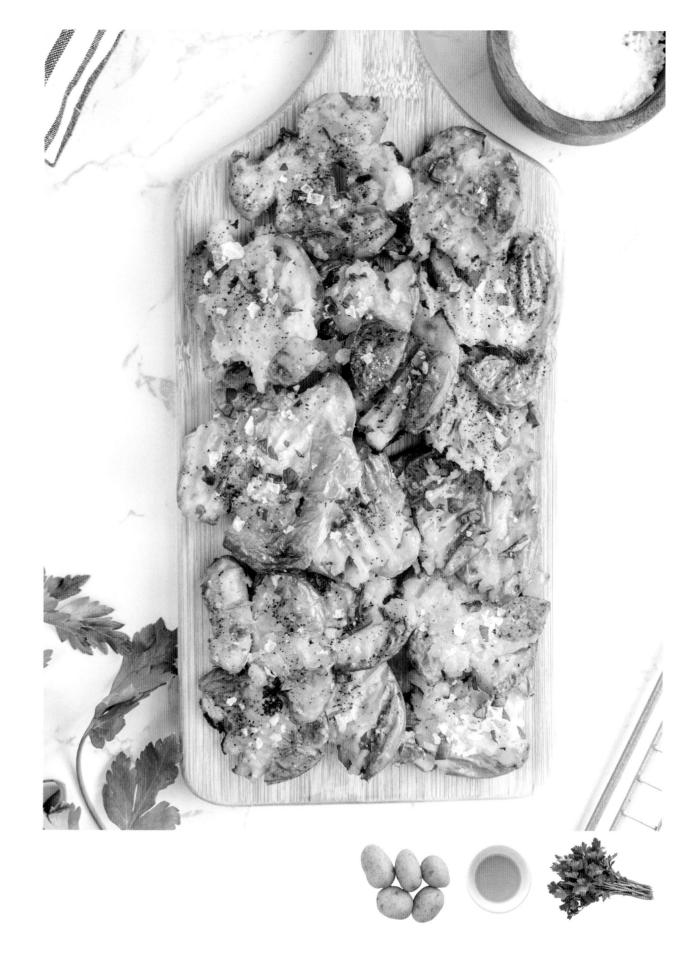

3-ingredient almond flour crackers

yield: **4 servings (5 crackers per serving)**   prep time: **20 minutes**   cook time: **10 minutes**

If you've ever turned over your cracker box to read the ingredient list, you know that most store-bought varieties are made with a long list of unpronounceable ingredients, including several fillers and preservatives. Forgo the store-bought crackers for homemade ones made with just three simple ingredients using an almond flour base.

cheesy almond flour crackers:

1 cup blanched almond flour

1 cup shredded sharp cheddar cheese (about 4 ounces)

Sea salt flakes, for topping

everything bagel almond flour crackers:

1½ cups blanched almond flour

1 large egg, beaten

2 tablespoons everything bagel seasoning

notes _____

Use a pizza cutter for easy cutting.

For dairy- and egg-free: Make the cheesy crackers, replacing the cheddar with a shredded plant-based cheese. I recommend Violife brand.

1. Preheat the oven to 350°F.

2. *To make the cheesy crackers,* place the almond flour and cheese in a food processor and process until combined. Add water 1 teaspoon at a time, pulsing to combine after each addition, until a dough forms. Divide the dough into two equal portions. Place one portion on a large sheet of parchment paper and cover with another sheet of parchment. Roll into a ¼-inch-thick rectangle using a rolling pin. Remove the top piece of parchment paper, cut the dough into twenty 1-inch squares, top with sea salt flakes, and place on a baking sheet. If desired, use a toothpick to poke a hole in the center of each cracker for a decorative touch. Repeat with the remaining dough and a second baking sheet. Bake both baking sheets until the edges of the crackers turn golden, 8 to 10 minutes. Let the crackers cool completely before serving.

3. *To make the everything bagel crackers,* place the almond flour, egg, and seasoning in a large bowl and combine using a rubber spatula until a dough forms. Divide the dough into two equal portions. Place one portion on a large sheet of parchment paper and cover with another sheet of parchment. Roll into a ¼-inch-thick rectangle using a rolling pin. Remove the top piece of parchment paper, cut the dough into twenty 1-inch squares, and place on a baking sheet. Repeat with the remaining dough and a second baking sheet. Bake both baking sheets until the edges of the crackers turn golden brown, 8 to 10 minutes. Let the crackers cool completely before serving.

4. Store in a sealed container in the pantry or on the counter for up to 3 days or in the refrigerator for up to 5 days.

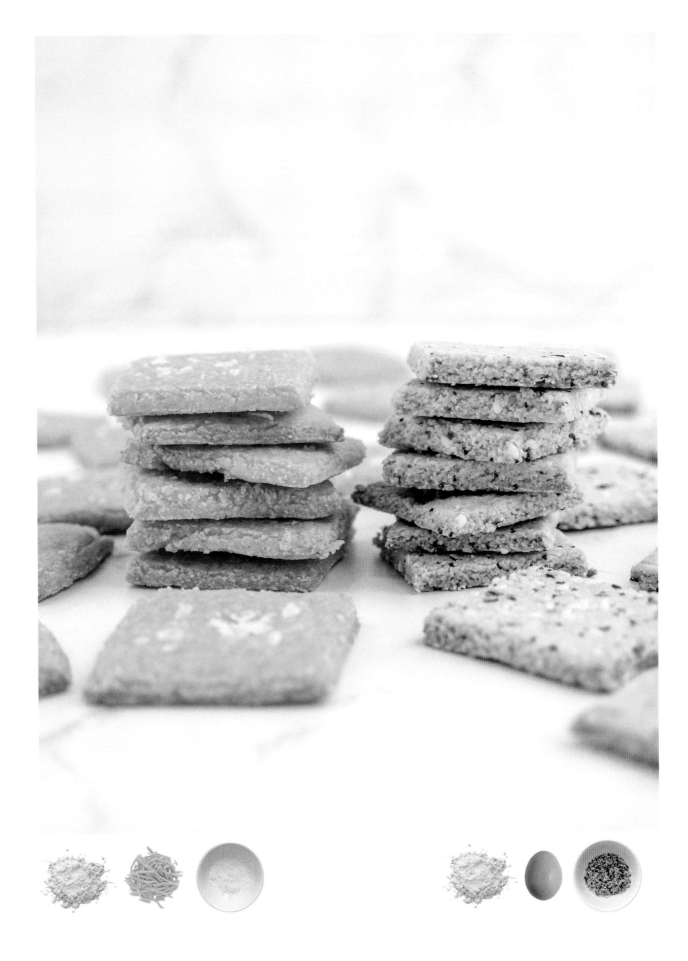

roasted vegetable pesto pasta

yield: **4 servings**   prep time: **10 minutes**   cook time: **20 minutes**

This quick and easy pesto pasta is a savory, earthy dish with bright, bold flavors that can be served as a side or a meal thanks to chickpea pasta rounding it out with protein and fiber. The vegetables can be grilled rather than roasted for quicker cooking and a smoky flavor profile. Serve this dish warm or cold.

1 pint cherry tomatoes

1 medium yellow squash, sliced into half-moons

1 medium zucchini, sliced into half-moons

1 cup frozen corn

1 tablespoon extra-virgin olive oil

¼ teaspoon finely ground Himalayan pink salt

⅛ teaspoon ground black pepper

1 (8-ounce) box short chickpea pasta, such as rigatoni, rotini, or fusilli

½ cup pesto, store-bought or homemade (page 114)

Juice of ½ lemon

¼ cup fresh basil leaves, for topping

1. Preheat the oven to 425°F.

2. In a large bowl, toss together the tomatoes, yellow squash, zucchini, corn, oil, salt, and pepper. Transfer the vegetables to a sheet pan and spread out in a single layer. Roast until the tomatoes have slightly burst and the vegetables are tender and slightly golden brown, 18 to 20 minutes.

3. Meanwhile, bring a large pot of salted water to a boil. Cook the pasta according to the package instructions until al dente. Drain the pasta, rinse under cold water, and return to the pot. Add the roasted vegetables and stir in the pesto and lemon juice. Top with the basil leaves before serving.

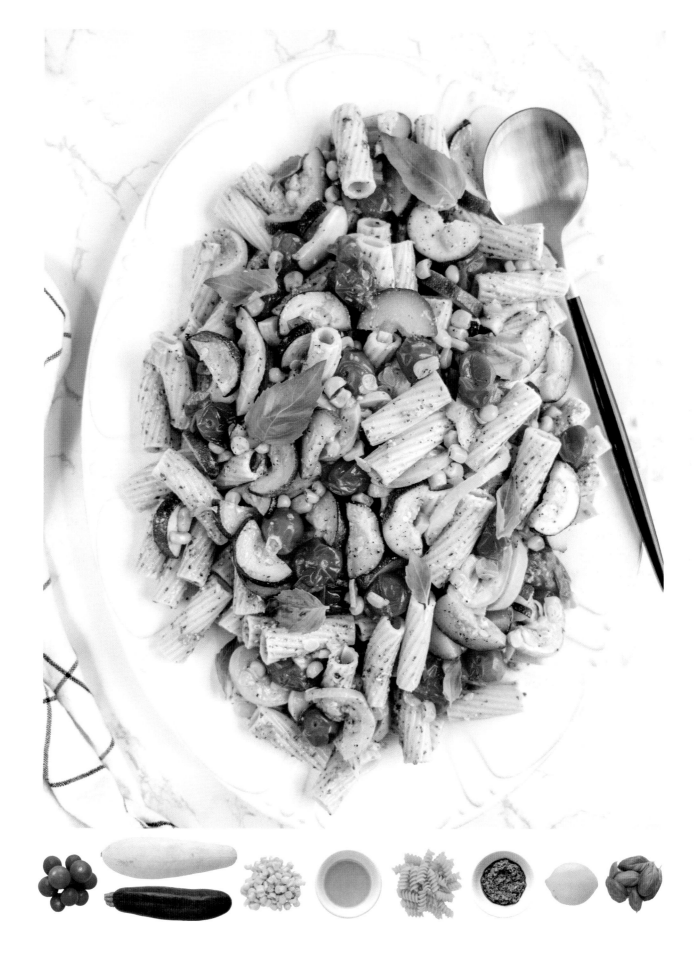

very veggie cauliflower fried rice

yield: **4 servings**   prep time: **10 minutes**   cook time: **15 minutes**

Not your typical takeout fried rice! This plant-forward version features a base of riced cauliflower, a naturally lower-calorie alternative to rice. While fried rice is traditionally served as a side dish, the addition of eggs makes it hearty enough to serve as a complete meal. Add a protein such as chicken, tofu, or an extra egg to bump up the staying power even more.

1 medium head cauliflower (about 1½ pounds), or 4 cups riced cauliflower

2 large eggs, whisked

2 tablespoons extra-virgin olive oil, divided

½ medium white onion, diced

2 cloves garlic, minced

2 cups sliced vegetables, such as carrots, broccoli, zucchini, red cabbage, and bell peppers, and/or whole sugar snap peas, snow peas, or frozen green peas

3 tablespoons low-sodium soy sauce

1 teaspoon finely ground Himalayan pink salt

Toasted sesame seeds, for topping (optional)

Sliced green onions, for topping (optional)

1. If using prericed cauliflower, skip ahead to Step 3. Otherwise, trim and discard the leaves and base of the cauliflower stalk. Cut the florets off the stalk.

2. Working in batches, pulse the cauliflower florets in a food processor until it resembles grains of rice. Set aside.

3. Scramble the eggs in a large skillet over medium heat with 1 teaspoon of the oil. Transfer the eggs to a small plate and set aside.

4. Pour 2 teaspoons of the oil into the skillet and increase the heat to medium-high. Add the riced cauliflower and cook, stirring often, until tender and slightly crisp, 5 to 6 minutes. Transfer to a plate and set aside to cool.

5. Pour the remaining tablespoon of oil into the skillet and increase the heat to high. Sauté the onion, garlic, and vegetables of your choice until the onion is translucent, the garlic is fragrant, and the veggies are tender, 4 to 6 minutes. Add the denser, longer-cooking vegetables such as carrots to the pan first, followed by the softer vegetables such as zucchini that take less time to cook.

6. Remove the pan from the heat and stir in the cauliflower, scrambled eggs, soy sauce, and salt. Top with toasted sesame seeds and/or green onions, if desired, and serve warm.

7. Store leftovers in a sealed container in the refrigerator for up to 3 days.

Make sure to cut the vegetables into very small, evenly sized pieces for quick cooking and to add the vegetables sequentially to the pan, starting with the denser, longer-cooking veggies followed by the softer, shorter-cooking ones.

For egg-free: Replace the eggs with scrambled firm tofu.

You can also make this recipe with chilled leftover cooked rice such as brown or short-grain white rice.

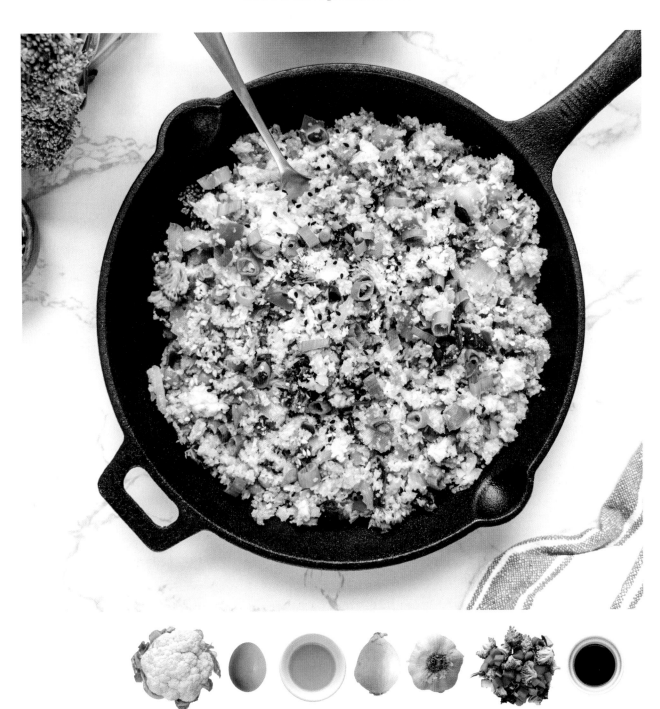

customizable no-bake granola bars

yield: **12 bars**   prep time: **10 minutes, plus 10 minutes to set in freezer**   cook time: **10 minutes**

Forget the store-bought granola bars you ate as a kid with their long lists of unrecognizable ingredients and make your own at home with a base of five simple ingredients plus the mix-ins of your choice. These bars are chewy, perfectly sweet, and easy to prepare—the perfect midday pick-me-up packed with filling fiber and plant-based protein.

2½ cups rolled oats

1 cup natural creamy cashew butter, warmed until liquid-y

⅓ cup raw manuka honey

1 teaspoon pure vanilla extract

¼ teaspoon finely ground Himalayan pink salt

mix-ins:

¼ cup chopped raw or roasted nuts, such as pecans, walnuts, almonds, or shelled pistachios

¼ cup seeds, such as chia, hemp, or shelled sunflower seeds

¼ cup dried berries, dark chocolate chips, or unsweetened coconut flakes

1. Preheat the oven to 350°F. Line an 8-inch square baking pan with parchment paper with the ends overhanging and line a sheet pan with parchment paper.

2. Spread the oats in a single layer on the prepared sheet pan. Toast in the oven until lightly golden, about 10 minutes.

3. Transfer the oats to a large bowl along with the cashew butter, honey, vanilla, and salt. Using a rubber spatula, stir until combined. Add the nuts, seeds, and flavor mix-ins and stir until combined.

4. Pour the mixture into the prepared baking pan and press down. Freeze for 10 minutes to set. Remove from the pan using the parchment paper and cut into 12 bars. Store in a sealed container in the refrigerator for up to 2 weeks.

note _____

You can use any creamy nut butter you have on hand in place of the cashew butter.

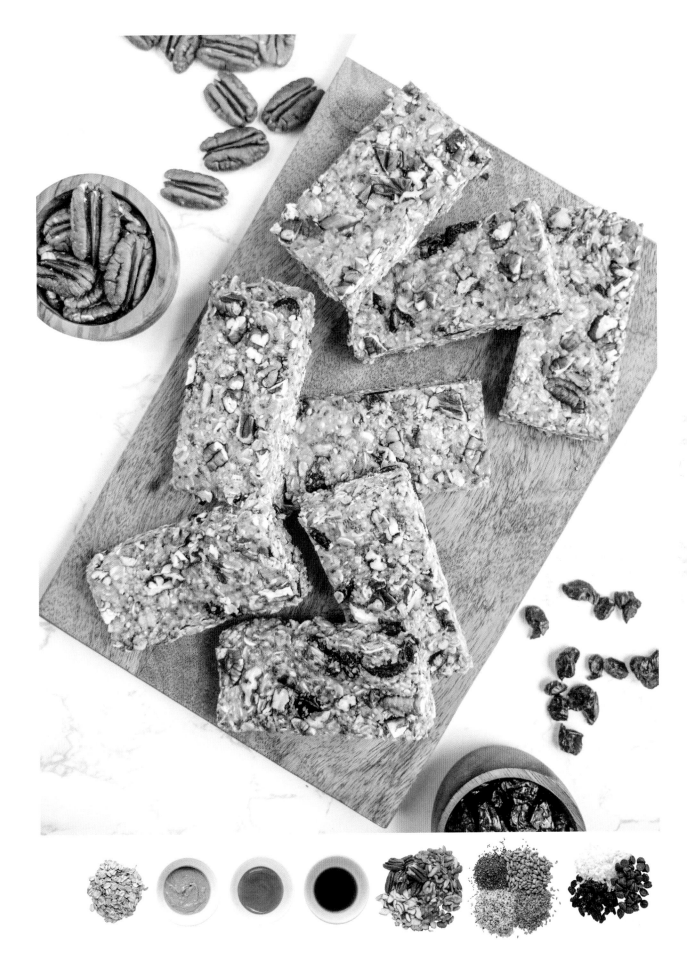

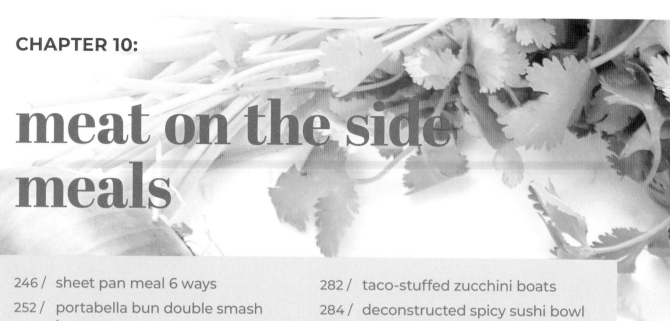

CHAPTER 10:

meat on the side meals

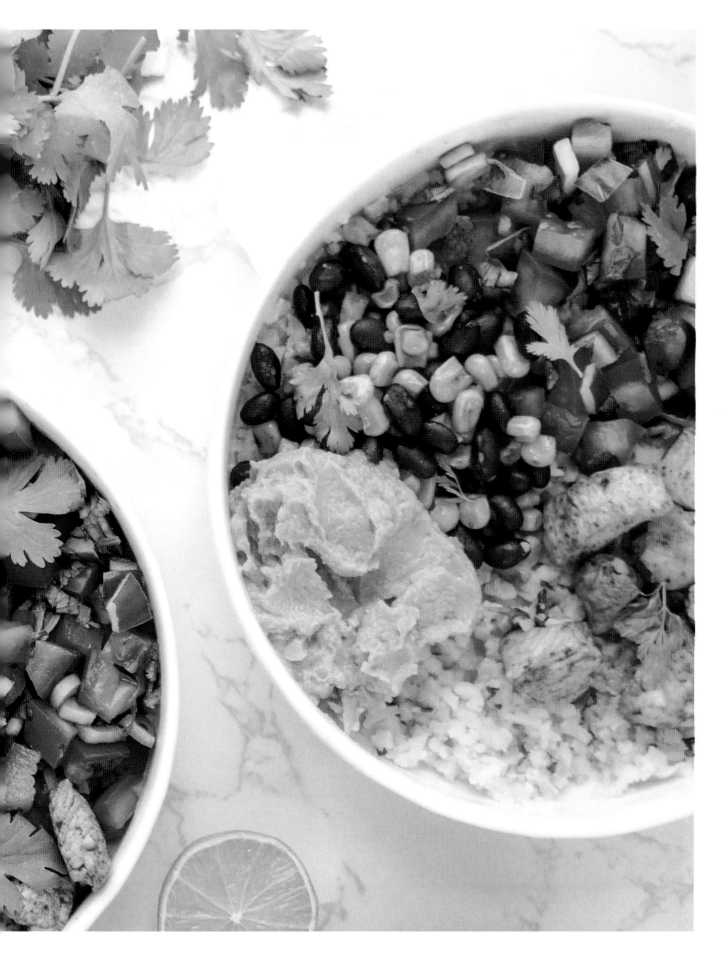

sheet pan meal

6 WAYS

yield: 2 servings   prep time: 15 minutes   cook time: 25 to 45 minutes, depending on version

With the benefits of hands-off cooking, easy cleanup, and endless nourishing use-up-the-contents-of-your-fridge options, sheet pan meals are sure to become a staple in your lazy weeknight dinner rotation, if they aren't already. I've included six flavorful combinations to satisfy a range of tastes, but the beauty of sheet pan meals is that they can be customized however you desire. Using the formula on pages 250 and 251, it's easy to make a balanced sheet pan meal using what you have on hand. Lemon juice, hot sauce, pesto, and tzatziki are great flavor additions after baking.

chicken fajitas:

8 ounces boneless, skinless chicken breasts, cut into 1½-inch-wide strips

½ medium red onion, cut into thin strips

1 medium red bell pepper, cut into thin strips

1 tablespoon avocado oil

2 teaspoons taco seasoning

4 (6-inch) corn tortillas, for serving

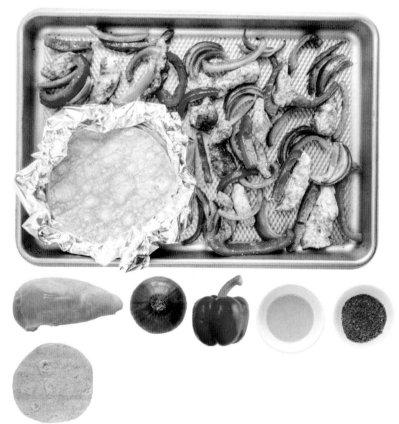

Preheat the oven to 400°F. Put the chicken, onion, and bell pepper on a sheet pan and toss with the oil and taco seasoning. Spread out in a single layer. Bake for 15 to 20 minutes, tossing halfway through cooking, until the vegetables are crisp-tender and the chicken is cooked through. While the sheet pan is in the oven, warm the tortillas in a skillet over medium heat to soften. Season the chicken and veggies with salt and pepper to taste and serve with the tortillas.

summer shrimp:

2 ears corn, husks removed

1 pound asparagus spears, ends trimmed

1 tablespoon extra-virgin olive oil, divided

1 teaspoon all-purpose seasoning, divided

8 ounces large shrimp, peeled and deveined

1 medium yellow squash, cut into ¼-inch rounds

Preheat the oven to 400°F. Wrap the corn in foil and place on a sheet pan. Spread the asparagus in a single layer on the pan and toss with half of the oil and half of the seasoning. Bake for 10 minutes. Remove from the oven, add the shrimp and squash, and toss with the remaining oil and seasoning. Bake for another 15 minutes, or until the vegetables are tender and the shrimp are pink and firm. Season with salt and pepper to taste and serve.

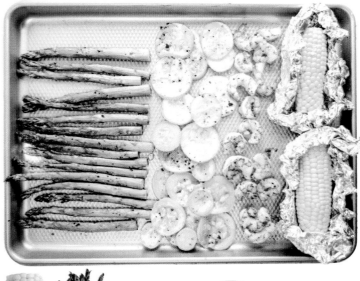

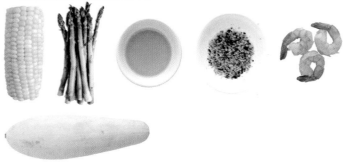

fall bounty:

2 (4- to 6-ounce) bone-in pork chops, about ½ inch thick

1 cup Brussels sprouts, halved

1 small acorn squash, peeled, seeded, and cut into quarter-moons

1 tablespoon extra-virgin olive oil

2 teaspoons herbes de Provence

Preheat the oven to 400°F. Put the pork chops, Brussels sprouts, and squash on a sheet pan and toss with the oil and herbes de Provence. Spread out in a single layer. Bake for 20 to 25 minutes, tossing the vegetables halfway through cooking, until the vegetables are tender and the pork reaches an internal temperature of 145°F. Season with salt and pepper to taste and serve.

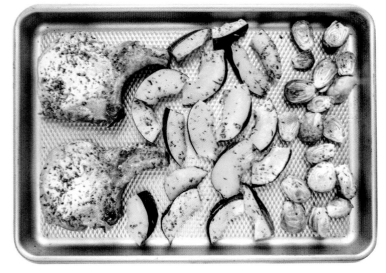

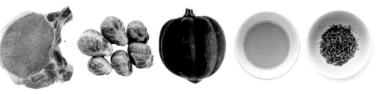

tikka:

2 cups small cauliflower florets

1 cup cooked chickpeas

½ medium red onion, thinly sliced

1 tablespoon extra-virgin olive oil

2 teaspoons tikka masala seasoning

2 whole-grain pita pockets, for serving

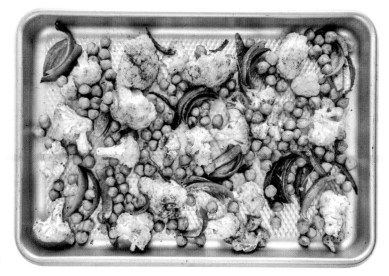

Preheat the oven to 400°F. Put the cauliflower, chickpeas, and onion on a sheet pan and toss with the oil and tikka seasoning. Spread out in a single layer. Bake, tossing halfway through cooking, for 30 minutes, or until the vegetables are tender and the chickpeas are crisp. While the sheet pan is in the oven, warm the pitas in a skillet over medium heat until softened. Season with salt and pepper to taste and serve with the pitas.

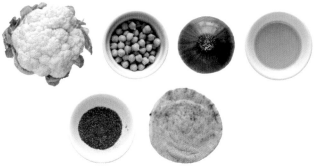

italian chicken:

2 bone-in chicken thighs (about 12 ounces)

1 tablespoon extra-virgin olive oil, divided

1 teaspoon Italian seasoning, divided

1 cup cherry tomatoes

1 cup broccoli florets

2 cups frozen cauliflower gnocchi (see note, page 304)

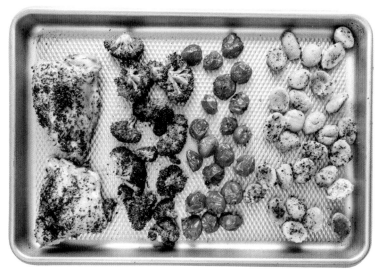

Preheat the oven to 400°F. Put the chicken thighs on a sheet pan and coat each with half of the oil and seasoning. Bake for 15 minutes. Remove from the oven and add the tomatoes, broccoli, and gnocchi. Toss with the remaining oil and seasoning. Bake for another 30 minutes, or until the vegetables are tender, the gnocchi are soft, and the chicken reaches an internal temperature of 165°F. Season with salt and pepper to taste and serve.

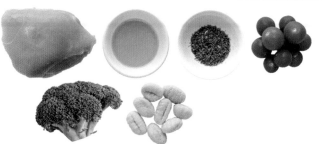

greek salmon:

1 pound baby potatoes, halved

1 pint cherry tomatoes

¼ medium red onion, thinly sliced

1 tablespoon extra-virgin olive oil, divided

1 teaspoon Greek seasoning, divided

2 (4-ounce) skin-on salmon fillets

1 medium zucchini, cut into ¼-inch rounds

Preheat the oven to 400°F. Put the potatoes, tomatoes, and onion on a sheet pan and coat with half of the oil and seasoning. Spread out in a single layer. Bake for 15 minutes. Remove from the oven and add the salmon fillets and zucchini. Brush on the remaining oil and sprinkle on the remaining seasoning. Bake for another 15 minutes, or until the vegetables are tender and the salmon reaches an internal temperature of 145°F. Season with salt and pepper to taste and serve.

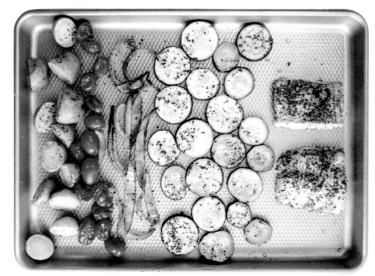

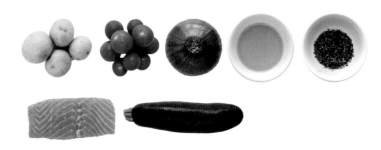

sheet pan meal formula (2 servings)

CHOOSE THE INGREDIENTS (see charts):

1 PROTEIN (8 oz. boneless or 1 lb. bone-in) **+** **2 NONSTARCHY VEGGIES** (1 to 3 cups total) **+** **1 STARCHY VEGETABLE OR CARB** (1 cup total)

CHOOSE A SEASONING BLEND (1 to 3 teaspoons each), such as

ALL-PURPOSE

CAJUN

EVERYTHING BAGEL

GREEK

HERBES DE PROVENCE

ITALIAN

TACO

TIKKA MASALA

PREPARE THE SHEET PAN MEAL:

Toss the protein and vegetables with 1 tablespoon of oil and season with the blend of your choice, plus finely ground Himalayan pink salt and ground black pepper. Omit or go light on the salt if the seasoning blend contains salt. Spread the ingredients in a single layer on a sheet pan and bake in a preheated 400°F oven until done, following the cook time guidelines in this chart. Serve with tortillas, pitas, or the cooked grain of your choice, if desired.

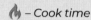 – Cook time

protein

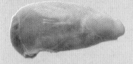

CHICKEN BREAST

Boneless whole breast halves
🔥 20 minutes
(internal temperature 165°F)

Cut into 1½-inch-thick strips
🔥 15–20 minutes

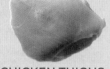

CHICKEN THIGHS

Bone-in whole thighs
🔥 45 minutes
(internal temperature 165°F)

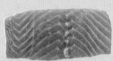

SALMON

4- to 6-ounce fillets
🔥 15 minutes
(internal temperature 145°F)

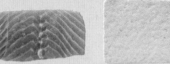

TOFU

Extra-firm, pressed and cubed
🔥 30 minutes, toss halfway

TEMPEH

Cubed
🔥 25–30 minutes

SHRIMP

Large, peeled and deveined
🔥 15 minutes
(until pink)

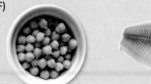

COOKED CHICKPEAS

Whole
🔥 30 minutes, toss halfway

TILAPIA

Whole fillet
🔥 15 minutes
(internal temperature 145°F)

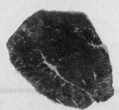

STEAK, BONELESS

Cut into 1-inch strips
🔥 20 minutes
(internal temperature 135°F for medium-rare)

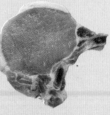

PORK CHOP, BONE-IN, ½ INCH THICK

Whole chops
🔥 20–22 minutes
(internal temperature 145°F)

nonstarchy vegetables

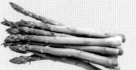 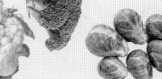

ASPARAGUS

Ends trimmed and cut into thirds (if leaving whole, use 8–10 spears)

🔥 20–25 minutes

BELL PEPPER

Cut into thin strips

🔥 25–30 minutes, toss halfway

BROCCOLI OR CAULIFLOWER

Cut into small florets

🔥 30 minutes

BRUSSELS SPROUTS

Halved

🔥 25–30 minutes

CHERRY TOMATOES

Whole

🔥 30 minutes

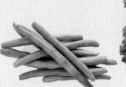 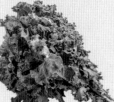 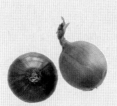 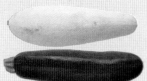

GREEN BEANS

Whole, ends trimmed

🔥 20–25 minutes

KALE

Stemmed and cut into small pieces

🔥 8–12 minutes

ONION

Cut into thin strips

🔥 25–30 minutes, toss halfway

ZUCCHINI OR YELLOW SQUASH

¼-inch rounds

🔥 10–15 minutes

starchy vegetables/carbs

 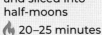 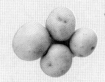 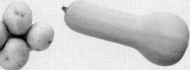 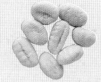 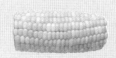

ACORN SQUASH

Peeled, seeded, and sliced into half-moons

🔥 20–25 minutes

BABY POTATOES

Quartered

🔥 25–30 minutes

BUTTERNUT SQUASH

Peeled, seeded, and chopped into 1-inch pieces

🔥 25–30 minutes

CAULIFLOWER GNOCCHI

Whole, frozen

🔥 20–25 minutes, flipping halfway

CORN ON THE COB

Whole, husked, wrapped in foil

🔥 25–30 minutes

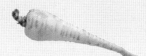 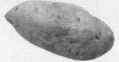

PARSNIPS

Peeled and cut into 2-inch strips

🔥 20–35 minutes

SWEET POTATO

Scrubbed and chopped into 1-inch pieces

🔥 25–30 minutes

portabella bun double smash burgers

yield: **4 burgers (1 per serving)**   prep time: **10 minutes**   cook time: **30 minutes**

Put a veggie-forward twist on burger night with roasted portabella mushroom "buns." Naturally grain-free, gluten-free, and lower in calories, this whole-food alternative to refined white-bread hamburger buns looks and acts like the real deal but with a juicier, meatier texture that complements hamburger patties seamlessly. Tip: You can cut the cook time in half by cooking the burgers while the buns are in the oven.

sauce:

2 tablespoons avocado oil mayonnaise

1 teaspoon spicy brown mustard

1 teaspoon dill relish

portabella buns:

8 equal-sized portabella mushrooms, about 4 inches in diameter, stems removed

1 tablespoon extra-virgin olive oil

¼ teaspoon finely ground Himalayan pink salt

⅛ teaspoon ground black pepper

1 tablespoon sesame seeds (optional)

smash burgers:

1 pound lean ground beef

½ teaspoon finely ground Himalayan pink salt

¼ teaspoon ground black pepper

suggested toppings:

Lettuce

Red onion slices

Pickle slices

Sliced cheese

Sliced tomatoes

1. To make the sauce, whisk together the mayonnaise, mustard, and relish in a small bowl.

2. To make the buns, wash the mushrooms and dry thoroughly. In a small bowl, whisk together the oil, salt, and pepper. Brush the mixture on both sides of the mushrooms.

If using the oven, preheat the oven to 450°F and line a sheet pan with parchment paper. Place the mushrooms gill side down on the prepared pan and roast until softened, 10 to 12 minutes.

If using a grill or grill pan, heat the grill or grill pan over medium-high heat. Cook the mushrooms gill side down for 3 to 4 minutes, flip, and cook for another 2 to 3 minutes, or until softened.

If using sesame seeds, sprinkle them on the tops of the buns before serving.

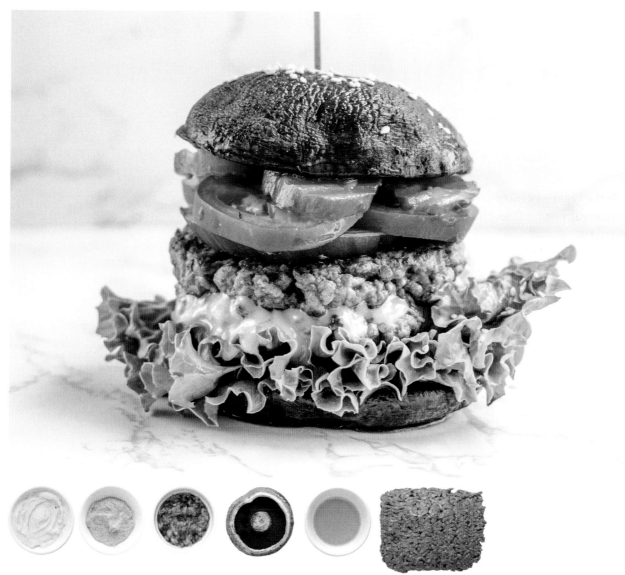

note

For meat-free: Replace the burger patties with Chickpea Carrot Burgers (page 278).

3. To make the burger patties, combine the beef with the salt and pepper in a large bowl. Divide into 8 equal portions. Heat a griddle or large cast-iron skillet over medium heat. Place 2 patties in the skillet and use a spatula to make them as flat as possible. Cook undisturbed until the bottoms are browned, 1½ to 2 minutes. Flip the patties and cook for another 1 to 2 minutes, or until the internal temperature is at least 160°F, for medium doneness; cook longer for more well-done patties. Repeat with the remaining patties.

4. To assemble the burgers, top four of the portabella buns with lettuce, if using, followed by a burger patty, a couple teaspoons of the sauce, and another burger patty. Add additional toppings of your choice, if desired, and top with another portabella bun.

simple cauliflower crust pizza

yield: 1 medium pizza (6 slices, 2 slices per serving)   prep time: 15 minutes
cook time: 30 to 40 minutes, depending on rice cooking method

Is there anything cauliflower can't do? This mild-tasting veggie can be made into rice, mashed potatoes, Buffalo "wings," and yes, even pizza crust. Compared to traditional pizza crust, cauliflower not only lowers the calories and carbohydrates, but also increases the fiber and key nutrients like vitamin C and potassium. And the taste is just about the same (some may even say better), making the switch from traditional pizza crust to cauliflower a no-brainer. Plus, it's all about the pizza toppings anyway, right?

1 medium head cauliflower (about 1½ pounds), cored and cut into small florets, or 4 cups riced cauliflower

1 tablespoon flaxseed meal

3 tablespoons water

½ cup blanched almond flour

1 teaspoon ground dried oregano

¼ teaspoon finely ground Himalayan pink salt

½ cup tomato sauce, store-bought or homemade (page 130), or store-bought marinara sauce

⅔ cup shredded cheese of choice

additional toppings (optional):

Diced bell peppers

Roasted vegetables of choice

Sliced olives

Sliced red onion

Chopped fresh basil

Arugula

1. Preheat the oven to 425°F and line a baking sheet with parchment paper.

2. If using prericed cauliflower, skip ahead to Step 3. Otherwise, place the cauliflower florets in a food processor and process into rice-sized pieces. Measure 4 cups of the rice for the crust; bag any remaining rice and refrigerate or freeze for later use.

3. Cook the rice using either a microwave or a steamer on the stovetop:

   If using the microwave, place the riced cauliflower in a large microwave-safe bowl, cover with a paper towel, and microwave on high for 4 to 5 minutes, or until soft.

   If using a steamer, set a steamer in a large pot, pour in a couple inches of water, keeping the level below the steamer, and bring the water to a boil. Place the riced cauliflower in the steamer, cover the pot, and steam until soft, about 15 minutes.

4. Allow the riced cauliflower to cool, then transfer it to a thin kitchen towel or piece of cheesecloth. Wrap the cloth around the rice and squeeze out as much water as possible. Removing the excess water will help ensure the pizza crust is crispy and sturdy.

5. Make a flax egg by combining the flaxseed meal and water in a small bowl; allow to sit for 5 minutes.

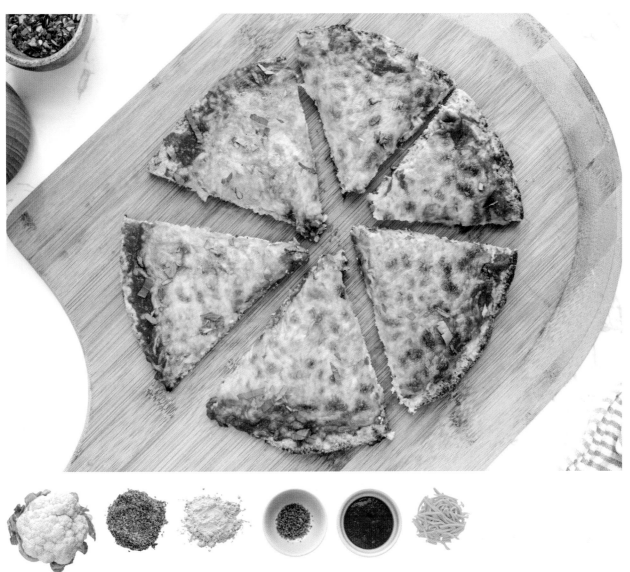

6. Put the cauliflower, flax egg, flour, oregano, and salt in a large bowl and stir until a dough forms. It won't be stretchy like your average pizza dough since it has no gluten.

7. Place the dough on the prepared baking sheet and, using your hands, press and shape it into a round, about ¼ inch thick. Par-bake until set, about 15 minutes. Remove from the oven and top with the sauce, cheese, and, if desired, other toppings of your choice. If using arugula or basil, add it to the pizza after it's fully baked. Return the pizza to the oven and bake until the cheese is melted, another 5 to 7 minutes. Set the oven to broil and broil until the top is golden, 1 to 3 minutes.

8. Let cool slightly before cutting into 6 slices. Top with arugula, if using. Store leftovers in a sealed container in the refrigerator for up to 3 days or in the freezer for up to a month.

rainbow veggie noodles

yield: **4 servings**   prep time: **10 minutes**   cook time: **15 minutes**

Comforting noodles meet nutrient-rich produce in this dish that helps you "eat the rainbow." Inspired by Thai flavors, these noodles are chock-full of phytonutrients thanks to an array of vegetables—like zucchini, red cabbage, bell peppers, and carrots—coated in a savory-sweet peanut sauce.

8 ounces brown rice noodles (optional)

1 cup frozen shelled edamame

1 tablespoon extra-virgin olive oil

3 cups zucchini noodles

2 cups shredded red cabbage

1 cup shredded or julienned carrots

1 medium red bell pepper, thinly sliced

12 ounces shredded rotisserie chicken

¼ cup sliced green onions

¼ cup peanut sauce, store-bought, or homemade Peanut Dressing/Dip (page 110)

suggested toppings:

Toasted sesame seeds

Chopped roasted peanuts

1. *If using rice noodles,* bring a large saucepan of salted water to a boil. Add the rice noodles and cook according to the package directions. Add the edamame in the last few minutes of cooking to defrost. Drain the noodles and edamame and run under cold water.

If not using rice noodles, cook the edamame in a medium saucepan of salted boiling water for 3 minutes, until defrosted, then drain and run under cold water.

2. Warm the oil in a large skillet over medium-high heat. Add the zucchini noodles, cabbage, carrots, and bell pepper and sauté until softened, about 5 minutes.

3. Place the rice noodles (if using), edamame, chicken, zucchini noodle mixture, and green onions in a large bowl. Pour the peanut sauce on top and toss to combine.

4. Top with toasted sesame seeds and/or peanuts, if desired.

notes _____

Store-bought rotisserie chicken is a tasty, convenient, and affordable meal solution that makes it easy to round out veggie-packed meals with high-quality complete protein throughout the week.

To make this dish even more veggie-packed, omit the brown rice noodles and add another 3 cups of zucchini noodles in Step 2.

For meat-free: Use a 14-ounce block of extra-firm tofu, pressed and then cubed, in place of the chicken. Before cooking the vegetables in Step 2, cook the tofu until slightly crisp on all sides, about 5 minutes total, then remove from the pan and proceed with the rest of Step 2.

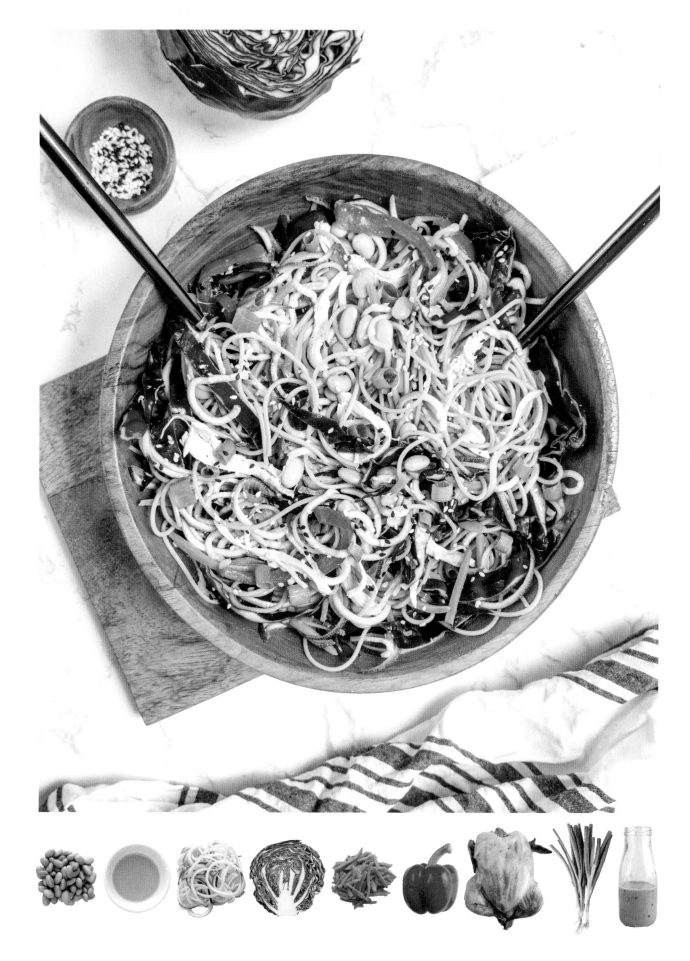

spaghetti squash lentil bolognese boats

yield: **2 boats (4 servings)**   prep time: **15 minutes**   cook time: **50 minutes**

If you are looking for comfort food with a plant-based twist, these Bolognese boats are the answer. Made with a hearty lentil mushroom Bolognese sauce and nature's own spaghetti, this dish is significantly lower in calories and carbohydrates than your traditional restaurant spaghetti Bolognese but has the same great flavor.

boats:

1 medium spaghetti squash (about 3 pounds)

1 tablespoon extra-virgin olive oil

¼ teaspoon finely ground Himalayan pink salt

⅛ teaspoon ground black pepper

quick bolognese sauce:

1 tablespoon extra-virgin olive oil

½ medium yellow onion, chopped

2 cloves garlic, minced

1 (28-ounce) can crushed tomatoes

¼ cup tomato paste

2 cups low-sodium vegetable broth

1 cup red lentils

2 teaspoons ground dried oregano

¼ teaspoon finely ground Himalayan pink salt

¼ teaspoon ground black pepper

suggested toppings:

¼ cup grated Parmesan cheese or plant-based parmesan, store-bought or homemade (page 124)

2 tablespoons chopped fresh basil

1. To cook the spaghetti squash, preheat the oven to 400°F and grease a sheet pan with cooking spray.

2. Slice the squash in half lengthwise, then scoop out and discard the seeds. In a small bowl, whisk together the oil, salt, and pepper. Brush the mixture onto the cut sides of the squash.

3. Place the squash cut side down on the prepared pan. Roast for 30 to 40 minutes, until the skin is lightly browned and the squash is fork-tender but still firm. Remove from the oven and let cool, then flip the squash over and use a fork to scrape and fluff the strands.

4. While the squash is roasting, make the sauce: Pour the oil into a large saucepan and set over medium heat. Add the onion and sauté until fragrant and translucent, 3 to 4 minutes. Add the garlic and sauté for 30 seconds.

5. Increase the heat to high and add the crushed tomatoes, tomato paste, broth, lentils, oregano, salt, and pepper. Bring to a boil, then lower the heat to medium and cook, stirring occasionally, until the sauce has thickened and the lentils are tender, 30 to 40 minutes. Serve over the spaghetti squash boats. Top with the Parmesan and/or basil, if desired.

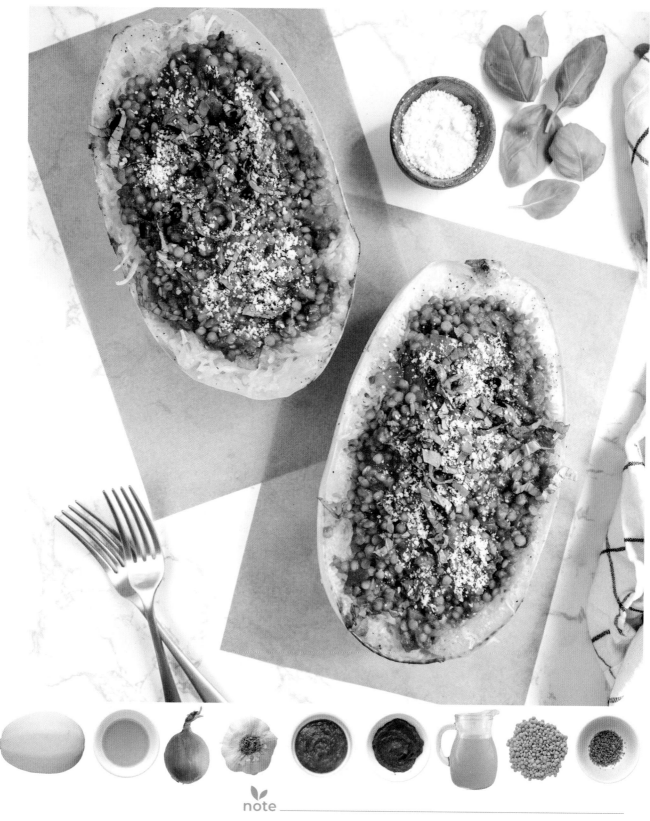

note

*For a more traditional meat-based Bolognese, use 8 ounces of lean
ground turkey or lean ground beef in place of the lentils. Brown and
crumble the meat, then add it to the sauce in Step 5.*

PART III: **10-ingredient or less mostly plant-based recipes**   259

chickpea tuna-less salad

yield: 2½ cups (4 servings)   prep time: 10 minutes

Whether you are a tuna lover or not, this plant-based take on tuna salad is one that all types of eaters can get on board with. Chickpeas are a source of plant protein and fiber and when mashed can take on the texture of tuna but remain mild in flavor. Enjoy it on its own, in a sandwich, or scooped onto a green salad.

1 (15-ounce) can no-salt-added chickpeas, drained and rinsed well, or 1½ cups cooked chickpeas (see page 44)

3 tablespoons avocado oil mayonnaise

½ cup diced celery (about 1 medium stalk)

¼ cup diced red onions (about ¼ medium red onion)

¼ cup dill relish

¼ teaspoon finely ground Himalayan pink salt

⅛ teaspoon ground black pepper

1. Put the chickpeas in a large bowl and mash using a fork.

2. Add the rest of the ingredients to the bowl and mix until incorporated. Serve immediately or store in a sealed container in the refrigerator for up to 3 days.

notes

For egg-free: Use 1 large avocado, mashed, in place of the mayonnaise.

If you miss the tuna, add a sprinkle of crumbled nori for some sea flavor.

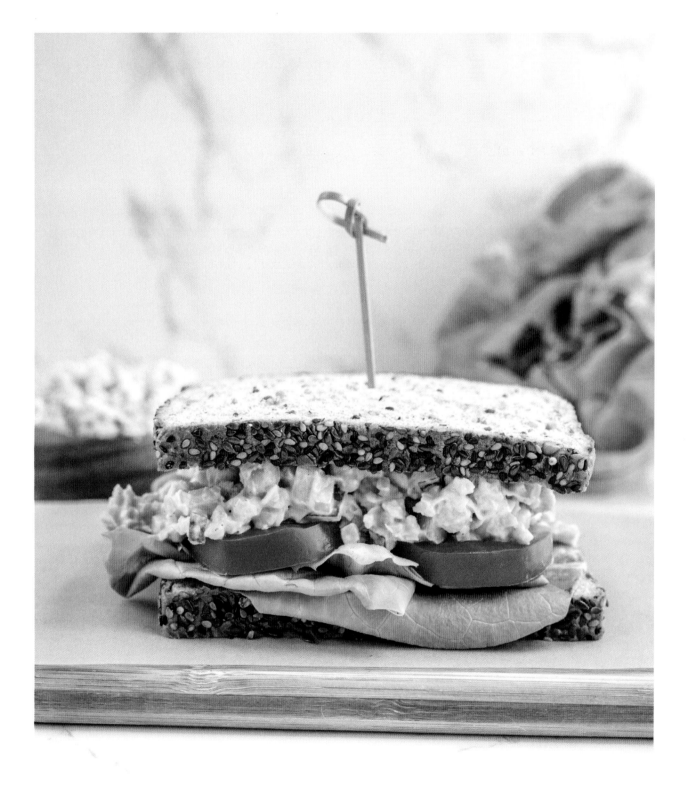

  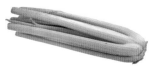

loaded cauliflower "chip" sheet pan nachos

yield: **4 servings**   prep time: **10 minutes**   cook time: **25 minutes**

I think we can all agree that nachos are all about the toppings. These loaded sheet pan nachos are made with a base of my favorite mild-tasting vegetable: cauliflower, of course! Lowering the calories significantly but increasing the fiber and key nutrients like vitamin C and potassium, cauliflower "chips" are the new tortilla chip.

1 large head cauliflower (about 2 pounds), cored and cut into 1-inch florets

2 tablespoons avocado oil, divided

1 tablespoon plus 2 teaspoons taco seasoning, divided

½ teaspoon finely ground Himalayan pink salt, divided

2 cloves garlic, minced

1 (15-ounce) can no-salt-added pinto beans, drained and rinsed well, or 1½ cups cooked pinto beans (see page 44)

⅔ cup shredded cheddar cheese

2 Roma tomatoes, seeded and diced

¼ small red onion, diced

1 large ripe avocado, peeled, pitted, and diced, or 1 cup guacamole, store-bought or homemade (page 118)

¼ cup fresh cilantro leaves

additional toppings (optional):

Sliced jalapeño

Shredded cooked chicken

Sour cream

Roasted corn kernels

1. Preheat the oven to 425°F. Line a sheet pan with parchment paper or spray it with cooking spray.

2. In a large bowl, toss the cauliflower florets with 1 tablespoon of the oil, 1 tablespoon of the taco seasoning, and ¼ teaspoon of the salt. Place the coated cauliflower in a single layer on the prepared baking sheet and bake for 20 minutes, or until tender and slightly crisp.

3. While the cauliflower is in the oven, prepare the refried beans: Put the remaining tablespoon of oil in a small saucepan and place over medium heat. Add the garlic and cook until fragrant, 1 to 2 minutes. Add the beans and the remaining 2 teaspoons of taco seasoning and cook until the beans are hot, 2 to 3 minutes. Smash the beans to the desired texture using a potato masher or fork. Stir in the remaining ¼ teaspoon of salt and a couple tablespoons of water to ensure the beans are not dry.

4. Spoon the refried beans onto the cauliflower "chips," spreading it evenly across, then top with the cheese. Bake until the cheese is melted, another 3 to 5 minutes. Top with the tomatoes, red onion, avocado, cilantro, and any additional toppings of choice before serving.

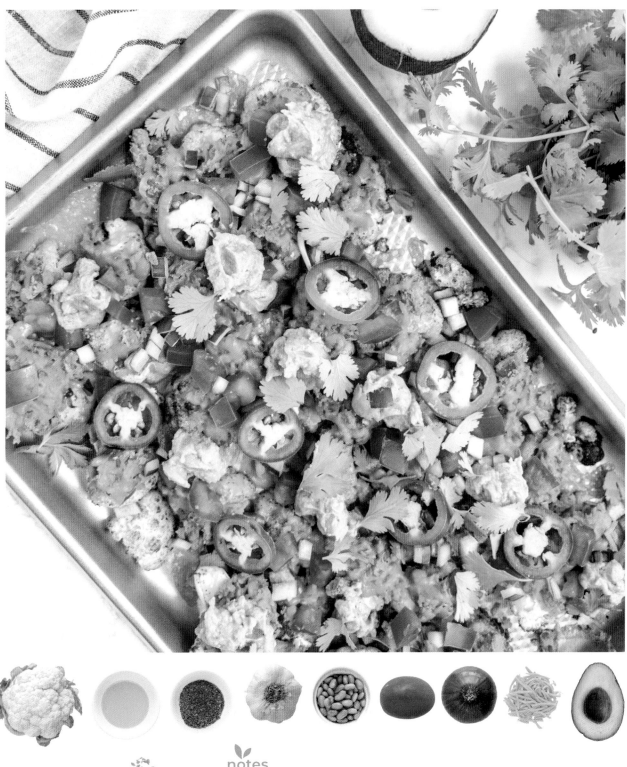

notes _____

Not a fan of cauliflower? Replace it with sweet potato "chips." Simply slice 2 large sweet potatoes into thin rounds using a sharp knife or mandoline and incorporate them in Step 2.

For dairy-free: Omit the cheese or use a dairy-free version.

one-skillet greek chicken and veggies

yield: **4 servings**   prep time: **15 minutes**   cook time: **13 or 20 minutes**, depending on whether orzo or riced cauliflower is used

One-skillet meals are the ultimate weeknight lifesaver. This dish is fresh, flavorful, and hearty but can be lightened up by opting for riced cauliflower instead of orzo.

2 tablespoons extra-virgin olive oil, divided

1 pound boneless, skinless chicken breasts, or 8 ounces tempeh, cut into bite-sized pieces

¼ teaspoon finely ground Himalayan pink salt

2 tablespoons balsamic vinegar

2 cloves garlic, minced

1 pint cherry tomatoes, halved

1⅓ cups orzo, or 2 cups riced cauliflower

1 cup canned artichoke hearts, chopped

½ cup kalamata olives, pitted and sliced

3 tablespoons chopped fresh flat-leaf parsley, for topping

additional toppings (optional):

Tzatziki, store-bought or homemade (page 128), for serving

Crumbled feta cheese

Lemon wedges

1. Heat 1 tablespoon of the oil in a 9-inch skillet over medium-high heat. Place the chicken in the pan, season it with the salt, and sauté until cooked through, 5 to 6 minutes. Stir in the vinegar and garlic and sauté for another 30 seconds, stirring often. Remove the chicken from the pan using a slotted spoon, leaving the juices in the pan, and set aside.

2. Heat the remaining tablespoon of oil in the same skillet and sauté the tomatoes until softened, 2 to 3 minutes.

3. *If using orzo,* add it and 1 cup of water to the pan. Cook, stirring occasionally, until the water is absorbed and the orzo is al dente, about 10 minutes.

If using riced cauliflower, add it to the pan and cook, stirring often, until the cauliflower is tender and slightly charred, 2 to 3 minutes.

4. Add the chicken, artichokes, and olives to the pan, stir to combine, and cook until heated through, 2 to 3 minutes. Top with the parsley and serve with tzatziki, crumbled feta, and/or lemon wedges, if desired.

notes _____

While I recommend orzo for this dish, you can substitute the grain of your choice.

For extra flavor, cook the orzo in broth instead of water.

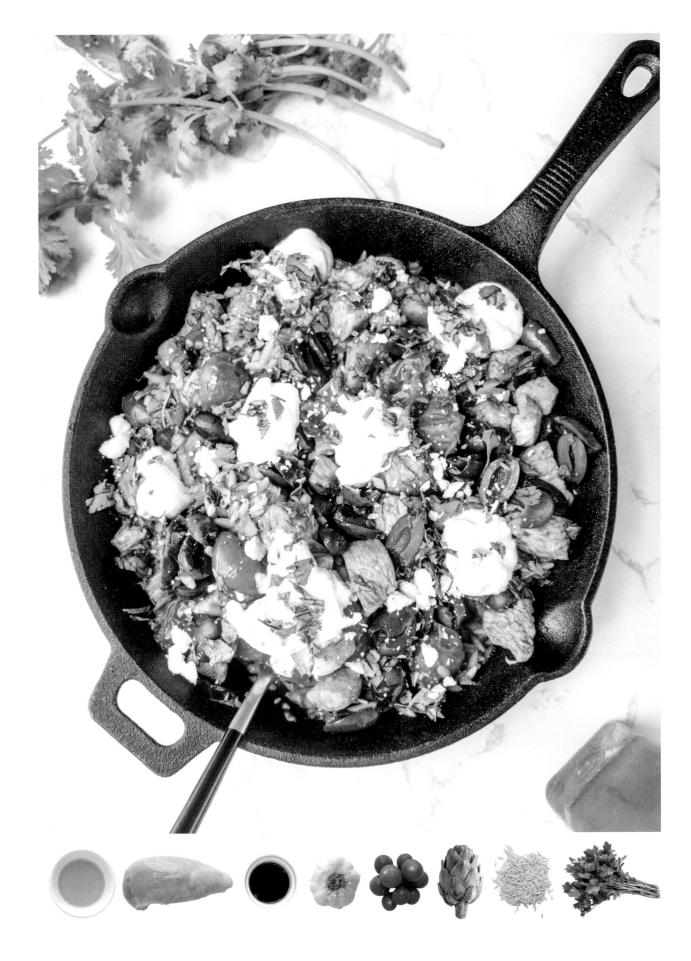

no-bread wrap

yield: **1 wrap**   prep time: **10 minutes**

It's all about the fixings—who agrees? This light and fresh no-bread sandwich picks you up without weighing you down. Wrapped in a crunchy romaine exterior, it can be customized to just about any classic sandwich combination you fancy. I've given you three of my favorites here.

5 to 6 romaine lettuce leaves

turkey avocado wrap:

1 tablespoon avocado oil mayonnaise

2 ounces low-sodium deli turkey (2 or 3 slices)

1 Roma tomato, sliced (about 3 slices)

½ medium avocado, sliced

¼ cup sprouts

hummus and veggie wrap:

¼ cup roasted red pepper hummus, store-bought or homemade (page 120)

1 Roma tomato, sliced (about 3 slices)

½ Persian cucumber, cut into matchsticks (about ¼ cup)

¼ cup sliced red onions (about ¼ red onion)

¼ cup shredded or julienned carrots

¼ cup microgreens

tempeh BLT wrap:

1 tablespoon avocado oil mayonnaise

3 or 4 slices Tempeh Bacon (page 126)

1 Roma tomato, sliced (about 3 slices)

½ medium avocado, sliced

1. Lay a piece of parchment paper on a large cutting board.

2. Cut out the stems of the lettuce leaves and lay the leaves in overlapping lines on the paper to form a large rectangle.

3. *To make the turkey avocado wrap,* spread the mayonnaise in an even layer on the lettuce and top with the turkey, tomato, avocado, and sprouts.

To make the hummus and veggie wrap, spread the hummus in a thin layer on the lettuce and top with the tomato, cucumber, onions, carrots, and microgreens.

To make the tempeh BLT wrap, spread the mayonnaise in a thin layer on the lettuce and top with the bacon, tomato, and avocado.

4. Use the parchment paper to roll the sandwich into a tight tube, folding in the ends as you roll. Slice the wrap in half.

note _____

You can use butter lettuce or little gem lettuce in place of the romaine.

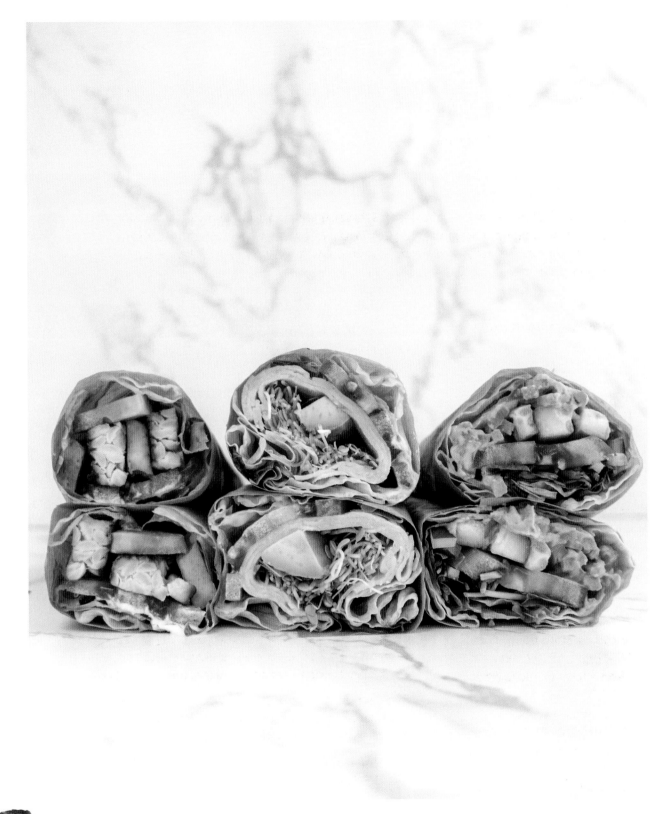
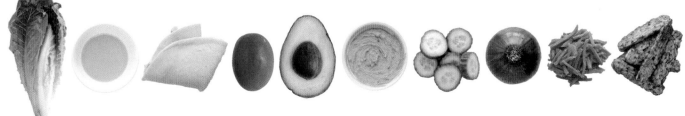

easy rotisserie chicken enchiladas

yield: 6 enchiladas (2 per serving)   prep time: 10 minutes   cook time: 35 minutes

Flavor meets convenience in these enchiladas made with precooked rotisserie chicken and a two-ingredient no-added-sugar enchilada sauce. Rotisserie chicken is a convenient and affordable source of flavorful protein that can be added to meals throughout the week for a boost of staying power.

filling:

1 tablespoon avocado oil

½ medium yellow onion, diced

1 pound shredded rotisserie chicken (about 1½ cups)

1 (15-ounce) can no-salt-added black beans, drained and rinsed well, or 1½ cups cooked black beans (see page 44)

1 cup fresh spinach

¼ cup water

2½ tablespoons taco seasoning

2-ingredient enchilada sauce:

1 (6-ounce) can tomato paste

1½ cups hot water

3 tablespoons taco seasoning

6 (10-inch) whole-grain tortillas

1 cup shredded sharp cheddar cheese

suggested toppings:

Fresh cilantro leaves

Sliced jalapeño pepper

Sliced avocado

Diced red onions

1. Preheat the oven to 375°F.

2. To make the filling, pour the oil into a large skillet. Add the onion and cook until tender and translucent, about 5 minutes. Stir in the chicken, beans, and spinach. Cook, stirring often, until the spinach has wilted and the ingredients are heated through, about 3 minutes.

3. Pour the water into the skillet and stir in the taco seasoning. Cook for another 1 to 2 minutes to let the flavors mingle.

4. To make the enchilada sauce, whisk together the tomato paste, water, and taco seasoning in a medium bowl. Pour ½ cup of the sauce into a 9 by 13-inch baking dish and spread out with a spoon to evenly coat the bottom.

5. To assemble the enchiladas, fill each tortilla with one-sixth of the filling, roll tightly, and arrange side by side in the baking dish, seam side down. Pour the remaining sauce over the enchiladas and sprinkle the cheese on top.

6. Bake until hot and bubbly, 20 to 25 minutes. Top with fresh cilantro, sliced jalapeño, sliced avocado, and/or diced red onions, if desired.

note _____

For meat-free: Use 2 cups of 100% Mushroom Base (page 133) instead of the chicken.

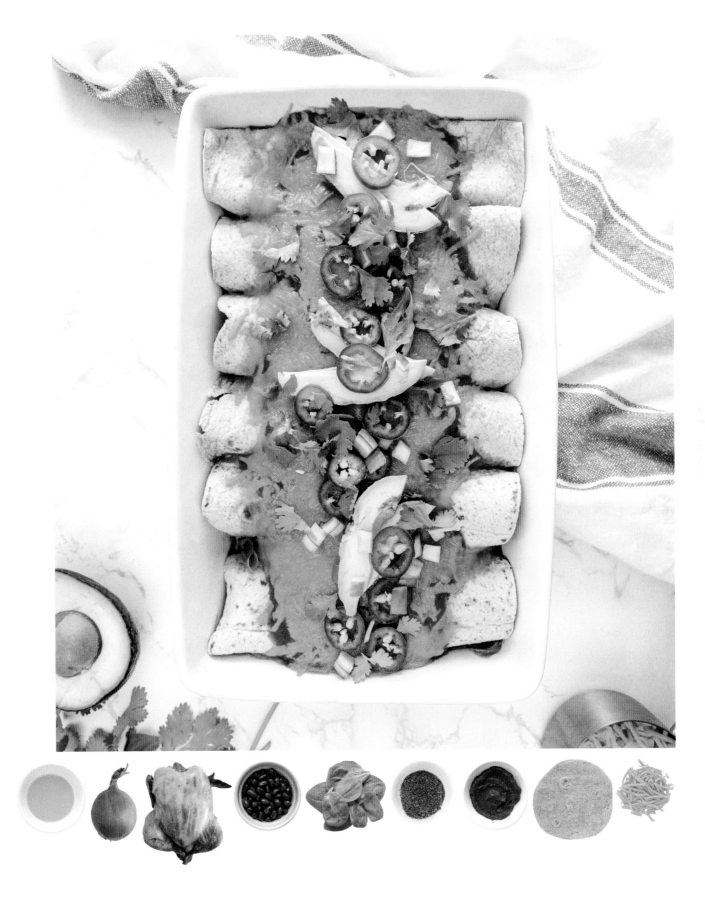

chipotle burrito bowl with cauliflower rice

yield: **2 servings**   prep time: **15 minutes**   cook time: **15 minutes**

Get all the goodness of a burrito at home for fewer calories and less sodium than the takeout variety. This lightened-up burrito bowl is made with a fluffy base of cilantro-lime cauliflower rice and topped with a balance of vegetable and protein toppings. Say hello to your new go-to satisfying weekday lunch—guac, not optional!

cilantro-lime cauliflower rice:

1½ teaspoons avocado oil

1 medium head cauliflower (about 1½ pounds), cored, cut into florets, and riced, or 4 cups prericed cauliflower

¼ cup fresh cilantro leaves, minced

Grated zest and juice of 1 lime

Finely ground Himalayan pink salt to taste

1½ teaspoons avocado oil

6 ounces boneless, skinless chicken breast or firm tofu, cut into bite-sized pieces

½ teaspoon chipotle powder

Finely ground Himalayan pink salt

1 cup frozen corn

⅔ cup cooked black beans

toppings:

⅔ cup pico de gallo, store-bought or homemade (page 116)

¼ cup guacamole, store-bought or homemade (page 118)

Fresh cilantro leaves

1. To make the rice, heat the oil in a large skillet over medium-high heat. Add the riced cauliflower and sauté until tender and slightly crisp, 2 to 3 minutes. Stir in the cilantro, lime zest and juice, and salt. Set aside.

2. To prepare the remaining ingredients, heat the oil in another large skillet over medium-high heat. In a large bowl, toss the chicken or tofu with the chipotle powder and salt, then add to the pan. Sauté until the chicken is no longer pink or the tofu is slightly crisp on all sides, about 5 minutes. Remove the chicken or tofu to a plate and set aside.

3. Put the corn in the skillet and cook until slightly charred, 2 to 3 minutes. Stir in the beans and cook until heated through, about 2 minutes.

4. To assemble, divide the cauliflower rice between two serving bowls and top with the chicken or tofu, corn and bean mixture, pico de gallo, guacamole, and more cilantro.

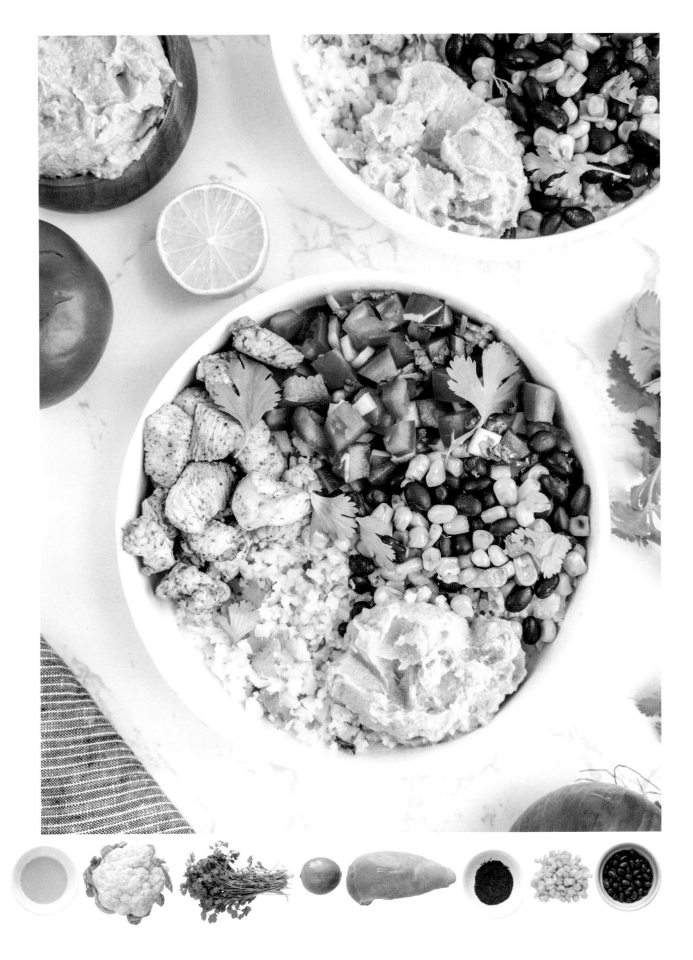

zucchini noodle lasagna

yield: **4 servings**   prep time: **15 minutes**   cook time: **52 minutes**

Level-up your lasagna! Made with wide planks of zucchini instead of pasta, this recipe is perfect for lasagna lovers looking to add more veggies to their life. Mild-tasting zucchini serves as an ideal blank canvas for the traditional fixings in this low-carb dish.

4 large zucchinis (about 2 pounds), trimmed

½ teaspoon finely ground Himalayan pink salt, divided

½ teaspoon ground black pepper

1 (15-ounce) container part-skim ricotta cheese

1 large egg, beaten

2 cloves garlic, minced

1 pound lean ground beef

2½ cups tomato sauce, store-bought or homemade (page 130), divided

¼ cup chopped fresh basil, plus extra for topping if desired

¼ cup chopped fresh flat-leaf parsley

½ cup shredded mozzarella cheese

notes

For dairy-free: Replace the ricotta filling with the Cauliflower Cashew Ricotta on page 286 and the mozzarella with a shredded plant-based cheese.

For meat-free: Replace the beef with a batch of 100% Mushroom Base (page 133).

1. Preheat the oven to 425°F. Line two sheet pans with parchment paper.

2. Using a chef's knife, slice the zucchinis lengthwise into ¼-inch-thick planks; you should get a total of 13 to 16. Transfer the zucchini planks to a large bowl and toss with ¼ teaspoon of the salt and the pepper.

3. Arrange the zucchini planks in a single layer on the prepared pans. Bake for 3 minutes, then flip and bake for another 3 minutes. This will help remove water from the zucchini so that the lasagna is not watery.

4. Lower the oven temperature to 400°F.

5. Put the ricotta, egg, garlic, and remaining ¼ teaspoon of salt in a medium bowl and mix until combined.

6. Brown the meat in a large skillet over medium-high heat until no longer pink, about 5 minutes. Drain the fat and stir in 1 cup of the tomato sauce. Cook for another 1 to 2 minutes, until heated through.

7. Using a rubber spatula, spread 1 cup of the tomato sauce on the bottom of a 9 by 13-inch (or 4-quart) baking dish. Layer half of the zucchini planks over the sauce, slightly overlapping.

8. Use the spatula to spread the ricotta mixture on top of the zucchini planks in an even layer. Top with the meat mixture, basil, and parsley. Layer the remaining zucchini planks on top, slightly overlapping.

9. Brush the remaining ½ cup of sauce over the zucchini and sprinkle the cheese on top.

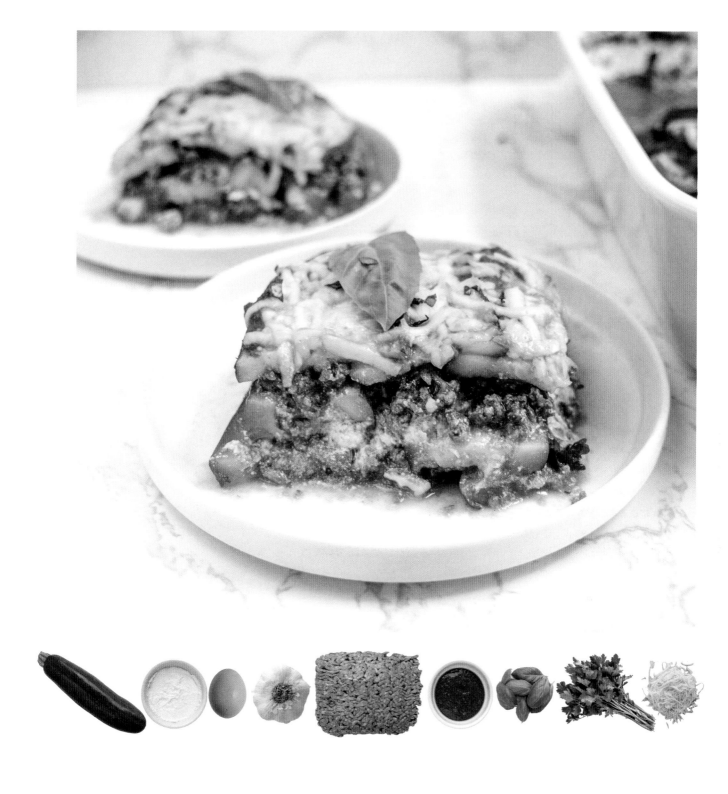

10. Bake, uncovered, until the cheese is golden and the zucchini is tender, 30 to 40 minutes. Top with more basil before serving, if desired.

all-in-one loaded sweet potato meal

3 WAYS

yield: **2 servings**   prep time: **15 minutes**   cook time: **50 minutes**

A baked sweet potato is more than just a starchy veggie on your dinner plate. It makes an excellent nutrient-rich canvas for protein, vegetables, and good-for-you fats. Build an all-in-one loaded sweet potato meal that's cozy, delicious, and satisfies your current cravings.

2 medium sweet potatoes

notes

To save time, you can cook the sweet potatoes in the microwave. Simply prick the outsides with a fork, place on a microwave-safe plate, and cook on high for 3 to 4 minutes, or until soft.

To make the BBQ filling meat-free, replace the chicken with 1 cup of cooked chickpeas.

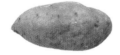

1. Preheat the oven to 425°F. Line a sheet pan with parchment paper.

2. Rinse and scrub the sweet potatoes, then pat dry. Prick the potatoes all over with a fork and place on the prepared pan. Bake until fork-tender, 40 to 50 minutes. Allow to cool before slitting open lengthwise along the top with a knife.

3. While the potatoes are baking, prepare the filling.

To make the burrito potatoes, heat the oil in a large skillet over medium-high heat. Add the onion to the pan and sauté until tender and fragrant, 3 to 4 minutes. Add the beef or tempeh and cook until combined with the onion and no longer pink. Add the corn, black beans, chili powder, cumin, and salt. Cook for another 2 to 3 minutes, stirring often, or until heated through. Transfer the mixture to the sweet potatoes and top with the guacamole and cilantro, if desired.

To make the chickpea hummus potatoes, fill each potato with ¼ cup of the hummus, ½ cup of the chickpea poppers, and half of the tomatoes and parsley.

To make the BBQ chicken potatoes, toss the chicken and BBQ sauce together, then transfer to the sweet potatoes. In a medium bowl, whisk together the mayonnaise, lemon juice, mustard, celery seeds, salt, and pepper until combined. Add the coleslaw mix to the bowl and toss to coat. Serve the coleslaw over the stuffed sweet potatoes.

Turn the page for FLAVOR OPTIONS.

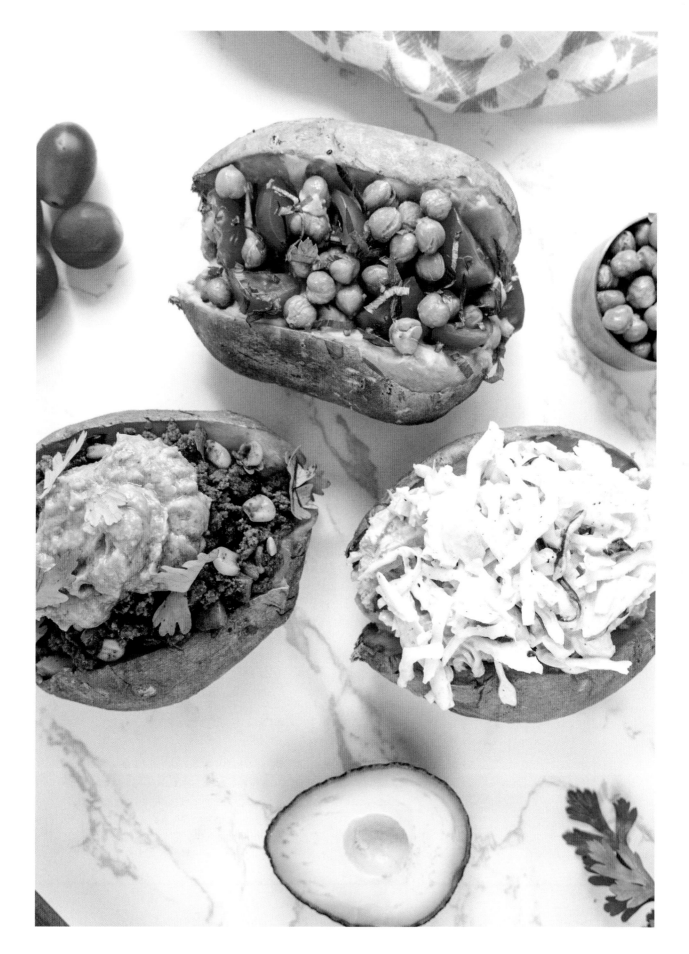

flavor options

burrito:

1 tablespoon avocado oil

¼ cup diced yellow onions

6 ounces lean ground beef or crumbled tempeh

½ cup frozen corn

½ cup cooked black beans

1 teaspoon chili powder

½ teaspoon ground cumin

¼ teaspoon finely ground Himalayan pink salt

¼ cup guacamole, store-bought or homemade (page 118)

Fresh cilantro leaves, for topping (optional)

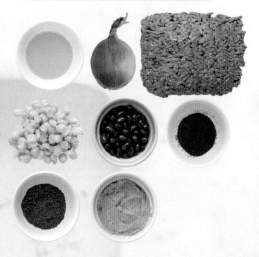

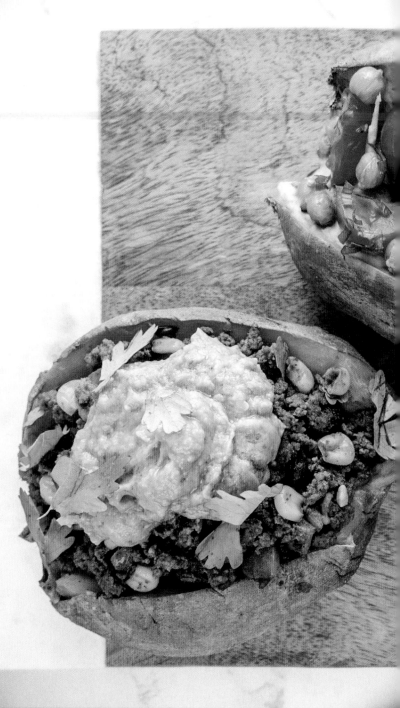

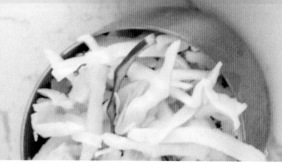

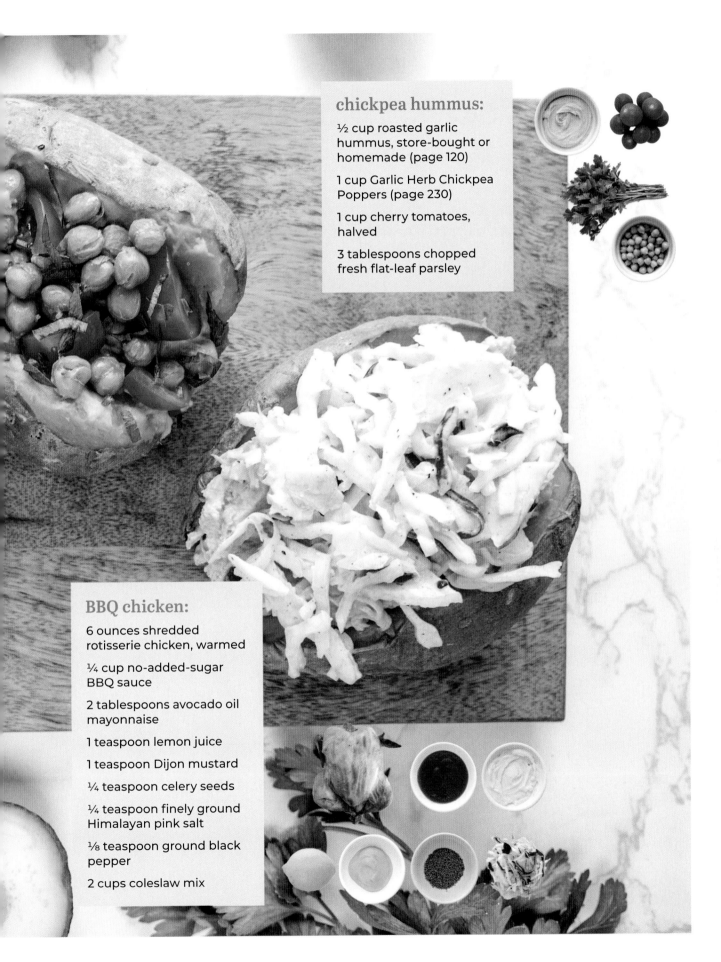

chickpea hummus:

½ cup roasted garlic hummus, store-bought or homemade (page 120)

1 cup Garlic Herb Chickpea Poppers (page 230)

1 cup cherry tomatoes, halved

3 tablespoons chopped fresh flat-leaf parsley

BBQ chicken:

6 ounces shredded rotisserie chicken, warmed

¼ cup no-added-sugar BBQ sauce

2 tablespoons avocado oil mayonnaise

1 teaspoon lemon juice

1 teaspoon Dijon mustard

¼ teaspoon celery seeds

¼ teaspoon finely ground Himalayan pink salt

⅛ teaspoon ground black pepper

2 cups coleslaw mix

chickpea carrot burgers

yield: **4 patties (1 per serving)**   prep time: **10 minutes, plus 15 minutes to set**
cook time: **7 to 20 minutes, depending on method**

These plant-powered patties give burger night a whole new meaning. You have the choice of cooking them in the oven, on a grill, or in a pan. Enjoy them on toasted whole-grain buns, on portabella buns (see page 252), or wrapped in lettuce. My favorite fixings are sliced red onions, sliced tomatoes, guacamole (see page 118 for my recipe), and lettuce.

1 (15-ounce) can no-salt-added chickpeas, drained and rinsed well, or 1½ cups cooked chickpeas (see page 44)

½ cup rolled oats

½ cup shredded carrots

¼ medium red onion, coarsely chopped

¼ cup shelled raw sunflower seeds

2 cloves garlic, peeled

1 tablespoon flaxseed meal

½ teaspoon finely ground Himalayan pink salt

⅛ teaspoon ground black pepper

1. Put all of the ingredients in a food processor and process for about 20 seconds, until a thick mixture forms. Do not overblend; retain some chickpea chunks for texture. Place the mixture in the refrigerator to firm up for 15 minutes, then divide it into 4 equal-sized portions and shape into patties.

2. *To bake,* preheat the oven to 375°F. Place the patties on a sheet pan lined with parchment paper and bake until crisp and lightly browned on both sides, 15 to 20 minutes.

To grill, preheat a grill to medium. Grill the patties until lightly browned on both sides, 5 to 7 minutes total.

To cook on the stovetop, cook the patties in a large greased skillet over medium-high heat until lightly browned on both sides, 3 to 4 minutes per side.

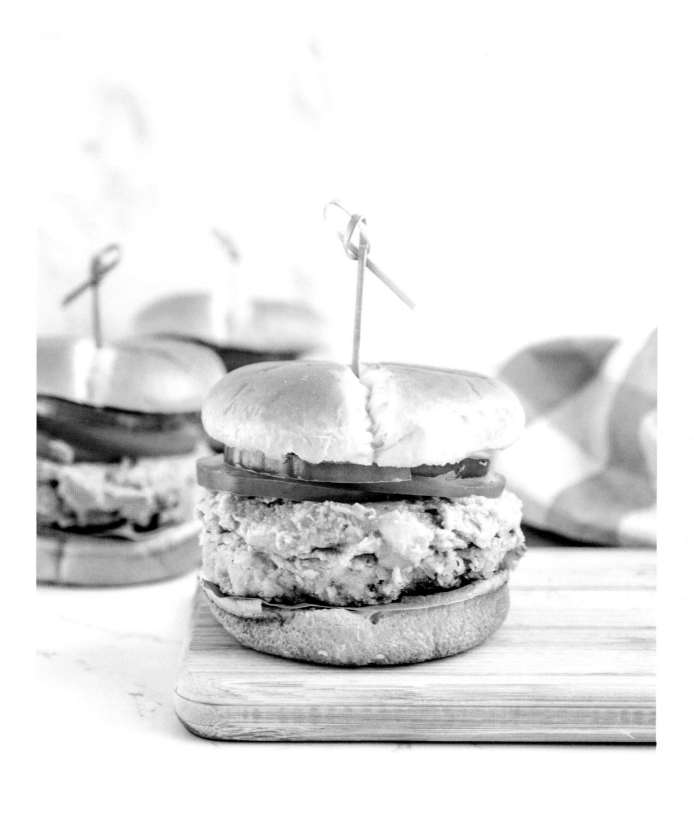

baked feta vegetable pasta

yield: **6 servings**   prep time: **10 minutes**   cook time: **40 minutes**

Pasta for dinner is always a good idea. This hands-off dish is made with a handful of fresh, flavorful ingredients: a base of protein-rich chickpea pasta combined with burst cherry tomatoes and roasted summer squash and eggplant, coated in creamy feta, and topped with fresh basil. Packed with protein, energizing carbohydrates, and veggie goodness, it makes for an easy, complete meal on busy weeknights.

1 pint cherry tomatoes

1 large yellow squash, sliced into half-moons

1 large zucchini, sliced into half-moons

½ small eggplant, chopped

1 tablespoon extra-virgin olive oil

½ teaspoon finely ground Himalayan pink salt

⅛ teaspoon ground black pepper

1 (8-ounce) block feta cheese

8 ounces chickpea rotini or penne pasta

2 cloves garlic, minced

¼ cup fresh basil leaves, torn if large

Red pepper flakes (optional)

1. Preheat the oven to 400°F.

2. Place the tomatoes, yellow squash, zucchini, and eggplant in a 9 by 13-inch baking dish. Toss with the oil, salt, and pepper. Make a space in the center and nestle the feta block in the space.

3. Bake until the tomatoes burst, the vegetables are tender, and the feta has melted, 35 to 40 minutes.

4. While the vegetables and feta are baking, cook the pasta: Bring a large pot of salted water to a boil and cook the pasta according to the package instructions until al dente. Drain and run the pasta under cold water to stop the cooking.

5. Remove the pan from the oven and stir in the pasta, garlic, basil, and red pepper flakes, if using.

notes _____

For dairy-free: Omit the cheese or use a plant-based feta (such as Violife).

Use another pasta of your choice if you can tolerate gluten.

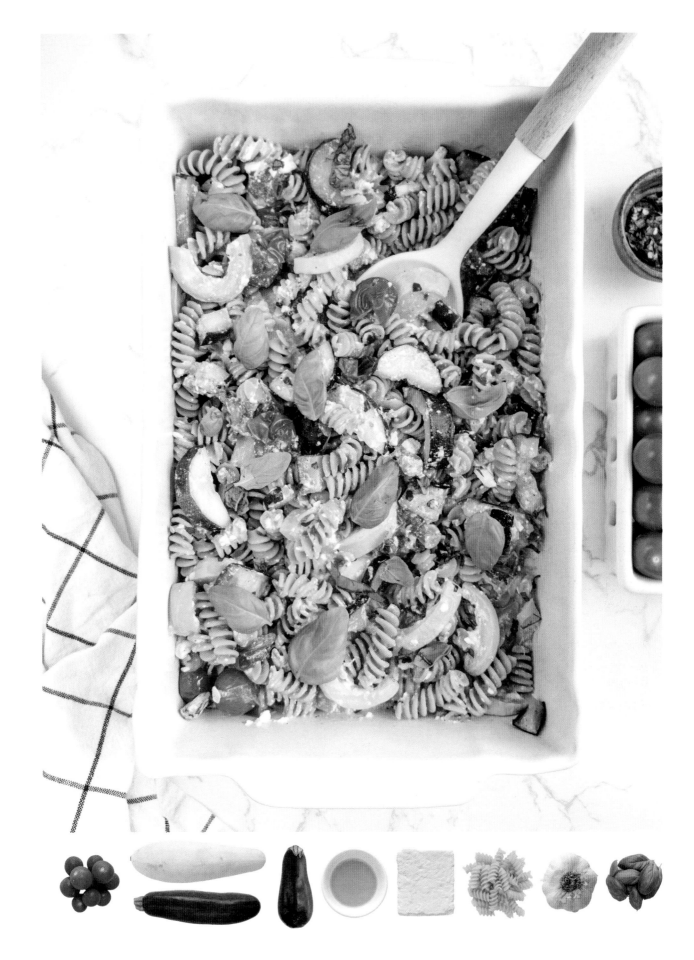

taco-stuffed zucchini boats

yield: **2 servings**   prep time: **10 minutes**   cook time: **30 minutes**

Taco night but with a veggie twist! If tacos make it into your weekly dinner rotation like mine, try this nutritious take. I love using vegetables such as zucchini, bell peppers, eggplant, and acorn squash as vehicles for flavorful protein and whole grains to build complete meals. Feel free to customize this recipe with your choice of protein and creamy topping; guacamole makes an excellent stand-in for cheese if you're looking for a dairy-free version.

4 medium zucchinis, cut in half lengthwise

1 tablespoon avocado oil

½ medium yellow onion, diced

6 ounces lean ground turkey

2 cloves garlic, minced

1 tablespoon taco seasoning

½ cup tomato sauce, store-bought or homemade (page 130)

1 cup cooked black beans

¼ cup shredded cheddar cheese or guacamole, store-bought or homemade (page 118)

suggested toppings:

Diced avocado

Sliced black olives

Sliced jalapeños

Fresh cilantro leaves

Lime juice

Sour cream

1. Preheat the oven to 400°F.

2. Use a ½-teaspoon measuring spoon to hollow out the centers of the zucchini halves, leaving about a ¼-inch-thick shell on each. Place cut side up in a 9 by 13-inch baking dish. Bake until tender, 15 to 20 minutes.

3. Meanwhile, prepare the filling: Heat the oil in a large skillet over medium-high heat. Add the onion and sauté until soft, about 3 minutes. Add the turkey and garlic and cook until the turkey is no longer pink, 5 to 6 minutes. Drain and return to the skillet. Stir in the taco seasoning, tomato sauce, and beans. Reduce the heat to medium and cook until heated through, 3 to 4 minutes.

4. Divide the mixture among the zucchini boats, top with the cheese, if using, and bake until heated through and the cheese has melted, about 10 minutes. If using guacamole, spoon it on top of the zucchini boats after baking.

5. Top as desired before serving.

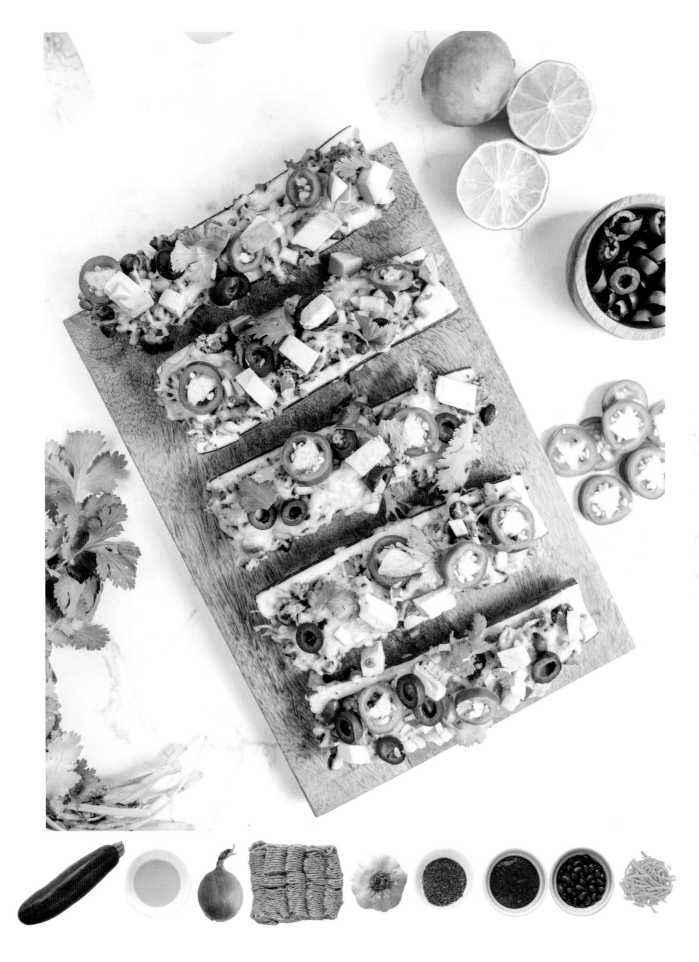

deconstructed spicy sushi bowl

yield: **2 servings**   prep time: **10 minutes**   cook time: **15 minutes**

Bring sushi night home without having to call in for takeout. This deconstructed sushi bowl is made with a base of light, fluffy riced cauliflower and topped with buttery salmon nuggets, crunchy produce, and a drizzle of two-ingredient spicy mayonnaise for some heat. Salmon is my favorite fish because of its melt-in-your-mouth flavor and brain-loving omega-3 fats, but you could use another fish of your choice if you prefer. For a plant protein replacement, I recommend shelled edamame (see the note, opposite).

8 ounces skinned salmon fillets

Finely ground Himalayan pink salt and ground black pepper

1 or 2 tablespoons avocado oil, divided

1 pound cauliflower florets (from about 1 large head), riced in a food processor, or 2 cups cooked brown rice, warmed

½ cup julienned carrots

1 Persian cucumber, sliced into half-moons (about ½ cup)

½ medium ripe avocado, thinly sliced

2 tablespoons low-sodium soy sauce

4 sheets roasted seaweed, torn or cut into small pieces or strips

suggested add-ins:

Sliced green onions

Steamed shelled edamame

Pickled ginger

Sliced radishes

Sesame seeds

Diced mango

easy spicy mayo:

¼ cup avocado oil mayonnaise

1 to 2 teaspoons Sriracha sauce, to taste

1. Cut the salmon into 1-inch chunks and season with salt and pepper.

2. Heat 1 tablespoon of oil in a large skillet over medium-high heat. Working in two or three batches, add the salmon to the skillet in a single layer and sear for 15 to 20 seconds per side, until all sides are golden and crisp and the internal temperature has reached 125°F to 130°F, about 3 minutes total per batch.

3. If using riced cauliflower, pour 1 tablespoon of oil into the skillet and sauté the cauliflower for 1 minute. Cover with a lid to let the cauliflower steam and become tender, 5 to 8 minutes. Season with salt and pepper to taste. If using brown rice, simply season it with salt and pepper.

4. Divide the rice between two bowls and top each with half of the salmon, carrots, cucumbers, avocado, and soy sauce. Divide the add-in ingredients, if using, between the bowls.

5. To make the spicy mayonnaise, combine the mayonnaise and Sriracha sauce in a small bowl. Drizzle over the bowls and top with the roasted seaweed.

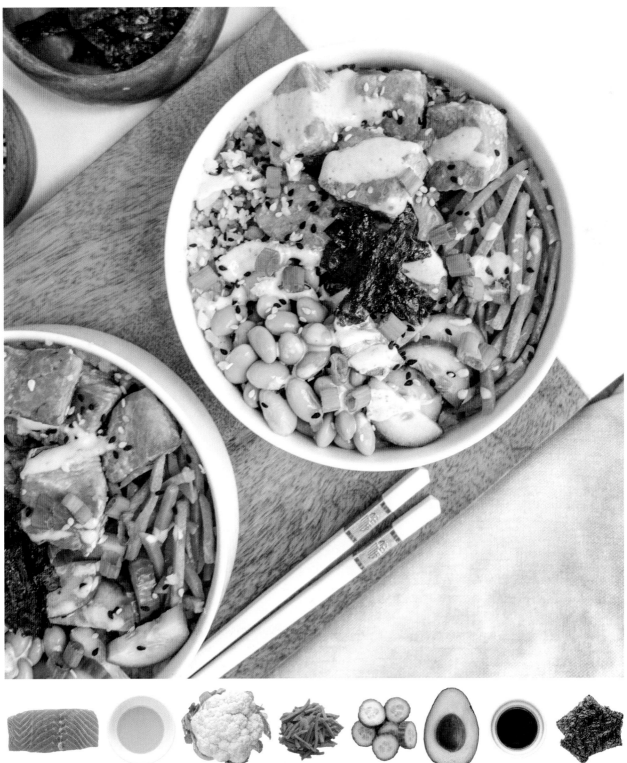

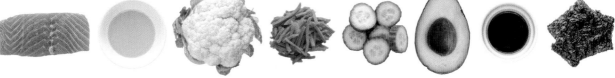

note

*For fish-free: Replace the salmon with 1 cup of frozen shelled edamame.
Cook according to the package instructions and divide between the
bowls in Step 4.*

cauliflower cashew ricotta–stuffed shells

yield: 4 servings   prep time: 10 minutes, plus 30 minutes to soak cashews   cook time: 55 minutes

This dish could trick even the pickiest eaters into eating their veggies. Say hello to saucy shells stuffed with a creamy cauliflower cashew plant-based ricotta for a cheesy flavor without the dairy, baked to golden brown perfection. To make this straightforward recipe even simpler, use real-deal ricotta and Parmesan cheese in the filling instead of the cashews and nutritional yeast; this swap will save you the step of soaking the cashews.

cauliflower cashew ricotta:

1 cup raw cashews

1 large head cauliflower (about 2 pounds), cut into bite-sized florets

3 tablespoons nutritional yeast

3 cloves garlic, minced

1 teaspoon onion powder

½ teaspoon finely ground Himalayan pink salt

⅛ teaspoon ground black pepper

24 jumbo whole-grain pasta shells

3 cups tomato sauce, store-bought or homemade (page 130), divided

¼ cup plant-based parmesan, store-bought or homemade (page 124), or grated Parmesan cheese

¼ cup minced fresh basil, for topping

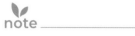

note _____

If you prefer, you can replace the cashews with 1 cup of ricotta and the nutritional yeast with 2 tablespoons of grated Parmesan.

1. Place the cashews in a large bowl and cover with water. Soak for at least 30 minutes or up to 1 hour, then drain.

2. Bring a large pot of salted water to a boil. Cook the pasta according to the package instructions until al dente; drain and rinse under cold water to stop the cooking.

3. Put 2 inches of water in a large pot and set a steamer basket inside the pot. Place the cauliflower in the basket and cover the pot with a tight-fitting lid. Steam over medium-high heat until the cauliflower is tender, 5 to 8 minutes.

4. Preheat the oven to 375°F.

5. Pour 1 cup of the tomato sauce into a 9 by 13-inch baking dish and spread with a spoon to evenly coat the bottom.

6. To make the ricotta filling, put the soaked cashews, steamed cauliflower, nutritional yeast, garlic, onion powder, salt, and pepper in a food processor and blend until the mixture has a ricotta-like texture. If needed, add water a tablespoon at a time and keep blending until the filling is thick and creamy.

7. Stuff the shells with the filling and place in a single layer in the baking dish. Pour the remaining 2 cups of sauce on top, cover the dish with foil, and bake for 25 minutes.

8. Remove the foil, top the shells with the Parmesan, and bake for another 10 minutes, or until the tops are golden. Top with the basil before serving.

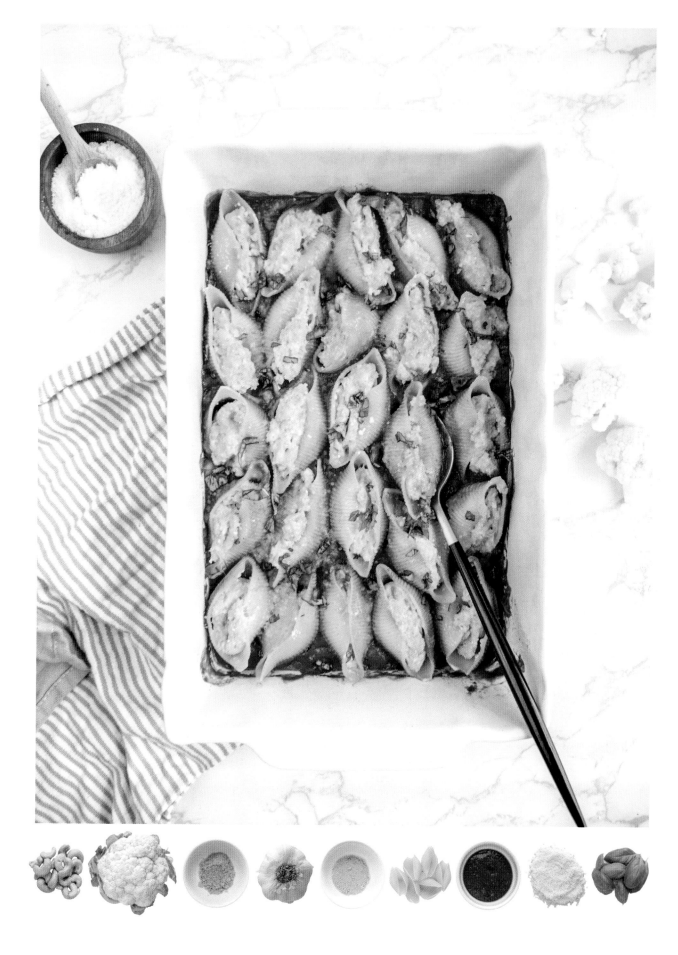

adult lunch box

yield: 1 serving   prep time: 10 minutes   cook time: 0 to 5 minutes, depending on box

Make work lunch fun and functional with preportioned bento boxes that encourage portion control and meet all of your food group needs in one meal. Once you check off the basic categories—produce, protein, whole grain, and good fats—the combinations are endless. I use a three-section lunch box with one large compartment and two equally sized smaller ones.

chicken avocado cups:

3 or 4 butter lettuce leaves

1 serving Avocado Chicken Salad (page 190)

1 cup sliced strawberries

¼ cup raw almonds

Fill the lettuce leaves with the chicken salad and place in the large compartment of the lunch box. Divide the strawberries and almonds between the two smaller compartments.

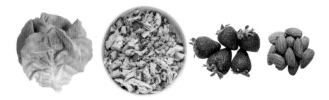

chickpea tuna-less salad melt:

1 cup mini bell peppers (any color), halved and seeds removed

1 cup Chickpea Tuna-Less Salad (page 260)

2 tablespoons shredded cheddar cheese

1 cup cassava chips

1 stalk celery, cut into 2- to 3-inch sticks

Preheat the oven to 400°F. Stuff the bell pepper halves with the chickpea salad and sprinkle the cheese on top. Bake until the cheese melts, 4 to 5 minutes. Transfer to the large compartment of the lunch box. Divide the chips and celery sticks between the two smaller compartments. Reheat the stuffed peppers in the microwave for 1 to 2 minutes or in a 350°F oven for 5 to 10 minutes.

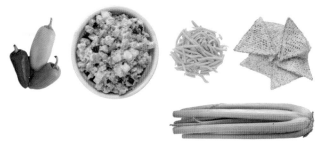

mediterranean:

¼ cup diced Persian cucumbers

¼ cup diced red onions

¼ cup diced tomatoes

¼ cup diced yellow bell peppers

2 tablespoons pitted kalamata olives

2 tablespoons chopped fresh flat-leaf parsley leaves

½ cup cooked quinoa

1 tablespoon balsamic vinaigrette, store-bought or homemade (page 110)

¼ cup tzatziki, store-bought or homemade (page 128)

½ cup Garlic Herb Chickpea Poppers (page 230) or cooked chickpeas

Combine the cucumbers, onions, tomatoes, bell peppers, olives, parsley, quinoa, and vinaigrette in a large bowl. Transfer to the large compartment of the lunch box. Divide the tzatziki and chickpeas between the two smaller compartments.

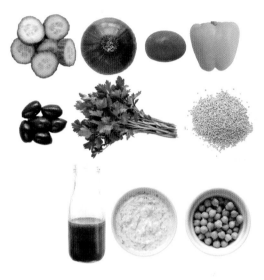

peanut noodles:

1 serving Rainbow Veggie Noodles (page 256)

¼ cup roasted peanuts

1 navel orange, sliced

Place the rainbow noodles in the large compartment of the lunch box and divide the peanuts and orange slices between the two smaller compartments.

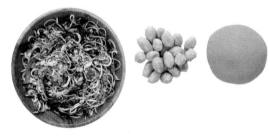

taco:

1 tablespoon avocado oil

3 ounces lean ground beef or crumbled tempeh

1 teaspoon taco seasoning

½ cup frozen corn

1 cup cooked cauliflower rice

¼ cup chopped romaine lettuce

1 Roma tomato, diced

¼ cup cooked pinto beans

1 tablespoon shredded cheese of choice (optional)

2 (5-inch) corn tortillas or butter lettuce leaves

¼ cup guacamole, store-bought or homemade (page 118)

Heat the oil in a medium skillet over medium-high heat. Sauté the beef with the taco seasoning until no longer pink, 5 to 6 minutes. Remove from the skillet and set aside. Add the corn to the pan and cook until slightly charred, about 5 minutes. To assemble, put the rice in the large compartment of the lunch box and layer with the corn, beef, romaine, tomato, beans, and cheese, if using. If using tortillas, warm them in a small skillet until softened. Place the guacamole and folded tortillas or lettuce leaves in the two smaller compartments. Before eating, place the tortillas and taco mixture on a microwave-safe plate and microwave for 1 to 2 minutes, or until warmed.

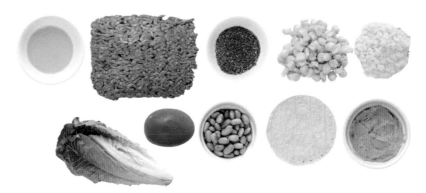

veggie lover's:

1 Spicy Hummus and Veggie No-Bread Wrap (page 266)

1 cup almond flour crackers, store-bought or homemade (page 236)

1 hard-boiled egg

1 apple or peach, sliced

Place the no-bread wrap in the large compartment of the lunch box and divide the crackers, egg, and fruit between the two smaller compartments.

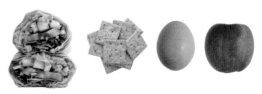

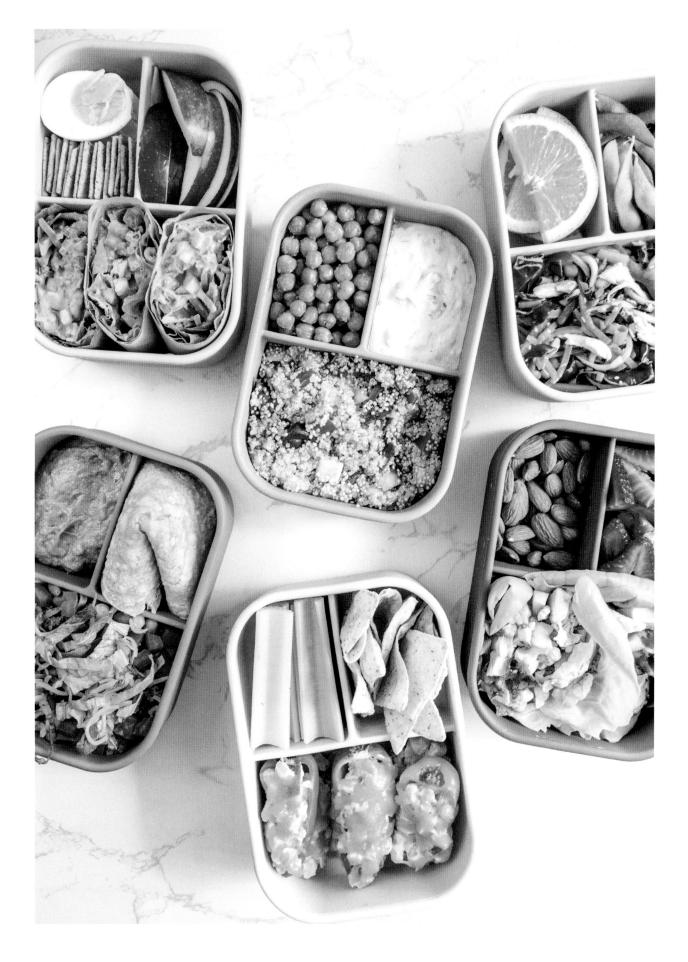

pizza-stuffed peppers

yield: **4 servings**   prep time: **10 minutes**   cook time: **45 minutes**

If you are craving pizza but not the heavy refined flour crust, try this super satisfying, nutrient-dense take. This dish packs all of the traditional pizza fixings in soft bell pepper shells that serve as a naturally gluten-free, lower-calorie, vitamin C–packed base. Did you know that bell peppers contain more vitamin C by weight than oranges? Meet 100 percent of your daily vitamin C needs with just one serving!

1 tablespoon extra-virgin olive oil

1 pound lean ground beef, or 8 ounces tempeh, crumbled

2 cloves garlic, minced

¼ teaspoon finely ground Himalayan pink salt

1 teaspoon Italian seasoning

2 cups tomato sauce, store-bought or homemade (page 130)

3 large bell peppers, any color, halved and seeds removed

⅔ cup shredded mozzarella cheese

¼ cup cherry tomatoes, sliced

2 tablespoons sliced olives

¼ cup chopped fresh basil leaves, for topping

1 tablespoon grated Parmesan cheese or plant-based parmesan, store-bought or homemade (page 124), for topping (optional)

1. Preheat the oven to 400°F. Grease a large casserole dish.

2. Heat the oil in a large skillet over medium-high heat. Add the meat or tempeh, garlic, and salt and cook until browned, about 5 minutes. Drain any excess grease. Season with the Italian seasoning, then stir in the sauce and simmer over medium-low heat until the sauce thickens, 5 to 8 minutes.

3. Divide the meat sauce evenly among the bell pepper halves, place in the prepared casserole dish, and bake for 20 minutes, or until the peppers soften. Remove from the oven and top the peppers with the cheese, tomatoes, and olives. Bake for another 10 minutes, or until the cheese is melted.

4. Top with fresh basil and Parmesan, if desired, before serving.

notes

To add extra vegetables to the filling, replace the ground beef with 2 cups of Italian Night Meaty Mushroom Grounds (page 132). Add the grounds in Step 2, when you add the sauce.

For dairy-free: Use a dairy-free shredded mozzarella (I recommend Violife brand) and plant-based parmesan.

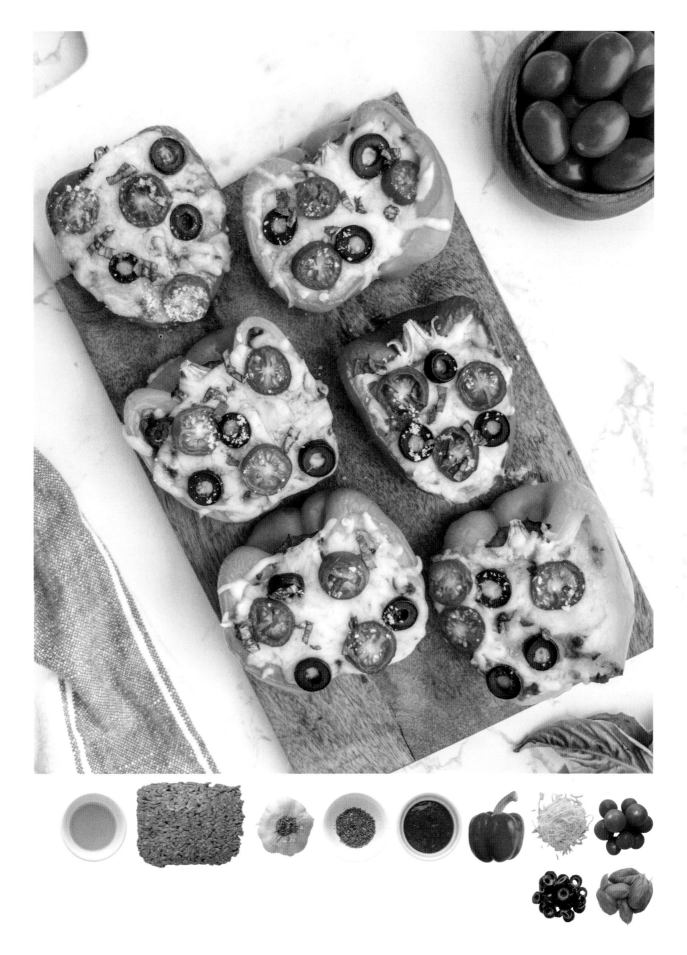

tempeh gyros

yield: **4 gyros (1 per serving)**   prep time: **10 minutes, plus 30 minutes to marinate**
cook time: **6 minutes**

This made-over classic captures the spirit of the traditional Greek street food but with a mostly plant-based twist. Tempeh's firm texture and adaptable flavor make it a great replacement for lamb. Enjoy flavorful tempeh, creamy tzatziki, and crisp fresh vegetables in each bite. If you don't care for tempeh or are craving a meat protein, you can replace the tempeh with chicken (see the note below).

marinade and tempeh:

3 tablespoons extra-virgin olive oil, divided

Juice of ½ lemon

2 cloves garlic, minced

2 teaspoons dried oregano leaves

¼ teaspoon finely ground Himalayan pink salt

⅛ teaspoon ground black pepper

1 (8-ounce) block tempeh, cut into ¼-inch strips

salad:

1 Roma tomato, diced

½ large English cucumber, diced

¼ medium red onion, diced

Juice of ½ lemon

Finely ground Himalayan pink salt and ground black pepper to taste

Coarsely chopped fresh dill fronds, to taste (optional)

¼ cup tzatziki, store-bought or homemade (page 128)

4 whole-grain pitas, warmed

1. To prepare the marinade, in a large shallow bowl, whisk 2 tablespoons of the oil with the lemon juice, garlic, oregano, salt, and pepper. Place the tempeh in the bowl and marinate for at least 30 minutes or up to 3 hours in the refrigerator.

2. To prepare the salad, in a large bowl, toss together the tomatoes, cucumber, onion, lemon juice, salt, pepper, and dill, if using. Set aside.

3. To cook the tempeh, warm the remaining tablespoon of oil in a large skillet over medium-high heat. Cook the tempeh until crisp, 1 to 3 minutes on each side.

4. To assemble the gyros, spread the tzatziki in a thin layer on each pita and top with the salad and tempeh.

note _____

In place of the tempeh, you can use 1 pound of boneless, skinless chicken breasts, cut into strips. Cook the marinated chicken in Step 3 until no longer pink in the center.

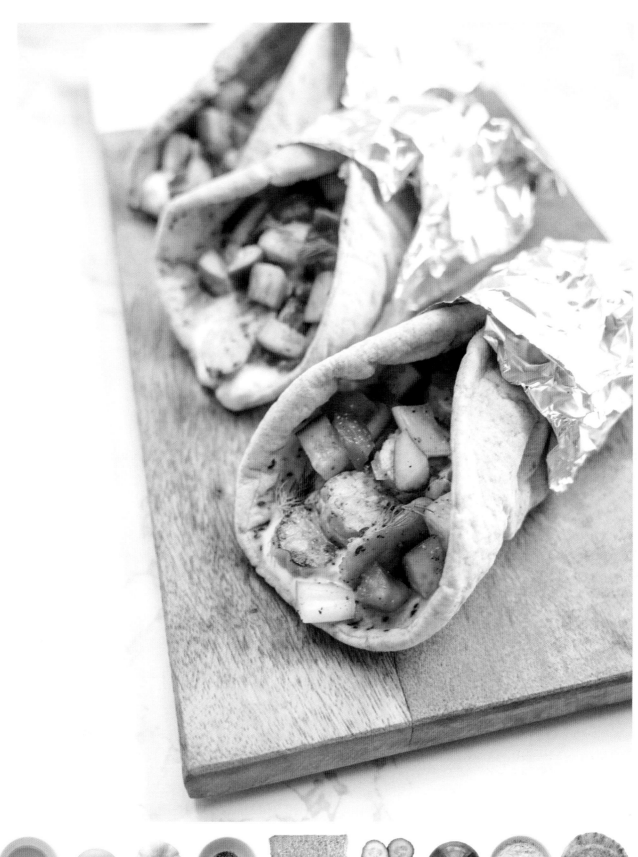

simple stir-fry

yield: **4 servings**   prep time: **10 minutes**   cook time: **10 minutes**

Having a simple stir-fry recipe in your weeknight repertoire makes healthy eating easy even when life gets busy. This dish is balanced with protein, vegetables, and good-for-you fat with the option to customize based on what's in your fridge. As a bonus, stir-frying rather than boiling results in tender-crisp vegetables that retain more nutrients.

1 tablespoon extra-virgin olive oil

1 pound boneless, skinless chicken breasts, cut into 1-inch pieces

Finely ground Himalayan pink salt and ground black pepper

2 cups broccoli florets

8 ounces white mushrooms, sliced

2 medium carrots, peeled and sliced into coins

1 medium red bell pepper, cut into 1-inch strips

4 cups cooked brown rice or cooked cauliflower rice, for serving (optional)

2 tablespoons low-sodium soy sauce

2 tablespoons garlic rice vinegar

⅛ teaspoon ginger powder

suggested toppings:

Sesame seeds

Sliced green onions

Red pepper flakes

1. Pour the olive oil into a wok or large skillet and place over medium-high heat. Add the chicken, season lightly with salt and pepper, and stir-fry until cooked through, 5 to 6 minutes. Remove the chicken from the pan.

2. Place the broccoli, mushrooms, carrots, and bell pepper in the pan and cook, stirring occasionally, until crisp-tender, 3 to 4 minutes. Return the chicken to the pan and stir to combine. Remove the pan from the heat and set aside.

3. Stir in the soy sauce, rice vinegar, and ginger powder until incorporated.

4. Serve over rice and top with sesame seeds, green onions, and/or red pepper flakes, if desired.

notes

Make sure the ingredients are cut to similar sizes to ensure even cooking.

Feel free to use other vegetables, such as baby corn, sugar snap peas, water chestnuts, and/or yellow bell pepper.

For meat-free: Use a 14-ounce block of extra-firm tofu, pressed and then cubed, in place of the chicken. Cook the tofu until slightly crisp on all sides, about 5 minutes total.

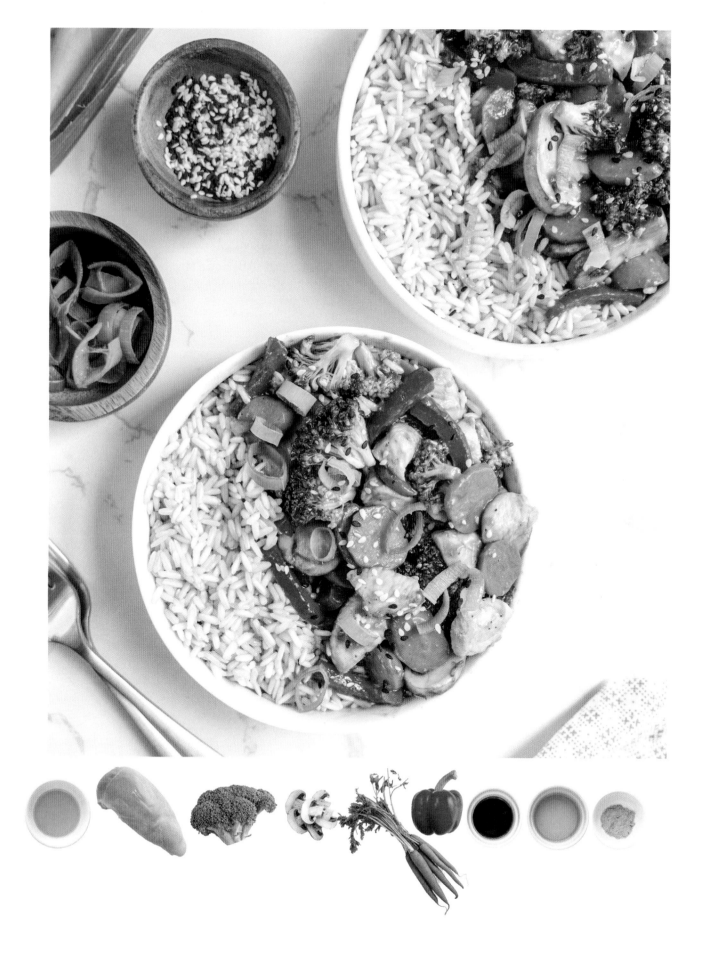

italian spaghetti squash casserole

yield: **4 servings**   prep time: **20 minutes**   cook time: **1 hour 10 minutes**

Comfort food with a veggie-forward twist! Spaghetti squash is one of nature's greatest creations for pasta lovers. When cooked, spaghetti squash strands serve as a mild-tasting canvas for your favorite traditional pasta fixings. It just so happens to be naturally lower in calories and carbohydrates than pasta, but rich in fiber, vitamins, and minerals.

1 medium spaghetti squash (about 3 pounds)

1 tablespoon extra-virgin olive oil

¼ teaspoon finely ground Himalayan pink salt

Pinch of ground black pepper

filling:

1 tablespoon extra-virgin olive oil

½ cup diced yellow onions

1 pound lean ground turkey

2 cloves garlic, minced

1 tablespoon Italian seasoning or dried oregano leaves

½ teaspoon finely ground Himalayan pink salt

⅛ teaspoon ground black pepper

1 (14.5-ounce) can diced fire-roasted tomatoes, drained

1 cup shredded mozzarella cheese or plant-based parmesan, store-bought or homemade (page 124), divided

¼ cup fresh basil leaves, chopped, for topping

1. Preheat the oven to 400°F. Line a sheet pan with parchment paper.

2. Slice the squash in half lengthwise. Remove and discard the seeds with a spoon.

3. In a small bowl, whisk together the oil, salt, and pepper. Brush the mixture onto the cut sides of the squash. Place the halves cut side down on the prepared pan and bake until fork-tender and lightly browned on the outside, 25 to 30 minutes. Let cool, then flip the halves over and remove the strands with a fork. Transfer the strands to a large bowl.

4. Reduce the oven temperature to 350°F. Grease a 9 by 13-inch baking dish with cooking spray.

5. To make the filling, heat the oil in a large skillet over medium-high heat, then cook the onions until softened, 1 to 2 minutes. Add the turkey and cook, using a wooden spoon to break up the clumps, until no longer pink, 5 to 6 minutes. Drain the fat, then stir in the garlic, Italian seasoning, salt, and pepper. Pour the tomatoes into the skillet and cook for another 3 minutes, stirring often.

6. Turn off the heat and stir in the squash and ½ cup of the cheese.

7. Transfer the mixture to the prepared baking dish and bake until the casserole is heated through and the mozzarella is melted, about 20 minutes.

8. Remove the pan from the oven and sprinkle the remaining ½ cup of cheese on top of the casserole. Set the oven to broil and broil the casserole until the cheese is melted, 2 to 3 minutes. Top with the basil before serving.

note _____

*For meat-free: Use 2 cups of
100% Mushroom Base (page 133)
instead of the turkey.*

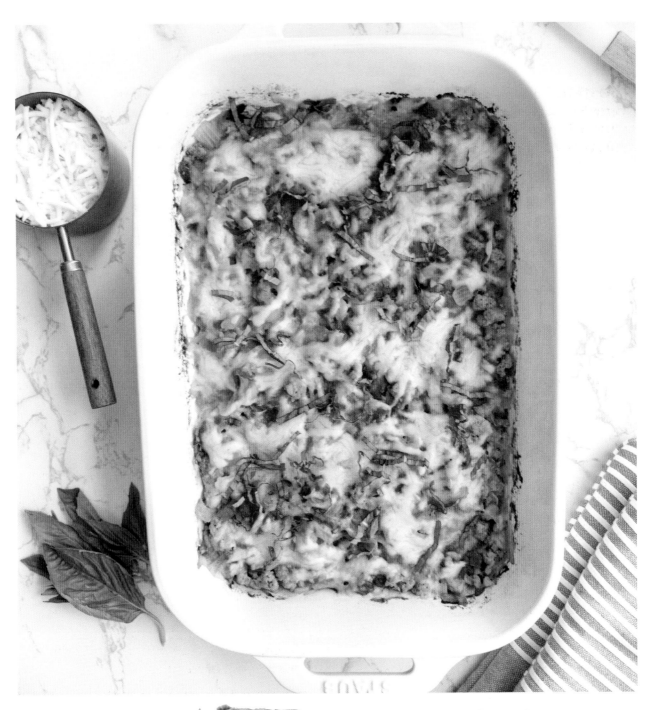

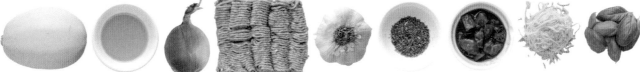

veggie lover's chickpea flatbread

yield: 4 servings   prep time: 15 minutes, plus 30 minutes to rest batter   cook time: 35 minutes

Socca, also referred to as farinata, is a naturally gluten-free pancake-like flatbread that hails from France and is surprisingly easy to make if you have chickpea flour on hand. It serves as the protein- and fiber-rich base of this veggie lover's flatbread topped with pesto, roasted mushrooms, zucchini, onion, and tomatoes.

flatbread:

1 cup chickpea flour

1 cup water

2 tablespoons extra-virgin olive oil, divided

½ teaspoon finely ground Himalayan pink salt

roasted vegetables:

1 cup white mushrooms

1 medium zucchini

¼ medium red onion

1 cup cherry tomatoes

2 cloves garlic

1 tablespoon extra-virgin olive oil

½ teaspoon finely ground Himalayan pink salt

toppings:

¼ cup pesto, store-bought or homemade (page 114)

2 tablespoons chopped fresh basil

Crumbled feta cheese (optional)

1. To make the flatbread batter, put the chickpea flour, water, 1 tablespoon of the oil, and the salt in a large bowl. Whisk until smooth, then set aside to rest for 30 minutes.

2. Meanwhile, prepare the roasted vegetables: Preheat the oven to 425°F. Slice the mushrooms, zucchini, and onion; halve the tomatoes; and mince the garlic. Place the vegetables in another large bowl and toss with the oil and salt.

3. Spread the vegetables in a single layer on a sheet pan and roast until softened, 18 to 20 minutes, tossing halfway through. Remove the pan from the oven.

4. Increase the oven temperature to 450°F.

5. To bake the flatbread, coat the bottom of a 10-inch oven-safe skillet with the remaining tablespoon of oil. Pour the batter into the pan and bake until well browned and crisp around the edges, 12 to 15 minutes.

6. Spread the pesto in a thin layer on the flatbread. Top with the roasted vegetables, basil, and feta, if using.

note _____

For dairy-free: Use a dairy-free pesto and omit the feta. If making the homemade pesto, use plant-based parmesan.

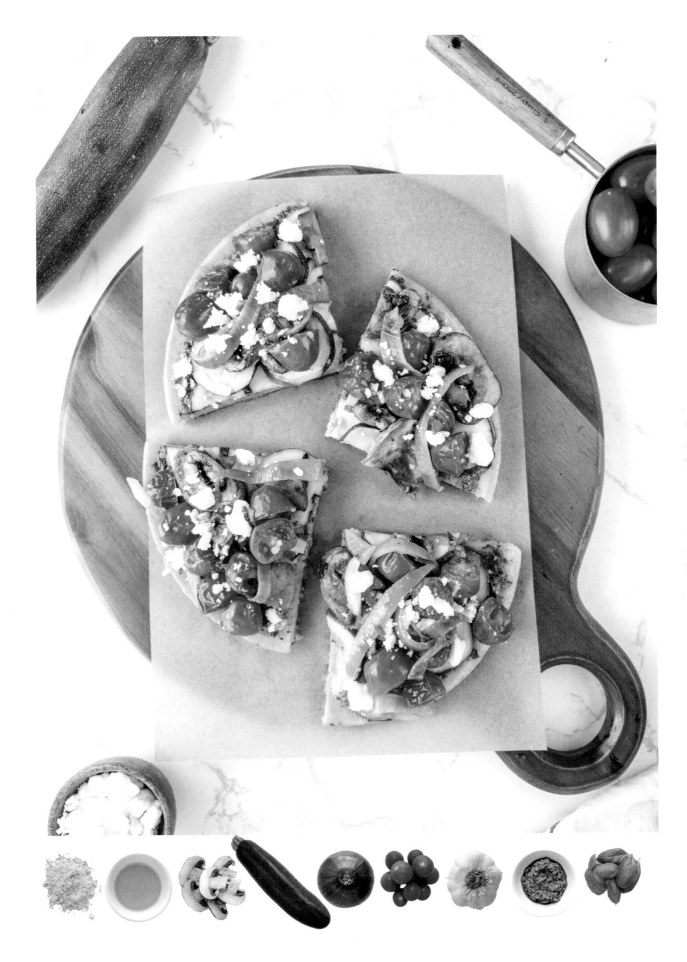

lemon tahini buddha bowl

yield: **2 servings**   prep time: **10 minutes**   cook time: **23 minutes**

Buddha bowls embody balance and are an aesthetically pleasing way to incorporate whole grains, lean proteins, and fresh vegetables accompanied by a flavorful sauce. Though optional, adding fermented vegetables such as kimchi or sauerkraut gives this dish a boost of microbiome-loving probiotics.

1 large sweet potato (about 8 ounces), scrubbed and cut into ½-inch cubes

1 tablespoon extra-virgin olive oil, divided

½ teaspoon finely ground Himalayan pink salt, divided

¼ teaspoon ground black pepper, divided

3 cups stemmed and coarsely chopped kale

1 cup cooked wild rice

1 cup cooked chickpeas

½ cup frozen shelled edamame, defrosted and steamed

½ medium avocado, pitted, peeled, and sliced

Fermented vegetables, such as kimchi or sauerkraut, for serving (optional)

tahini sauce:

2 tablespoons tahini

1 teaspoon lemon juice

1 tablespoon extra-virgin olive oil

¼ teaspoon finely ground Himalayan pink salt

⅛ teaspoon ground black pepper

1. Preheat the oven to 400°F. Line a sheet pan with parchment paper.

2. In a large bowl, toss the sweet potato cubes with ½ tablespoon of the oil, ¼ teaspoon of the salt, and ⅛ teaspoon of the pepper. Transfer to the prepared pan and spread out in a single layer. Roast until tender and slightly crisp, about 20 minutes, tossing halfway through cooking.

3. In the same bowl, toss the kale with the remaining ½ tablespoon of oil, ¼ teaspoon of salt, and ⅛ teaspoon of pepper.

4. Arrange the kale on top of the sweet potatoes and return the pan to the oven. Bake for another 2 to 3 minutes, until the kale is softened.

5. To make the sauce, whisk together the tahini, lemon juice, oil, salt, and pepper in a small bowl. Add water a teaspoon at a time until the sauce reaches the desired consistency. Set aside.

6. To assemble, divide the rice, sweet potatoes, kale, chickpeas, edamame, avocado, and fermented vegetables, if using, evenly between two serving bowls. Drizzle the sauce on top.

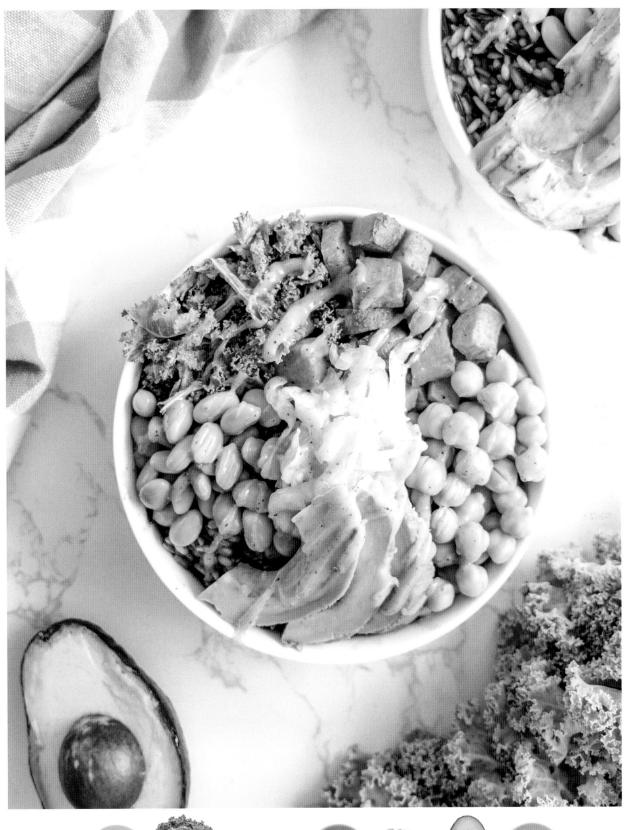

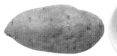

caprese cauliflower gnocchi skillet

yield: **3 servings**   prep time: **10 minutes**   cook time: **15 minutes**

Pillows of thick and soft cauliflower gnocchi pair perfectly with blistered tomatoes, buttery white beans, and fresh basil in this one-skillet supper. Compared to traditional potato gnocchi, the cauliflower version is lower in calories and higher in fiber.

1 tablespoon extra-virgin olive oil

1 (10-ounce) package frozen cauliflower gnocchi or regular gnocchi

4 cloves garlic, minced

1 pint cherry tomatoes

¼ cup water

½ cup cooked white beans

1 teaspoon dried oregano leaves

½ teaspoon finely ground Himalayan pink salt

¼ teaspoon ground black pepper

¼ teaspoon red pepper flakes (optional)

4 ounces fresh mozzarella cheese pearls

1 cup arugula

¼ cup chopped fresh basil leaves, for topping

1. Heat the oil in a large oven-safe skillet over medium-high heat. Add the gnocchi in a single layer and cook undisturbed until golden brown on one side, 2 to 3 minutes. Flip the gnocchi with a spatula and continue to cook, turning often, until browned and crisp all over, 2 to 3 more minutes. Remove the gnocchi from the skillet and set aside; place an oven rack in the top position and set the oven to broil.

2. Put the garlic in the skillet and cook until fragrant, about 30 seconds. Add the tomatoes and water and cook until the tomatoes have softened, 4 to 5 minutes, stirring occasionally and smashing the tomatoes as they burst.

3. Return the gnocchi to the skillet. Stir in the beans, oregano, salt, black pepper, and red pepper flakes, if using, until the ingredients are combined. Top with the mozzarella pearls.

4. Transfer the skillet to the oven and broil until the cheese is slightly melted, 2 to 3 minutes. Stir in the arugula and top with the basil.

notes

For a smoky and richer take on this dish, replace the beans with sliced fully cooked low-sodium chicken sausage.

For dairy-free: Omit the cheese.

Cauliflower gnocchi is an increasingly popular ingredient that you can find in the frozen foods section of the grocery store. Unlike potato gnocchi, which is typically boiled, cauliflower gnocchi can be prepared in several ways, including boiling, sautéing, and microwaving.

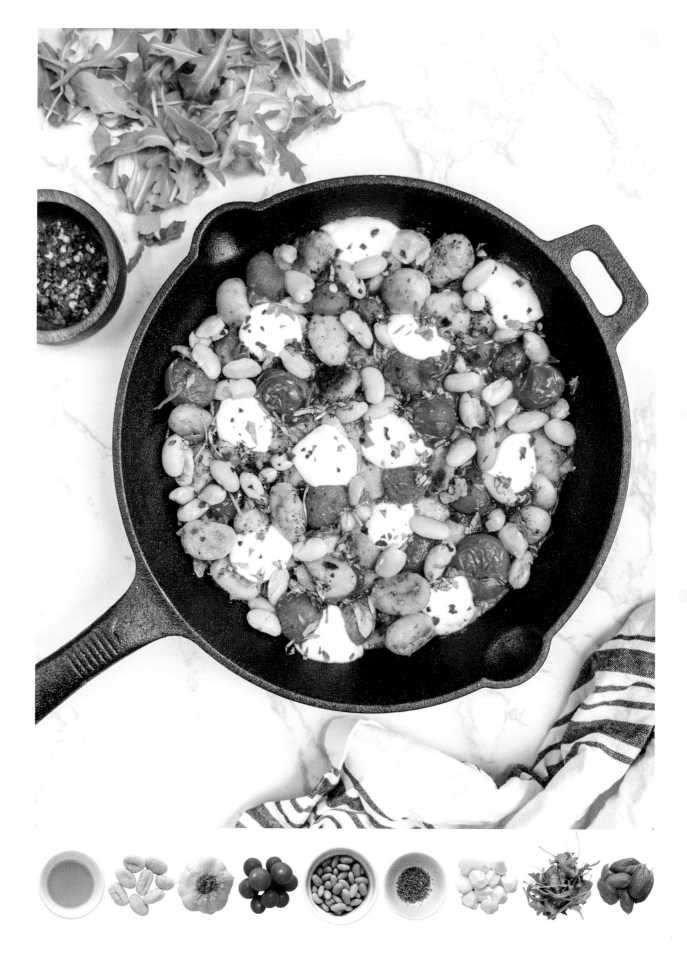

baked eggplant parmesan stacks

yield: 6 stacks (1 per serving)   prep time: 15 minutes, plus 20 minutes to drain eggplant
cook time: 35 minutes

This dish is a lighter, easier, and faster take on traditional eggplant Parm. While the Italian classic is typically made with eggplant coated in both flour and breadcrumbs and then fried, the eggplant in this recipe is breaded with simple homemade whole-grain breadcrumbs, which add texture and a boost of fiber and B vitamins, and then baked. To make it even simpler, you can omit the breading altogether.

12 (¼-inch thick) eggplant rounds (from 2 large eggplants)

1 teaspoon finely ground Himalayan pink salt

3 cups tomato sauce, store-bought or homemade (page 130), divided

1 pound fresh mozzarella cheese, sliced into 6 thin rounds

¼ cup grated Parmesan cheese or plant-based parmesan, store-bought or homemade (page 124)

¼ cup chopped fresh basil, for topping

breading:

2 slices whole-grain bread

¼ cup grated Parmesan cheese or plant-based parmesan, store-bought or homemade (page 124)

1 teaspoon garlic powder

1 teaspoon ground dried oregano

¼ teaspoon finely ground Himalayan pink salt

1 large egg

1. Line a sheet pan with parchment paper or grease it with cooking spray.

2. Sprinkle both sides of the eggplant slices with the salt and place in a colander in the sink or in a single layer on a wire rack set over a sheet pan. Set aside for at least 20 minutes to draw out moisture.

3. Once beads of moisture start to appear, rinse the eggplant slices under water to remove the excess salt. Dry the slices with a paper towel and place in a single layer on the prepared sheet pan. Preheat the oven to 350°F.

4. To bread the eggplant slices, toast the bread and place in a food processor with the Parmesan, garlic powder, oregano, and salt. Process until crumbly, then transfer to a large shallow bowl. Whisk the egg in another large shallow bowl. Coat each eggplant slice in the egg, then dip into the breadcrumbs and place on the prepared pan in a single layer. Bake until golden, 15 to 20 minutes.

5. Pour 2 cups of the tomato sauce into a 9 by 13-inch baking dish and spread in a thin layer. Arrange half of the baked eggplant slices on the sauce. Top each slice with a spoonful of the remaining sauce, a slice of mozzarella, and another eggplant slice. Pour the remaining sauce over the stacks and sprinkle the Parmesan cheese on top.

6. Bake until heated through and the cheese is bubbling, 10 to 12 minutes. Top with fresh basil before serving.

notes

For dairy-free: Use plant-based parm in the breading and replace the mozzarella with a shredded vegan cheese. Or, omit the cheese and breading altogether and make eggplant marinara stacks.

For egg-free: Replace the egg used for breading with 3 tablespoons of unsweetened plant milk mixed with 1 tablespoon of flaxseed meal.

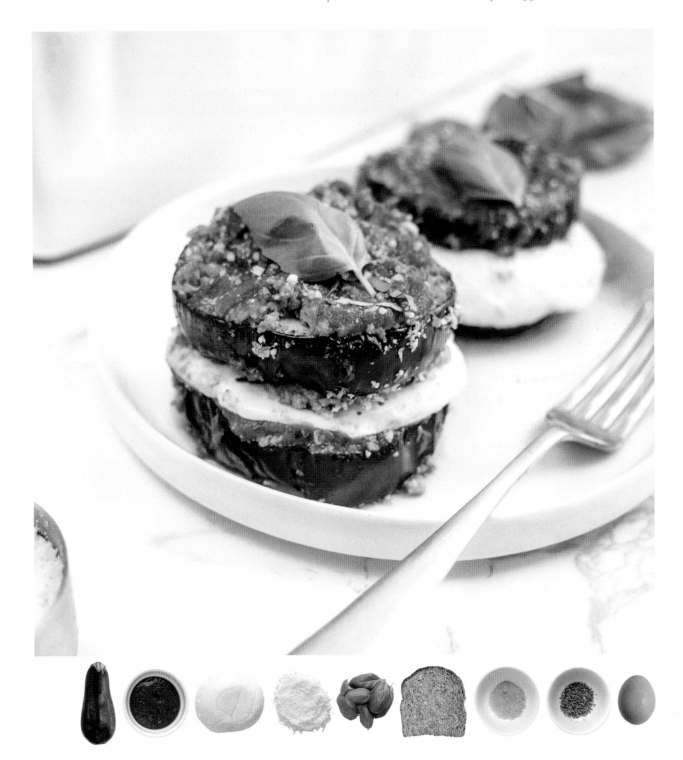

asian-inspired lentil lettuce cups

yield: **4 servings**   prep time: **10 minutes**   cook time: **16 minutes**

Humble but mighty lentils take center stage in these crunchy meat-free lettuce cups. Lentils are among the highest-protein legumes with around 12 grams per ½-cup serving; they also provide the key nutrients potassium, folate, iron, and manganese. Ready in just 25 minutes with no presoaking required, lentils win in both the convenience and the nutrition departments.

1 cup red lentils, rinsed and drained

3 cups water

⅛ teaspoon finely ground Himalayan pink salt

1 tablespoon extra-virgin olive oil

1 medium red bell pepper, chopped

1 cup julienned carrots

1 clove garlic, minced

1 tablespoon unseasoned rice vinegar

1 tablespoon low-sodium soy sauce

⅛ teaspoon ginger powder

1 (8-ounce) can water chestnuts, drained, rinsed, and chopped

1 head butter lettuce, leaves separated

suggested toppings:

Toasted sesame seeds

Sliced green onions

1. Place the lentils, water, and salt in a medium saucepan. Bring to a boil over medium-high heat, then reduce the heat to low, cover, and simmer until the lentils are tender, 8 to 10 minutes. Drain the lentils.

2. Pour the oil into a large skillet over medium-high heat. Add the bell pepper and cook, stirring frequently, until soft, about 5 minutes. Add the carrots and garlic and cook for another 30 seconds.

3. Remove the pan from the heat and stir in the lentils, rice vinegar, soy sauce, ginger powder, and water chestnuts.

4. Serve the lentil mixture in the lettuce leaves and top with toasted sesame seeds and/or green onions, if desired.

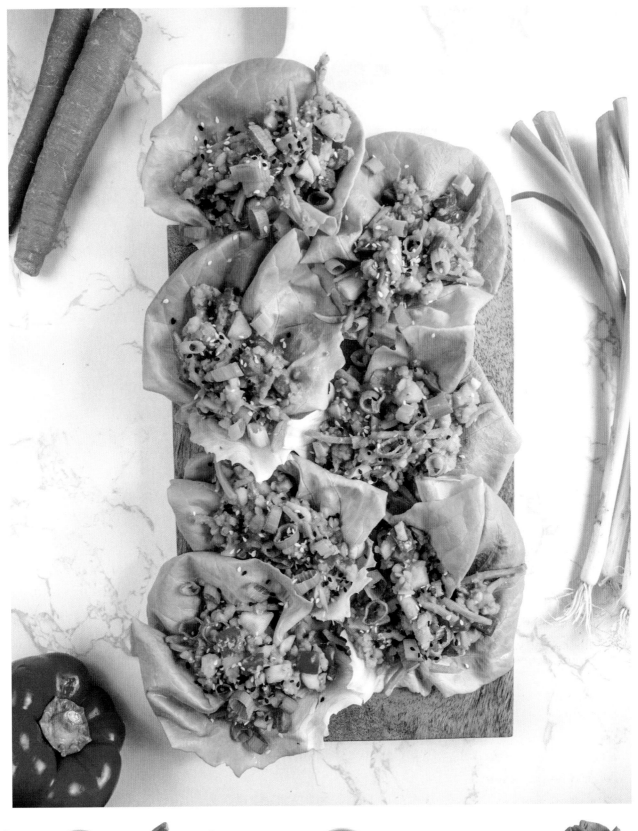

cauliflower potato shepherd's pie

yield: **4 servings**   prep time: **10 minutes**   cook time: **35 minutes**

This recipe puts a lightened-up, veggie-forward twist on a classic comfort food. While traditional shepherd's pie is made with a potato topping blended with butter and milk, this topping calls for half cauliflower, which not only lowers the calories and carbohydrates but also ups the nutrition by adding more vitamin C, antioxidants, and fiber. Also, if you love shepherd's pie but not the typically long list of ingredients or numerous steps, this recipe is for you.

cauliflower potato mash:

2 cups small cauliflower florets

2 large russet potatoes, scrubbed and chopped

1 teaspoon finely ground Himalayan pink salt

filling:

1 tablespoon extra-virgin olive oil

¼ cup diced yellow onions

1 pound lean ground beef

1 (12-ounce) bag frozen mixed vegetables, such as peas, corn, carrots, and green beans

¼ cup tomato paste

1 teaspoon ground dried thyme

1 teaspoon finely ground Himalayan pink salt

¼ teaspoon ground black pepper

Chopped fresh flat-leaf parsley, for topping (optional)

1. Preheat the oven to 400°F.

2. To make the mash, place the cauliflower and potatoes in a large pot and cover with water. Bring to a boil, then cover with a lid and lower the heat to maintain a simmer. Cook until the vegetables are tender, 10 to 15 minutes. When done, drain the vegetables and transfer them to a blender or food processor. Add the salt and blend until smooth.

3. While the cauliflower and potatoes are cooking, prepare the filling: Heat the oil in a 12-inch oven-safe skillet over medium heat. Add the onions and cook, stirring frequently, until softened, about 5 minutes. Add the beef and cook, breaking it up into crumbles and stirring frequently, until browned, about 5 minutes.

4. Add the frozen vegetables and cook, stirring frequently, until soft, 4 to 6 minutes.

5. Stir in the tomato paste, thyme, salt, and pepper. Smooth the mixture with a rubber spatula.

6. Pour the cauliflower-potato mixture over the meat mixture, smooth with the spatula, and bake until the topping is golden brown and the filling is bubbling, 20 to 25 minutes. Top with parsley before serving, if desired.

notes _____

For meat-free: Replace the beef with 2 cups of cooked lentils or 100% Mushroom Base (page 133). Add in Step 3, stirring it into the softened onion until heated through.

To add extra veggie goodness to the cauliflower potato mash, add a peeled and chopped parsnip in Step 2.

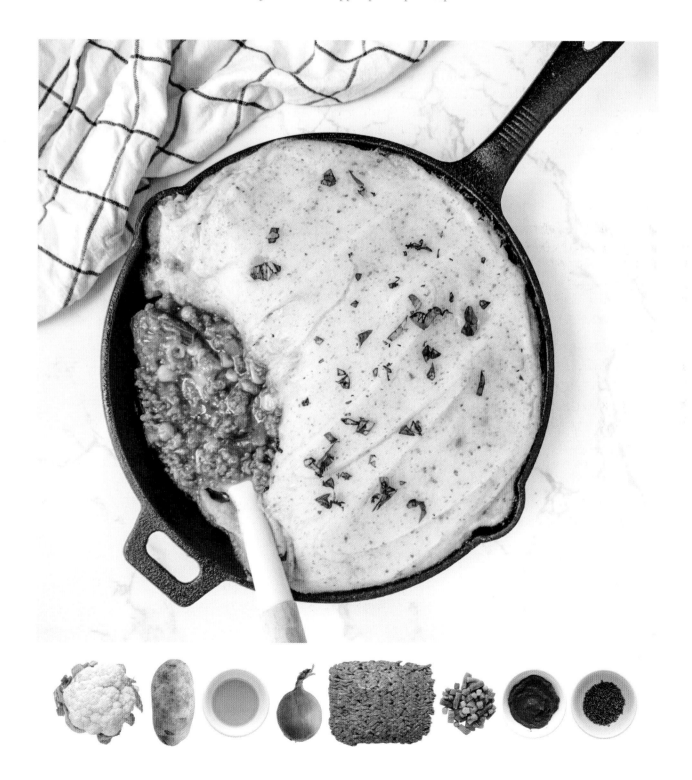

black bean "meatball" subs

yield: 3 sandwiches (1 per serving)   prep time: 10 minutes   cook time: 30 minutes

Black beans are an excellent plant-based swap for meat because they are hearty and packed with protein. When mixed with oats and savory spices, these "meatballs" take on the flavor and texture of classic meatballs. If you don't have rolls, they can also be served over zucchini noodles or brown rice pasta.

meatballs:

1 tablespoon flaxseed meal

3 tablespoons water

1 (15-ounce) can no-salt-added black beans, drained and rinsed well, or 1½ cups cooked black beans (see page 44)

½ cup rolled oats

¼ cup grated Parmesan cheese or plant-based parmesan, store-bought or homemade (page 124)

1 clove garlic, minced

1 teaspoon Italian seasoning

½ teaspoon finely ground Himalayan pink salt

1½ cups tomato sauce, store-bought or homemade (page 130)

3 (6-inch) whole-grain sub, hero, or hoagie rolls, toasted

⅓ cup shredded mozzarella cheese or plant-based parmesan, store-bought or homemade (page 124)

2 tablespoons chopped fresh basil, for topping

1. Preheat the oven to 400°F. Line a sheet pan with parchment paper.

2. Make a flax egg by combining the flaxseed meal and water in a small bowl; allow to sit for 5 minutes.

3. To prepare the meatballs, pulse the beans, oats, Parmesan, garlic, Italian seasoning, salt, and flax egg in a food processor until mostly smooth and evenly blended. Use a 2-tablespoon cookie scoop to drop the mixture onto the prepared sheet pan, spacing the meatballs 1 inch apart. Bake for 10 minutes, then turn each ball over and bake for another 10 minutes, until the meatballs are crisp on the outside.

4. Heat the tomato sauce in a medium saucepan over medium-high heat. Add the meatballs and stir to coat.

5. Place the toasted rolls on the sheet pan, divide the meatballs and sauce between them, and sprinkle the mozzarella over the meatballs. Bake until the cheese is melted, 3 to 4 minutes. Top with the basil before serving.

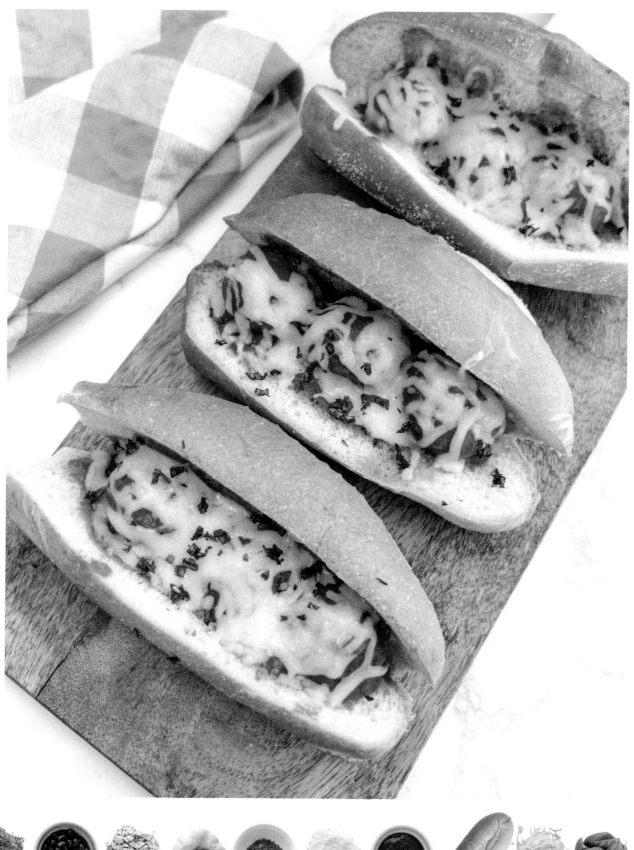

       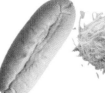

pesto salmon packets

yield: **4 servings**   prep time: **10 minutes**   cook time: **18 minutes**

Foil packets are the ultimate fast, mess-free meal that can conveniently be made in the oven or on the grill (see the notes below). Earthy pesto perfectly complements flaky, buttery salmon and fresh summer vegetables in this meal that cooks up in under 20 minutes. Salmon is a smart lower-mercury fish option that boasts bioavailable DHA omega-3 fats, which are essential for brain and heart health.

1 pound asparagus, ends trimmed

1 pint cherry tomatoes

2 medium zucchinis, sliced into half-moons

Juice of 1 lemon

1 tablespoon extra-virgin olive oil

2 cloves garlic, minced

½ teaspoon finely ground Himalayan pink salt

¼ teaspoon ground black pepper

1 (1-pound) salmon fillet, cut into 4 portions

⅓ cup pesto, store-bought or homemade (page 114)

1. Preheat the oven to 400°F.

2. In a large bowl, toss together the asparagus, tomatoes, zucchinis, lemon juice, oil, garlic, salt, and pepper.

3. Lay out four 12-inch square pieces of foil and place a salmon fillet in the center of each. Spread 1 heaping tablespoon of pesto on top of each fillet.

4. Divide the vegetables evenly among the foil pieces, arranging them around the salmon fillets.

5. Fold the foil over and seal to form packets. Place on a sheet pan.

6. Bake until the vegetables are tender and the salmon flakes easily with a fork, 15 to 18 minutes.

notes _____

For fish-free: Replace the salmon with a 15-ounce can of no-salt-added chickpeas, drained and rinsed well, or 1½ cups of cooked chickpeas (see page 44). Toss the chickpeas with the other ingredients in Step 2.

To grill the packets, preheat a grill to high. Grill the packets until the vegetables are tender and the salmon flakes easily with a fork, about 10 minutes.

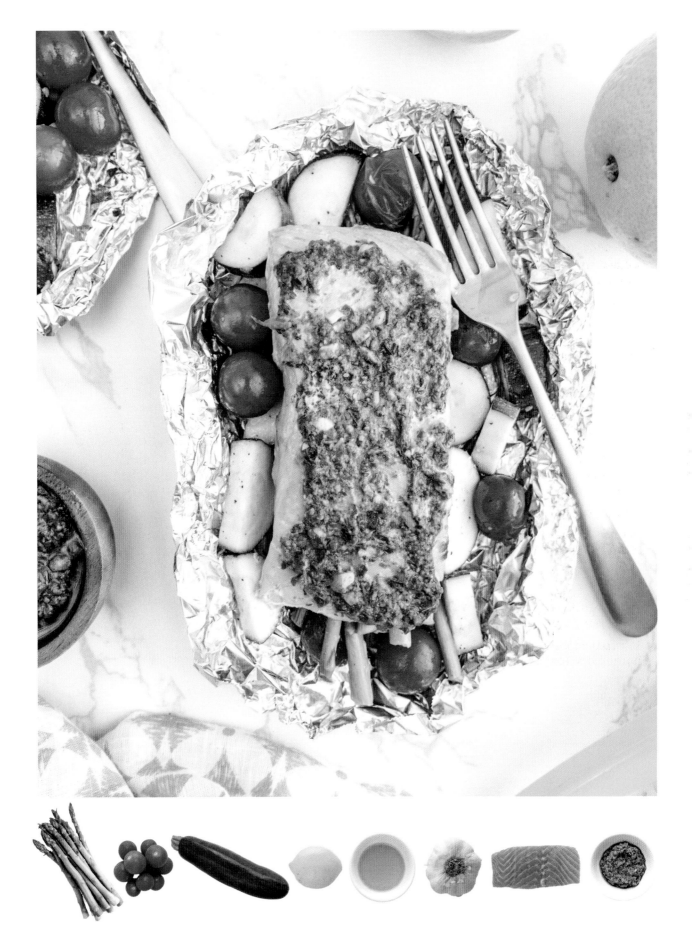

better-than-takeout orange chicken bowls

yield: **4 servings**   prep time: **10 minutes**   cook time: **10 minutes**

Savor the flavor of your favorite takeout meal with less sugar and sodium. Made with a zesty six-ingredient sauce that gets its sweetness from pure orange juice and coconut sugar, this is a meal that loves you back. You even have the option to make it meat-free if you like (see the note below). To build a complete meal, the orange chicken is served over brown rice or riced cauliflower with steamed broccoli.

1 tablespoon extra-virgin olive oil

1 pound boneless, skinless chicken breasts, cut into bite-sized pieces

¼ teaspoon finely ground Himalayan pink salt

⅛ teaspoon ground black pepper

4 cups cooked brown rice, or 8 cups cooked riced cauliflower

2 cups broccoli florets, steamed

sauce:

⅓ cup pure orange juice

1 tablespoon low-sodium soy sauce

1 tablespoon unseasoned rice vinegar

¼ cup coconut sugar

½ teaspoon garlic powder

1 tablespoon cornstarch

suggested toppings:

Toasted sesame seeds

Sliced green onions

Orange slices

1. Warm the oil in a large skillet over medium-high heat. Season the chicken with the salt and pepper and sauté until cooked through, about 4 minutes.

2. To make the sauce, bring the orange juice, soy sauce, rice vinegar, coconut sugar, and garlic powder to a boil in a small saucepan, then reduce to a simmer. Cook for 3 minutes, stirring every minute or so. Whisk in the cornstarch and continue cooking until thickened.

3. Pour the thickened sauce over the chicken and stir to coat.

4. To assemble, fill each serving bowl with one-quarter of the rice, broccoli, and orange chicken. Top with sesame seeds, green onions, and/or an orange slice, if desired.

note _____

For meat-free: Use a 14-ounce block of extra-firm tofu, pressed and then cubed, in place of the chicken. After seasoning the tofu cubes with salt and pepper, sauté them in the oil until crisp on all sides, 1 to 2 minutes per side.

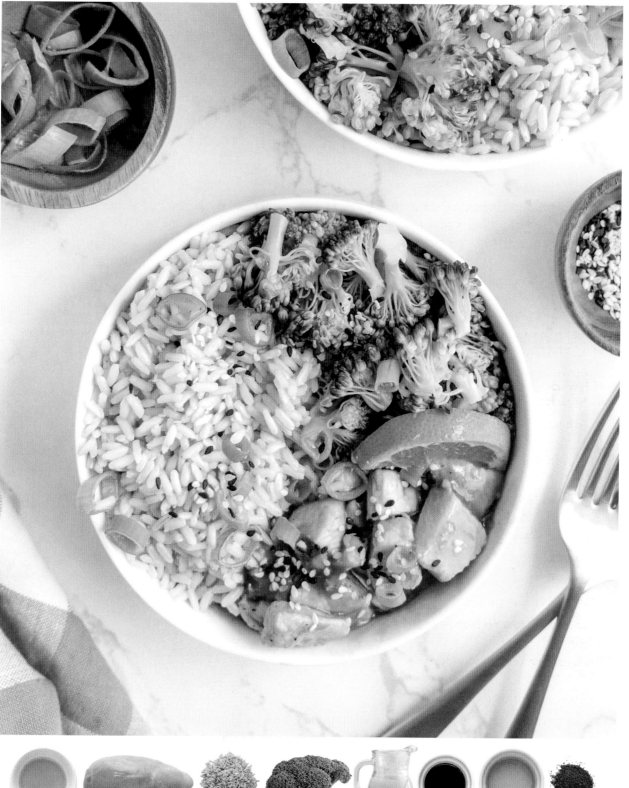
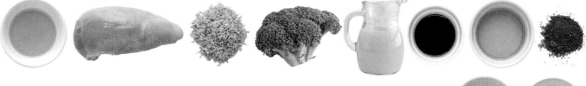
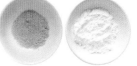

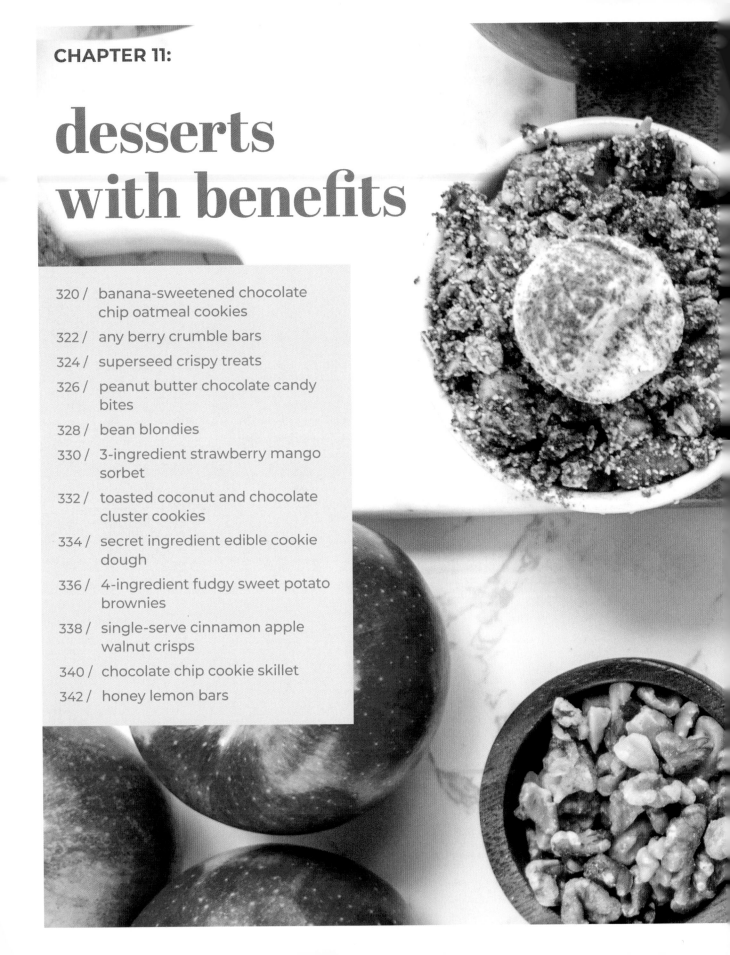

CHAPTER 11:

desserts with benefits

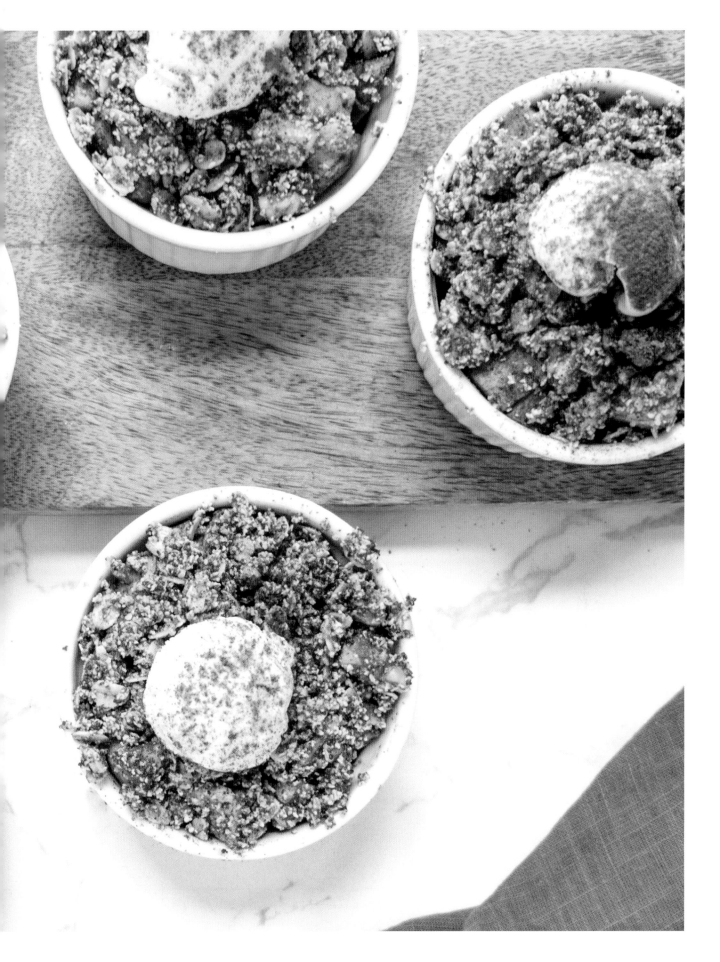

banana-sweetened chocolate chip oatmeal cookies

yield: **12 cookies (1 per serving)**   prep time: **10 minutes**   cook time: **10 minutes**

Who knew that cookie dough could be made without flour, eggs, or added sugar? These soft, chewy cookies are made with just a handful of pantry staples plus the two ripe bananas you may have on your counter right now. While I think chocolate chips are essential in this better-for-you dessert, feel free to omit them for a no-added-sugar cookie that is healthy enough for breakfast!

2 large ripe bananas, mashed (about 1 cup)

¼ cup natural creamy peanut butter

1 cup quick oats (see notes)

½ cup rolled oats

1 teaspoon pure vanilla extract

¼ cup dark chocolate chips

Sea salt flakes, for topping

1. Preheat the oven to 350°F. Line a baking sheet with parchment paper.

2. Put the bananas, peanut butter, oats, and vanilla in a large bowl and use a rubber spatula to mix until a sticky, gooey dough forms. Gently fold in the chocolate chips.

3. Use a 2-tablespoon cookie scoop to drop the dough onto the prepared baking sheet, leaving 2 inches between cookies. Press down with your fingers to flatten. Bake until slightly golden on the edges, 8 to 10 minutes.

4. Remove from the oven, top with sea salt flakes, and let cool on the pan for 5 minutes before transferring to a wire rack to cool completely.

5. Store in a sealed container in the refrigerator for up to 5 days.

notes _____

You can use any creamy nut butter you have on hand in place of the peanut butter.

Quick oats (not to be mistaken for instant oats) are rolled oats that are cooked, dried, and then pressed. As a result, the grains are thinner. The combination of rolled and quick oats in this recipe makes for a perfectly chewy cookie. If you don't have quick oats on hand, simply blitz 1 cup of rolled oats in a food processor for 10 to 15 seconds.

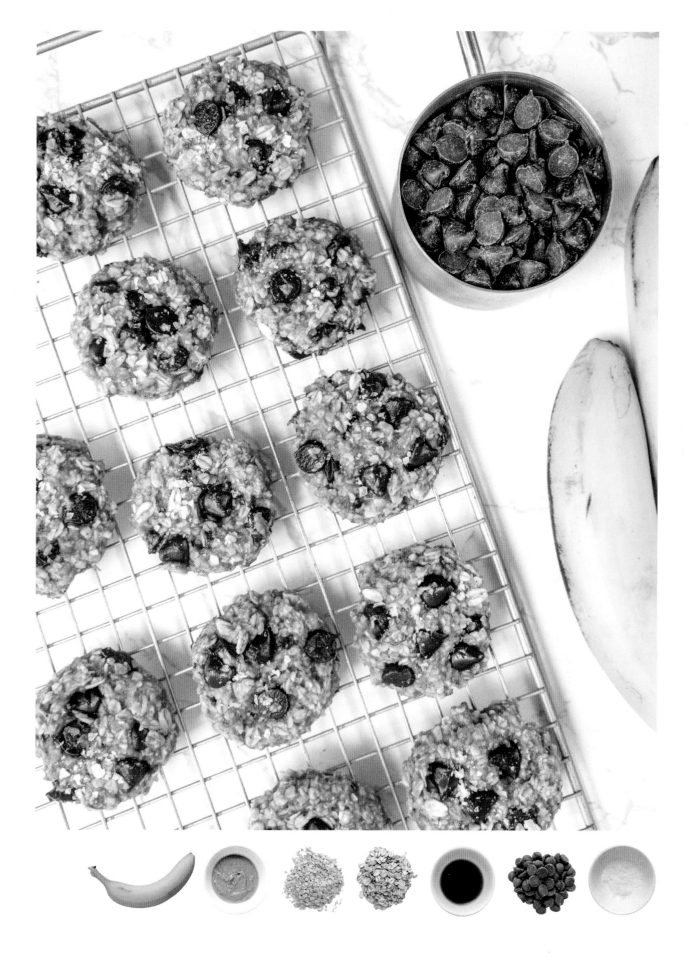

any berry crumble bars

yield: 9 bars (1 per serving)   prep time: 10 minutes   cook time: 35 minutes

Gooey, crumbly, and perfectly sweet. It doesn't have to be summer to enjoy this dessert as long as you have a bag of frozen berries on hand. Frozen berries are not only a more affordable option that lasts longer; research shows that they are just as nutritious as fresh berries (and sometimes more so) since they are frozen at peak ripeness, which helps lock in their nutrients. Small but mighty, berries add filling fiber, natural sweetness, and a boost of antioxidants to this feel-good dessert.

filling:

2 cups frozen berries, such as blueberries, raspberries, blackberries, and/or chopped strawberries

2 teaspoons lemon juice

2 tablespoons pure maple syrup

2 tablespoons chia seeds

crumble topping and base:

1½ cups rolled oats

1 cup blanched almond flour

⅓ cup coconut oil, melted

⅓ cup pure maple syrup

1 teaspoon pure vanilla extract

⅛ teaspoon finely ground Himalayan pink salt

1. Preheat the oven to 350°F. Line an 8-inch square baking pan with parchment paper, leaving some paper overhanging the sides for easy removal of the bars.

2. To make the filling, heat the berries and lemon juice in a small saucepan over medium heat, stirring and crushing the berries periodically to encourage them to break down. Cook until the berries are mashed and bubbling, about 5 minutes.

3. Turn off the heat and stir in the maple syrup and chia seeds. Let the mixture thicken while you prepare the crumble.

4. To make the crumble topping and base, put all of the ingredients in a food processor and pulse until well combined and crumbly, about 45 seconds.

5. Press three-quarters of the crumble mixture into the bottom of the prepared pan and par-bake for 10 minutes, or until set.

6. Pour the filling over the par-baked crust and use your fingers to sprinkle the remaining crumble on top. Bake for another 15 to 20 minutes, or until the topping is golden brown and the filling is bubbling. Let cool completely before lifting from the pan and slicing into bars.

7. Store leftover bars covered in the refrigerator for up to 6 days.

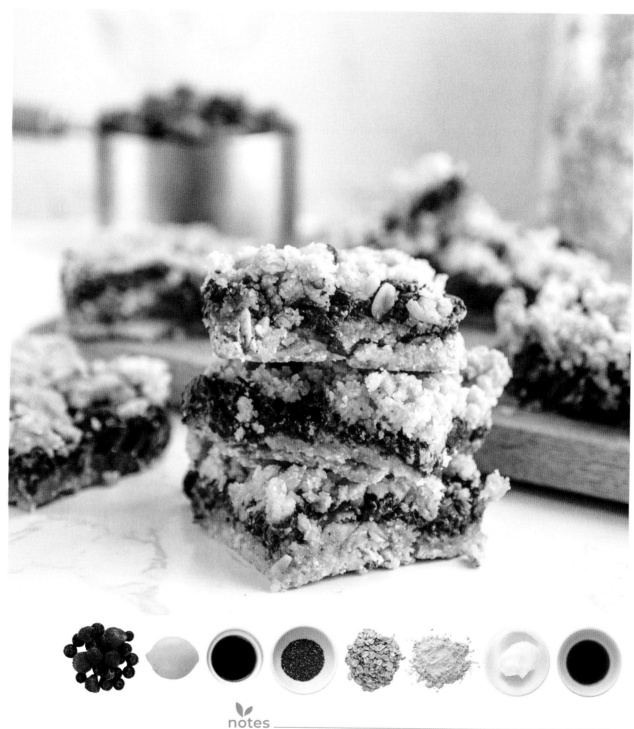

notes _____

You can use fresh berries instead of frozen.

For a subtly sweet dessert that is lower in added sugar, feel free to omit the maple syrup from the filling.

To speed up the cooling process, place the bars, once mostly cooled, in the refrigerator or freezer for 10 to 15 minutes. If you can't wait, you can enjoy this crumble straight out the oven, spooned into a bowl (with a scoop of ice cream, if you like). It will be messier but still delish!

superseed crispy treats

yield: 9 bars (1 per serving)   prep time: 15 minutes, plus 30 minutes to set in freezer   cook time: 7 minutes

This made-over classic treat packs the same sweetness and crispiness, but without the marshmallows, butter, or refined sugar. Plus, the pumpkin, sunflower, and chia seeds not only add to the crunch factor but also provide a boost of plant protein and good fats.

2½ cups puffed brown rice cereal

¼ cup pepitas

¼ cup shelled sunflower seeds

2 tablespoons chia seeds

¼ cup plus 1 tablespoon coconut oil, melted, divided

¼ cup pure maple syrup

¼ cup natural creamy cashew butter or other nut butter of choice

1 teaspoon pure vanilla extract

1 cup dark chocolate chips

Sea salt flakes, for topping

1. Line an 8-inch square baking pan with parchment paper with the ends overhanging for easy removal of the bars.

2. In a large bowl, combine the puffed brown rice, pepitas, sunflower seeds, and chia seeds.

3. In a small saucepan, heat ¼ cup of the oil, the maple syrup, cashew butter, and vanilla over medium heat, stirring frequently, until combined and liquid, 45 to 60 seconds.

4. Pour the wet ingredients over the dry and use a rubber spatula to mix them together, making sure the cereal is evenly coated.

5. Pour the mixture into the prepared pan and use the spatula to spread in an even layer. Press down firmly to make sure everything sticks together.

6. Place the chocolate chips and remaining tablespoon of coconut oil in a microwave-safe bowl and microwave on high in 30-second increments, stirring after each increment, until melted, about 90 seconds total. Pour the melted chocolate over the brown rice mixture to coat and smooth into an even layer using a rubber spatula. Top with sea salt flakes.

7. Place the pan in the freezer to set for 30 minutes. Once set, remove from the pan and cut into squares. Store in a sealed container in the refrigerator for up to a week or in the freezer for up to a month. Let frozen bars sit out for 10 to 15 minutes before consuming.

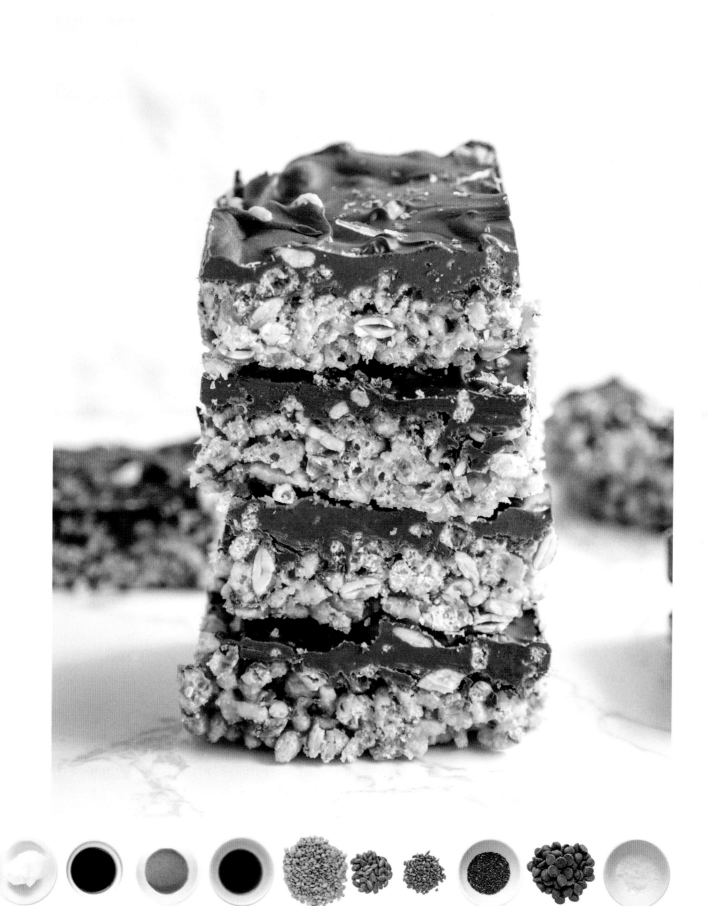

peanut butter chocolate candy bites

yield: 12 candy bites (1 per serving)   prep time: 10 minutes, plus 20 minutes to set

Dark chocolate and peanut butter meet medjool dates in these crazy delicious candy bites. Dates are among the sweetest fruits in the world, earning them the title "nature's candy." However, because they are a fruit, they also add fiber and key nutrients like potassium and magnesium, making this recipe a dessert with benefits.

12 soft pitted medjool dates

⅓ cup natural creamy peanut butter

2 tablespoons chopped raw or dry roasted peanuts

2 ounces coarsely chopped dark chocolate (about ¼ cup), melted

Sea salt flakes, for topping

1. Line a sheet pan with parchment paper.

2. Place the dates on the prepared pan and stuff each date with 1 heaping teaspoon of peanut butter. Transfer to the freezer for 10 minutes to set.

3. Top the peanut butter filling in each date with ½ teaspoon of peanuts. Drizzle the melted chocolate on top and sprinkle with sea salt flakes. Return the pan to the freezer for another 10 minutes to set the chocolate.

4. Enjoy immediately or store in a sealed container in the refrigerator for up to a week.

note _____

Feel free to replace the peanut butter and peanuts with any nut/seed butter and nut/seed combination you like, such as sunflower seed butter and sunflower seeds or almond butter and almonds.

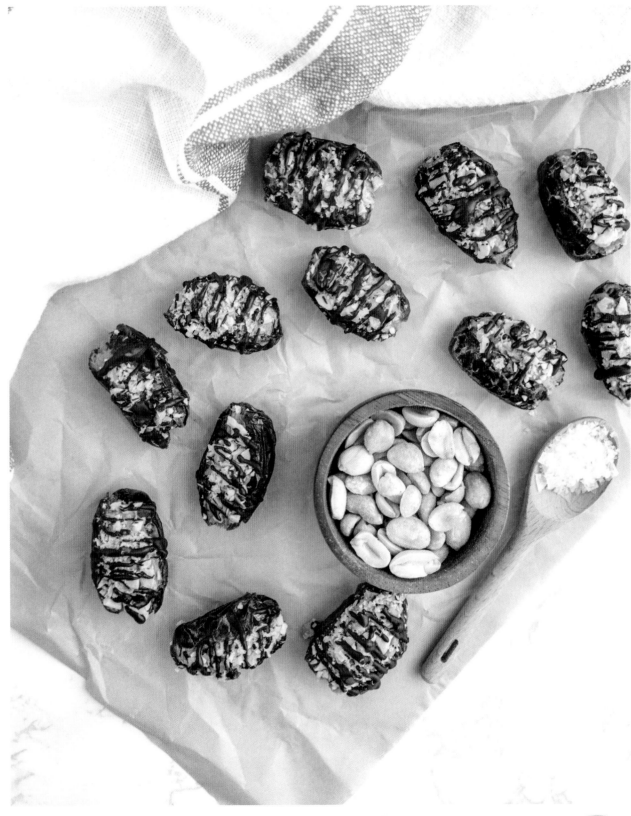

bean blondies

yield: 9 blondies (1 per serving)   prep time: 10 minutes   cook time: 30 minutes

Feeling hesitant about beans in dessert? Don't knock it 'til you try it! When cooked and rinsed well, beans can add moisture and fudginess to baked goods like brownies and blondies while cutting back on the amount of fat and flour needed. Not only that, but beans add nutrients such as plant protein, B vitamins, and fiber, making this another dessert with benefits. While I prefer using chickpeas in this recipe, white beans would work as well.

1 tablespoon flaxseed meal

3 tablespoons water

1 (15-ounce) can no-salt-added chickpeas, drained and rinsed well, or 1½ cups cooked chickpeas (see page 44)

½ cup rolled oats

⅔ cup coconut sugar

3 tablespoons coconut oil, melted

1 teaspoon pure vanilla extract

1 teaspoon baking powder

¼ teaspoon baking soda

½ cup dark chocolate chips

1. Preheat the oven to 350°F and grease an 8-inch square baking pan with cooking spray.

2. Make a flax egg by combining the flaxseed meal and water in a small bowl; allow to sit for 5 minutes.

3. Place the flax egg along with the rest of the ingredients, except the chocolate chips, in a food processor and blend until smooth. Fold in the chocolate chips by hand.

4. Scoop the batter into the prepared pan using a rubber spatula, smooth the top, and bake for 30 minutes. It will look a little underbaked when you take it out of the oven but will firm up as it cools.

5. Let cool completely before slicing into 9 squares.

6. Store leftovers in a sealed container in the refrigerator for up to a week.

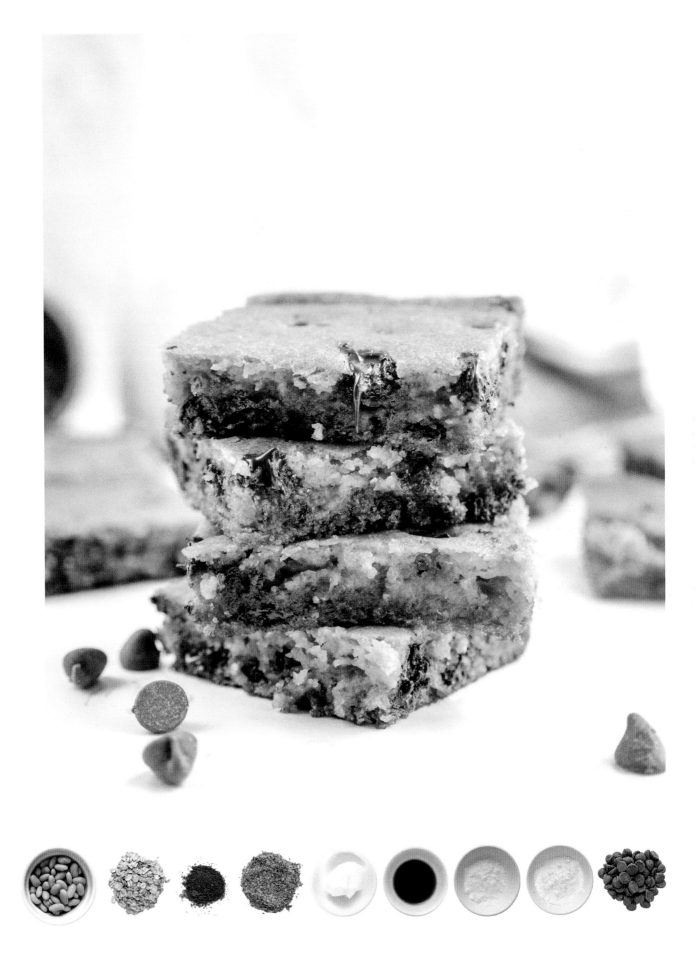

3-ingredient strawberry mango sorbet

yield: **2 servings**   prep time: **5 minutes**

This simple sorbet makes eating fruit more fun. While store-bought sorbets are typically high in added sugar, this one is naturally sweetened with just fruit.

1 (10-ounce) bag frozen strawberries (about 2 cups)

1 (10-ounce) bag frozen mango chunks (about 2 cups)

1 teaspoon lemon juice

1. Place the strawberries and mango chunks in a food processor and process until you achieve small shreds, about 15 seconds.

2. Add the lemon juice and mix for another 15 seconds. Add water a tablespoon at a time and blend until a creamy texture develops; you will likely need about 3 tablespoons total.

3. Enjoy immediately or freeze in a sealed container. To enjoy, remove and thaw for 10 to 15 minutes for easy scooping.

note

For a sweeter sorbet, add 2 tablespoons of raw manuka honey in Step 2.

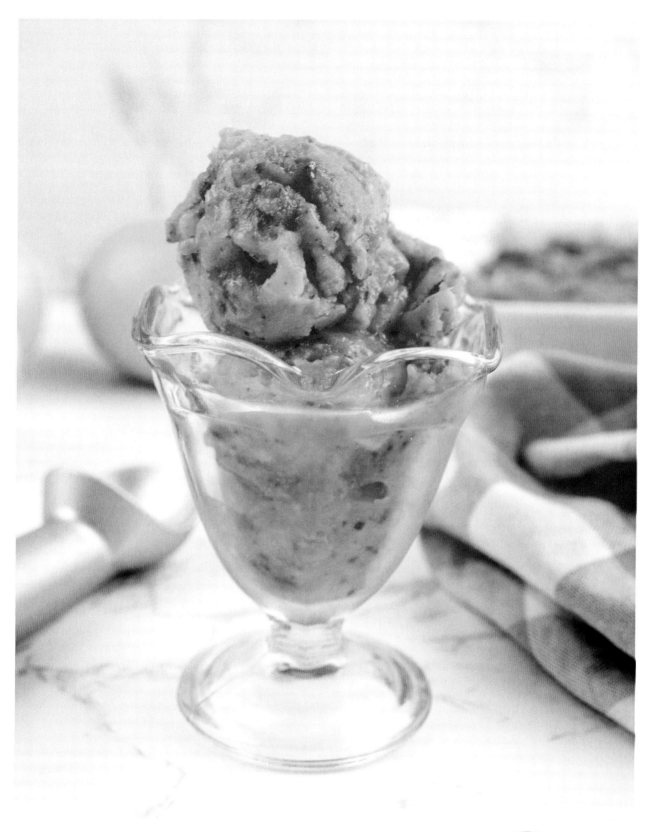
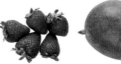

toasted coconut and chocolate cluster cookies

yield: 12 cookies (1 per serving)   prep time: 15 minutes, plus 20 minutes to soak dates and 10 minutes to set   cook time: 10 minutes

Try this simple whole-food take on nostalgic chewy chocolate coconut cookies. Sweetened with dates instead of refined sugar and made with a base of walnuts instead of white flour, this is a feel-good dessert.

12 soft pitted medjool dates

1¼ cups unsweetened shredded coconut

1 cup raw walnuts

½ cup dark chocolate chips

1 teaspoon coconut oil

Sea salt flakes, for topping

notes

Coconut burns easily, so keep a close eye on it. Alternatively, you can toast the coconut in a skillet on the stovetop.

Another way to melt the chocolate is to use the double boiler method. Bring a few inches of water to a boil in a pot on the stovetop, then reduce the heat to a low simmer. Place the chocolate and coconut oil in a metal bowl that fits snugly over the top of the pot of water. Stir often until the chocolate is melted.

1. Place the dates in a large bowl and cover with warm water. Set aside to soak for 20 minutes, then drain.

2. Meanwhile, toast the coconut: Preheat the oven to 350°F and line a sheet pan with parchment paper. Spread the coconut in a thin layer on the prepared pan. Bake until slightly golden brown and toasted, 2 to 4 minutes.

3. Put the walnuts in a food processor and pulse until finely ground, about 15 seconds. Add the drained dates and 1 cup of the toasted coconut and blend until a slightly sticky dough forms. Pour the remaining ¼ cup of toasted coconut into a small bowl and set aside.

4. Remove the food processor blade and, using your hands, roll about 2 tablespoons of the dough at a time into 1-inch balls. Place the balls on the same prepared sheet pan, spacing them about 2 inches apart. Flatten them using the bottom of a cup or small bowl, then use a straw or chopstick to poke a hole in the center of each cookie.

5. Place the pan in the freezer for 10 minutes to allow the cookies to harden.

6. When the cookies are nearly ready to come out of the freezer, melt the chocolate. Place the chocolate chips and coconut oil in a microwave-safe bowl. Microwave on high for 30 seconds. Stir and return the bowl to the microwave. Continue heating in 30-second intervals until all of the chips are just about melted. Continue to stir until the last pieces have melted.

7. Remove the pan from the freezer and use a fork to dip the bottom of each cookie into the chocolate. Place the

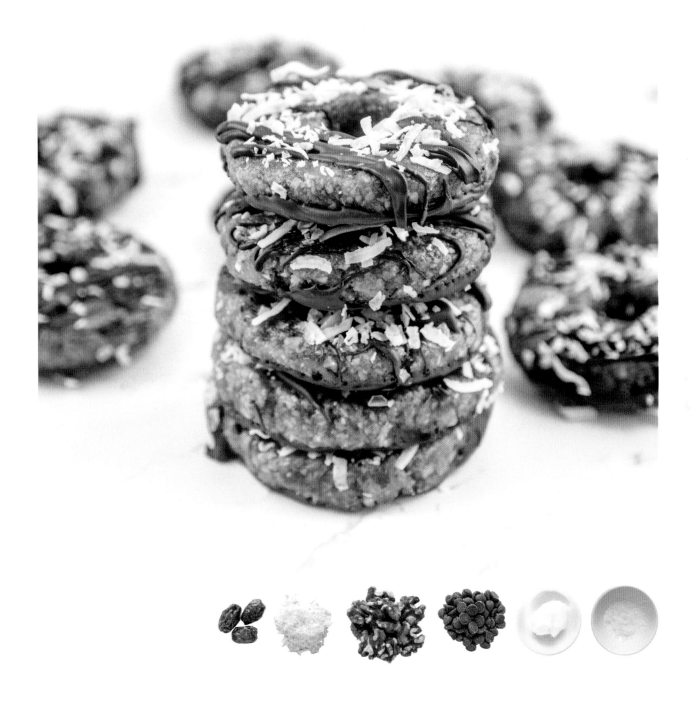

dipped cookies, dipped side up, back on the pan. Freeze for another 5 minutes, until the chocolate is set, then flip the cookies over and use a spoon to drizzle or spread additional chocolate over the cookies. Top with the remaining toasted coconut and sea salt flakes.

8. Store in a sealed container in the refrigerator for up to 2 weeks.

secret ingredient edible cookie dough

yield: 1 cup (2 tablespoons per serving)   prep time: 5 minutes

If you think licking cookie dough off the spatula is the best part about baking cookies, then this recipe is for you. Satisfy your cookie dough fix without having to turn on the oven with this no-bake recipe. This edible cookie dough is made with a secret ingredient that you can't taste: chickpeas! These mild-flavored beans add a smooth creaminess to this recipe while also bumping up the protein and fiber—two nutrients you won't find in traditional cookies. Enjoy this cookie dough by the spoonful or serve it as a dessert dip with fresh strawberries or apple slices.

1 (15-ounce) can no-salt-added chickpeas, drained and rinsed well, or 1½ cups cooked chickpeas (see page 44)

⅓ cup coconut sugar

¼ cup natural creamy cashew butter

¼ cup rolled oats

2 teaspoons pure vanilla extract

⅓ cup dark chocolate chips

1. Put all of the ingredients except the chocolate chips in a food processor and blend until smooth. Fold in the chocolate chips by hand.

2. Serve immediately or store in the refrigerator for up to 5 days.

note _____

I prefer the taste of cashew butter in this recipe, but feel free to use any creamy nut or seed butter you like.

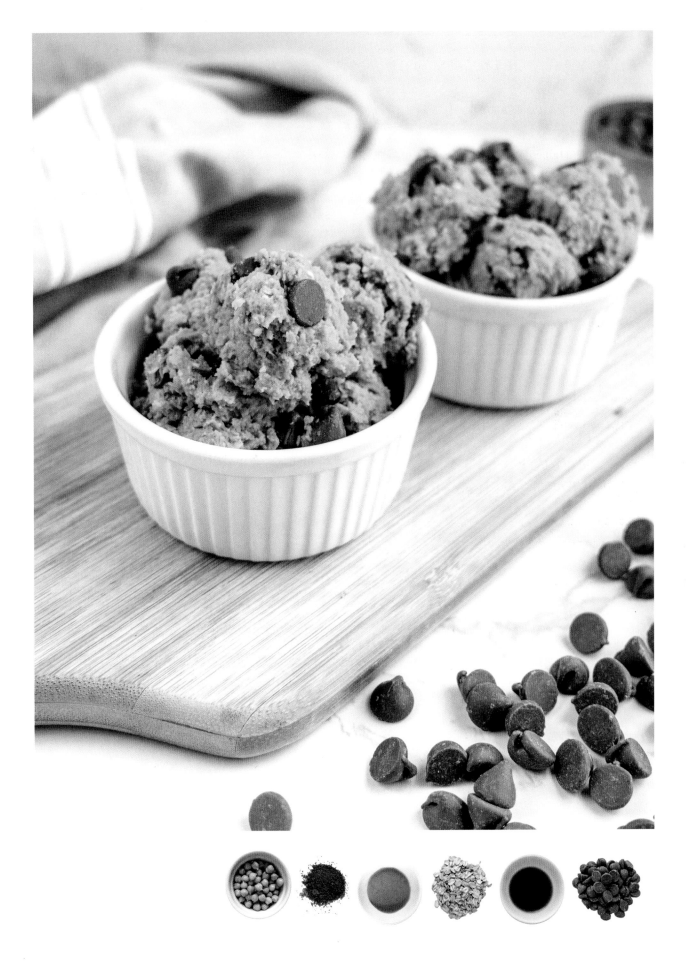

4-ingredient fudgy sweet potato brownies

yield: 8 brownies (1 per serving)   prep time: 15 minutes   cook time: 35 to 45 minutes

These brownies with a veggie twist are made with sweet potatoes, a filling root vegetable packed with fiber and beta-carotene antioxidants that our bodies convert to vitamin A, which is important for skin and immune health. Using sweet potatoes adds moisture and a melt-in-your-mouth texture that also allows you to cut back on the amount of fat and added sweetener used in traditional brownie recipes. This recipe calls for tahini, a sesame seed paste, but can be made with any unsweetened, unsalted nut or seed butter.

2 large sweet potatoes (about 1 pound), peeled and cut into 1-inch chunks

⅔ cup tahini

⅓ cup unsweetened cocoa powder

⅓ cup pure maple syrup

1. Preheat the oven to 350°F. Line an 8-inch square baking pan with parchment paper.

2. Put the sweet potato chunks in a large pot and cover with water. Bring to a boil, then reduce to a simmer. Boil the potatoes until fork-tender, 10 to 15 minutes.

3. Drain the potatoes in a colander and transfer to a food processor. Add the remaining ingredients and blend until the batter is well combined and smooth.

4. Transfer the batter to the prepared pan and smooth the top with a rubber spatula. Bake until a toothpick comes out clean when inserted into the center, 25 to 30 minutes. Allow to cool for about 15 minutes before slicing into 8 squares. Remove the brownies using a spatula.

5. Store in a sealed container in the refrigerator for up to 5 days.

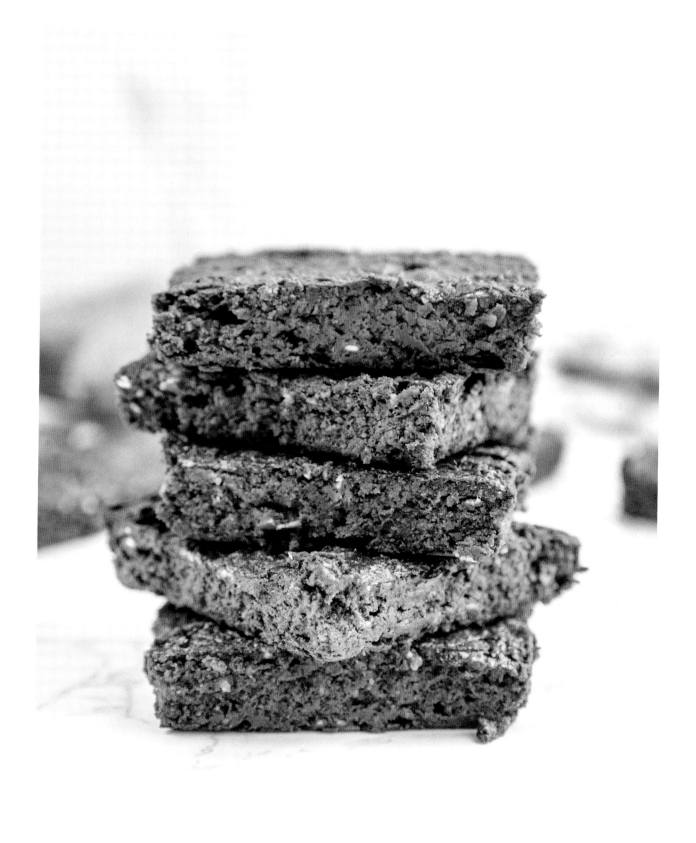

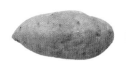

single-serve cinnamon apple walnut crisps

yield: **4 servings**   prep time: **10 minutes**   cook time: **30 minutes**

Nothing says fall like warm, baked cinnamon apples topped with a crunchy, crumbly walnut oat topping. Contrary to popular belief, not all apples are made equal. For this recipe, I recommend firm apples that hold up during cooking, such as Granny Smith, Honeycrisp, or Pink Lady. If apples are sweet enough on their own for you, feel free to omit the sugar from the filling for a minimal-added-sugar recipe that barely qualifies as dessert (because it's so nutritious!).

filling:

4 medium-sized firm apples, peeled and chopped

2 tablespoons coconut sugar

1 teaspoon lemon juice

½ teaspoon ground cinnamon

topping:

¼ cup rolled oats

¼ cup blanched almond flour

2 tablespoons coconut oil, melted

2 tablespoons coconut sugar

2 tablespoons chopped raw walnuts

Pinch of Himalayan pink salt

1. Preheat the oven to 350°F. Grease four 6-ounce ramekins with cooking spray and set on a sheet pan.

2. To make the filling, combine the apples, sugar, lemon juice, and cinnamon in a large bowl. Divide the mixture among the prepared ramekins.

3. To make the topping, put the oats, flour, oil, sugar, walnuts, and salt in another large bowl and use a rubber spatula to mix until crumbly. Sprinkle the mixture on top of the apples.

4. Bake until the apples are tender and the crumb topping is crisp and golden brown, 25 to 30 minutes.

notes

If you don't have ramekins, you can bake this in a greased 9-inch pie dish.

Serve warm with a scoop of ice cream or a dollop of whipped cream and a sprinkle of cinnamon.

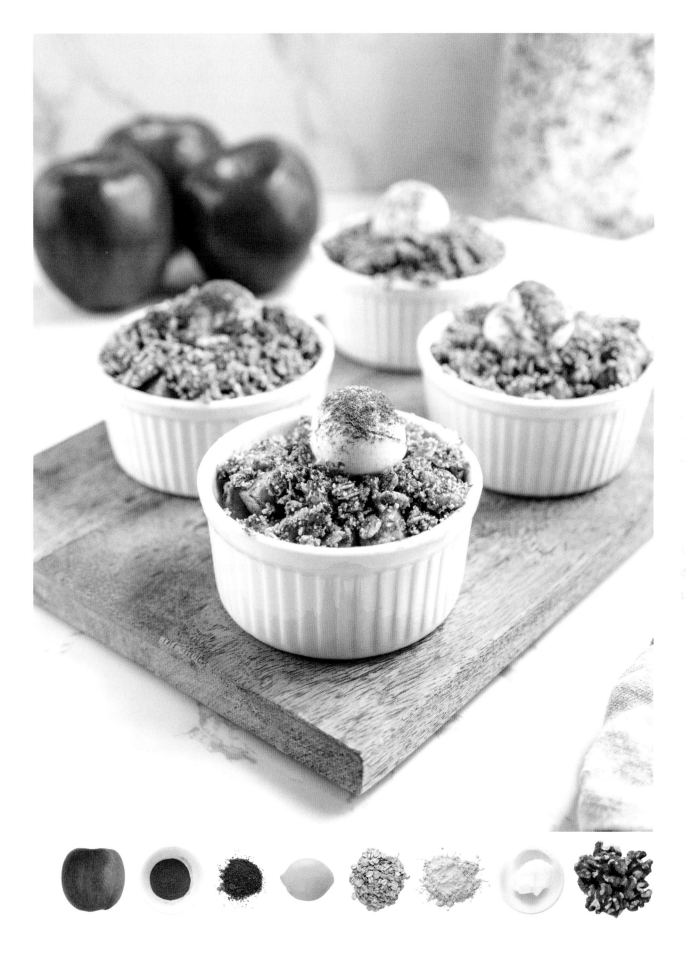

chocolate chip cookie skillet

yield: **6 servings**   prep time: **15 minutes**   cook time: **30 minutes**

Put a crowd-pleasing twist on chocolate chip cookies with this one-pan dessert. It's made with naturally gluten-free flours and is completely plant-based to meet a variety of dietary needs. Enjoy it on its own or with whipped cream or a scoop of ice cream on top!

2 tablespoons flaxseed meal

6 tablespoons water

1 cup blanched almond flour

¼ cup tapioca flour

⅓ cup coconut sugar

1 teaspoon baking powder

¼ teaspoon finely ground Himalayan pink salt

⅓ cup natural creamy cashew butter

¼ cup coconut oil, melted

1 teaspoon pure vanilla extract

⅔ cup dark chocolate chips, divided

Sea salt flakes, for topping (optional)

1. Preheat the oven to 350°F and grease a 9-inch oven-safe skillet with cooking spray.

2. Make 2 flax eggs by combining the flaxseed meal and water in a large bowl; allow to sit for 5 minutes.

3. In a small bowl, whisk together the almond flour, tapioca flour, sugar, baking powder, and salt.

4. Add the cashew butter, coconut oil, and vanilla to the bowl with the flax eggs and whisk to combine.

5. Add the dry ingredients to the wet ingredients and stir until combined. Gently fold in ½ cup of the chocolate chips.

6. Scoop the batter into the prepared skillet using a rubber spatula, smooth the top, and top with the remaining chocolate chips.

7. Bake until a toothpick inserted in the center comes out clean, 25 to 30 minutes.

8. Top with sea salt flakes, if desired, and let cool in the pan before cutting into 6 slices.

9. Store leftovers in a sealed container in the refrigerator for up to 5 days or in the freezer for up to 3 months.

note _____

In place of the cashew butter, you can use peanut butter or any creamy nut butter, such as almond butter.

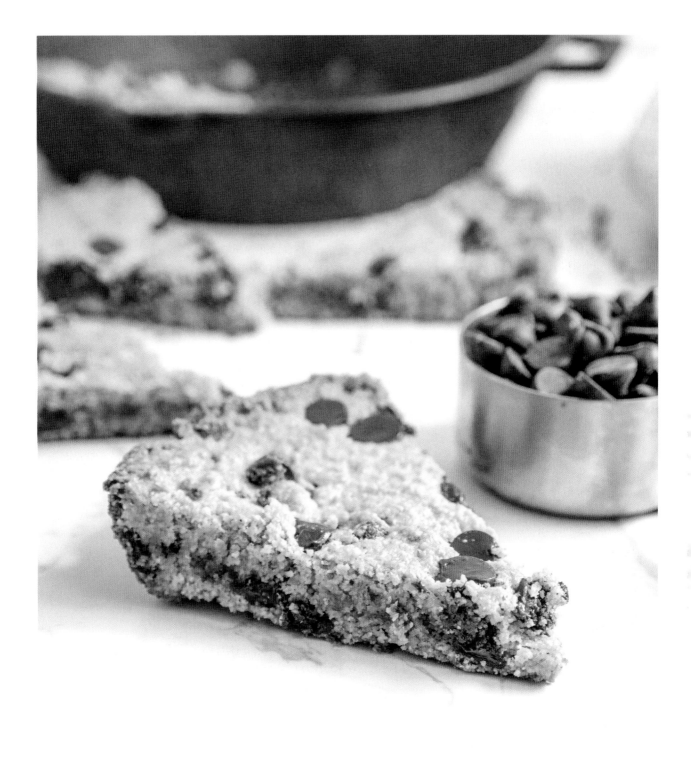

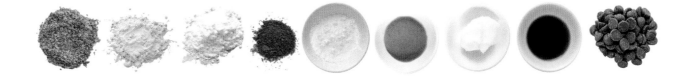

honey lemon bars

yield: 9 bars (1 per serving)   prep time: 10 minutes   cook time: 35 minutes

Lemon bars are the quintessential sweet and tart spring treat. These bars are made with a chewy oat flour crust and topped with a light and luscious four-ingredient lemon filling. Keeping with tradition, this recipe uses eggs, though you can replace them with raw cashews and coconut cream to impart a plant-based creaminess (see the note below).

crust:

3 cups rolled oats, processed into flour

⅓ cup raw manuka honey

3 tablespoons coconut oil, melted

1 teaspoon pure vanilla extract

¼ teaspoon finely ground Himalayan pink salt

filling:

3 large eggs, beaten

⅓ cup raw manuka honey

2 tablespoons tapioca flour

½ cup lemon juice

1. Preheat the oven to 350°F. Line an 8-inch square baking pan with parchment paper with the ends overhanging for easy removal of the bars.

2. To make the crust, put the oat flour, honey, oil, vanilla, and salt in a large bowl and mix using a rubber spatula until a crumbly dough forms. Scoop the mixture into the prepared baking dish, press down with your hands, and par-bake until golden brown around the edges and set in the middle, 12 to 15 minutes.

3. While the crust is baking, make the filling: In a blender or food processor, pulse the eggs, honey, tapioca flour, and lemon juice until smooth. Pour over the par-baked crust and bake until the filling has set, another 15 to 20 minutes.

4. Allow to cool for 30 minutes before removing from the pan and slicing into 9 squares. Store in a sealed container in the refrigerator for up to a week.

notes _____

You can use pure maple syrup instead of honey.

If you don't have tapioca flour, you can use cornstarch, arrowroot flour, or all-purpose flour.

For egg-free: Replace the eggs with ½ cup of raw cashews plus ½ cup of coconut cream. Blend with the rest of the filling ingredients in a food processor until smooth.

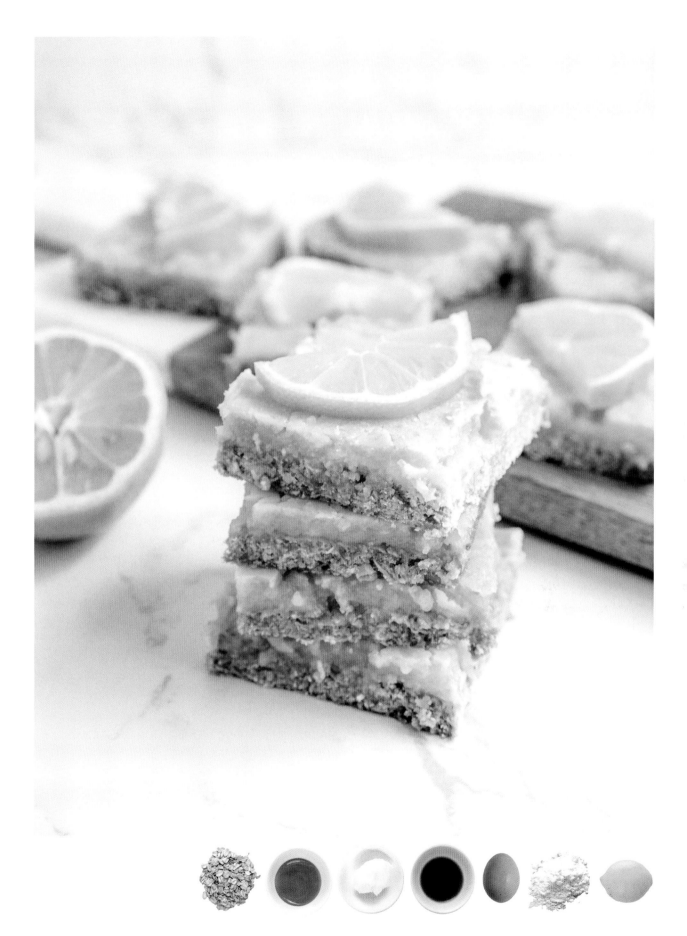

acknowledgments

To Ryan, for being my unwavering support system. Even after working 12-hour shifts, you have been there to source last-minute ingredients and help wash a never-ending pile of dishes from recipe testing, all while never complaining about our two constantly filled-to-the-brim fridges and freezers of ingredients and recipes marked "do not eat yet."

To my parents, Meng and Gina, whose endless love and support have made it possible for me to follow my dreams.

To my brother, Mark, and sister-in-law, Phoebe, thank you for being my biggest cheerleaders in work and in life.

To Carol, my future mother-in-law, you have believed in and supported me since the day we met. You are always the first person to share my recipes and TV segments, and I know you will be the first person to buy this book.

To Kelley Martin, my dietetic internship director at the Medical University of South Carolina, for taking a chance on a girl from California and matching me to your dietetic internship program in a city that I'd never once been to. Charleston, South Carolina, changed the trajectory of my life, and I will forever be grateful.

To my interns, Bridget, Jahaira, Madison, Caroline, Kylie, and Mackenzie, thank you for being my right-hand ladies and second set of eyes in all things mostly plant-based recipes and evidence-based nutrition.

To my 19-pound furry best friend, Maizy, the best thing to come out of 2020, who kept me company and was on my lap or by my side as I wrote every word of this book and cooked each recipe.

To Pam Mourouzis, Holly Jennings, Lance Freimuth, Susan Lloyd, Kat Lannom, Justin Velasco, Yordan Terziev, Boryana Yordanova, and everyone else at Victory Belt, thank you for believing in me, supporting me every step of the way, and bringing my dream book to life.

And last but not least, thank you to the readers, viewers, and followers of Nutrition By Mia. Your loyalty and support of my recipes since I started in 2014 have made it possible for me to bring this book into the world.

helpful resources

conversion charts

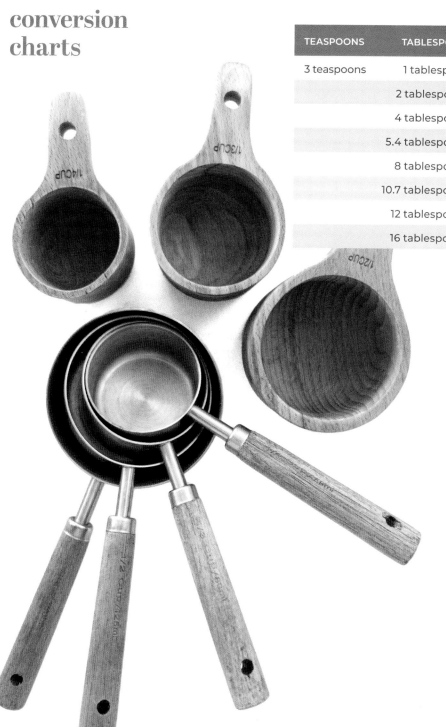

TEASPOONS	TABLESPOONS	CUPS	MILLILITERS
3 teaspoons	1 tablespoon		15 ml
	2 tablespoons	⅛ cup	30 ml
	4 tablespoons	¼ cup	60 ml
	5.4 tablespoons	⅓ cup	80 ml
	8 tablespoons	½ cup	120 ml
	10.7 tablespoons	⅔ cup	160 ml
	12 tablespoons	¾ cup	180 ml
	16 tablespoons	1 cup	240 ml

CUPS	FLUID OUNCES
¼ cup	2 fl. oz.
½ cup	4 fl. oz.
¾ cup	6 fl. oz.
1 cup	8 fl. oz.

FAHRENHEIT	CELSIUS
200°F	95°C
300°F	150°C
325°F	165°C
350°F	175°C
375°F	190°C
400°F	205°C
425°F	220°C
450°F	230°C

my favorite food companies

A2 Milk

www.thea2milkcompany.com

Real cow's milk that offers the same nutrition but comes from cows that produce only the A2 protein (and no A1), which some people find is easier to digest and prevents stomach discomfort.

Barilla

www.barilla.com

Red lentil and chickpea pastas made with just one ingredient.

BareOrganics Superfoods

www.bareorganics.com

Organic "superfood" ingredients for smoothies, baked goods, and more, including cacao nibs, spirulina powder, wheatgrass, and unsweetened cacao powder.

Bob's Red Mill

www.bobsredmill.com

Alternative flours like almond, coconut, cassava, chickpea, and tapioca, along with other baking essentials, including coconut sugar and flaxseed meal.

Cali'flour Foods

www.califlourfoods.com

Delicious premade pizza crusts made from cauliflower.

Enjoy Life Foods

www.enjoylifefoods.com

I keep their mini chocolate chips on hand for baking. All their chocolate is free of 14 common food allergens, including the top 8 (milk, eggs, fish, shellfish, peanuts, soy, tree nuts, and wheat), plus gluten, mustard, and sesame.

Food For Life

www.foodforlife.com

Sprouted breads found in the grocery store freezer section.

Fresh Cravings

www.freshcravings.com

Salsa made without preservatives that tastes homemade, found refrigerated in the produce section.

Green Giant

www.greengiant.com

I keep their frozen riced cauliflower, zucchini noodles, and cauliflower gnocchi on hand for time-saving convenience.

Kite Hill

www.kite-hill.com

Dairy-free cream cheese that tastes like the real deal.

Mary's Gone Crackers

www.marysgonecrackers.com

Crunchy plant-based whole-grain and seed crackers.

Otamot

www.otamotfoods.com

Thick, delicious pizza and pasta sauces made with more than nine organic vegetables.

Pacific Foods

www.pacificfoods.com

Broths and stocks made with real-food ingredients.

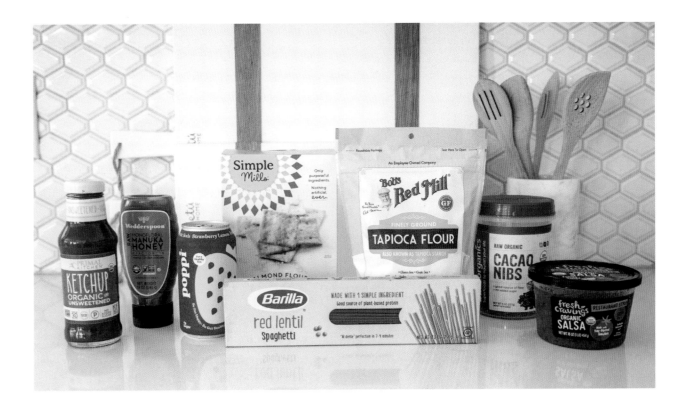

Poppi

www.drinkpoppi.com

Prebiotic sodas made with apple cider vinegar and 5 grams of sugar or less that can help satisfy a soda fix.

Primal Kitchen

www.primalkitchen.com

Sauces and condiments made with real-food ingredients, nutritious oils like avocado oil, and no dairy or refined sugar. Some of my favorites are their avocado oil mayonnaise, unsweetened ketchup, and salad dressings like balsamic vinaigrette, Caesar, green goddess, and avocado oil ranch.

Safe Catch

www.safecatch.com

Low-mercury canned fish including tuna, salmon, and sardines.

Siete Foods

www.sietefoods.com

Grain-free tortillas and tortilla chips made with alternative flours like almond, coconut, and cassava.

Simple Mills

www.simplemills.com

Crackers, cookies, and other products made with real-food ingredients. I like their almond flour crackers, seed flour crackers, and baking mixes.

Spiceology

www.spiceology.com

Unique spice blends including sugar-free and salt-free options.

Violife

www.violifefoods.com

Vegan cheeses, including Just Like Feta Block and Just Like Parmesan Grated.

Vital Farms

www.vitalfarms.com

One of the only brands of pasture-raised eggs available in the United States. You can taste (and see) the difference.

Wedderspoon Honey

www.wedderspoon.com

Raw manuka honey for sweetening baked goods and meals.

ingredient brand recommendations

BBQ SAUCE
Primal Kitchen
True Made Foods

BREADS
Base Culture
Food For Life Ezekiel 4:9

BROTH
Bonafide Provisions
Pacific Foods

CAULIFLOWER GNOCCHI
Green Giant
Trader Joe's

CHOCOLATE CHIPS
Enjoy Life

COCONUT SUGAR
Bob's Red Mill
Nutiva

CRACKERS
Mary's Gone Crackers
Simple Mills

EGGS
Vital Farms

FLAXSEED MEAL
Bob's Red Mill
Trader Joe's

FLOURS
Bob's Red Mill

MANUKA HONEY
Comvita
Wedderspoon

MAYONNAISE
Primal Kitchen

PASTA
Banza
Barilla

PICO DE GALLO AND SALSA
Fresh Cravings

PLANT-BASED PARMESAN AND OTHER CHEESES
Violife

RICE VINEGAR
Nakano

SALAD DRESSINGS
Primal Kitchen

SEA SALT FLAKES
Maldon

SPICE BLENDS
Simply Organic
Spiceology

SUPERFOODS
BareOrganics
Navitas Organics

TOMATO SAUCE
Otamot
Primal Kitchen
Rao's Homemade

TORTILLAS AND TORTILLA CHIPS
Food For Life Ezekiel 4:9
Siete Foods

kitchen appliances and cookware

Bento lunch boxes for adults
www.bentgo.com
www.ecolunchboxes.com
thedearestgrey.co
These bento boxes are stylish and functional lunch box options for adults (with kid versions available as well).

Brava Smart countertop oven
shop.brava.com
Save precious counter space with an appliance that does it all, including bake, toast, reheat, air-fry, sear, and dehydrate.

Caraway Home nontoxic ceramic-coated cookware and bakeware
www.carawayhome.com
These pans are not only beautiful, but also offer a healthier way to cook foods that might otherwise stick, such as eggs and animal proteins, requiring little to no oil.

Instant Pot
www.instanthome.com
A pressure cooker, slow cooker, rice cooker, and yogurt maker all in one. This is a great investment if "set it and forget it" dinners are your jam.

KitchenAid food processor
www.kitchenaid.com
KitchenAid makes mini food processors (3½-cup capacity) that are ideal for making smaller-volume recipes like sauces and dressings in addition to their larger (10- to 13-cup) options.

Lodge cast-iron skillet
www.lodgecastiron.com
These pans are affordable, durable, multifunctional, and long-lasting. Use them on the stovetop, oven, or grill to cook proteins, veggies, eggs, and even skillet cookies.

Ninja Kitchen air fryer
www.ninjakitchen.com
This is an affordable, high-quality air fryer option.

Vitamix blender
www.vitamix.com
Vitamix is the gold standard of high-powered blenders.

my website

www.nutritionbymia.com

For more mostly plant-based recipes, meal ideas, and evidence-based nutrition tips

endnotes

Chapter 1

1. USDA, Dietary Guidelines for Americans 2020–2025, 9th Edition, December 2020, https://www.dietaryguidelines.gov/sites/default/files/2021-03/Dietary_Guidelines_for_Americans-2020-2025.pdf.

2. Yunsheng Ma et al., "Single-Component Versus Multicomponent Dietary Goals for the Metabolic Syndrome: A Randomized Trial," *Annals of Internal Medicine* 162, no. 4 (2015): 248–57, https://doi.org/10.7326/M14-0611.

3. Molly J. Higgins and John E. Hayes, "Regional Variation of Bitter Taste and Aftertaste in Humans," *Chemical Senses* 44, no. 9 (2019): 721–32, https://www.ncbi.nlm.nih.gov/pmc/articles/PMC6872973/.

4. Julieanna Hever, "Plant-Based Diets: A Physician's Guide," *The Permanente Journal* 20, no. 3 (2016): 15-082, https://www.ncbi.nlm.nih.gov/pmc/articles/PMC4991921/.

5. USDA, Dietary Guidelines for Americans 2020–2025, 9th Edition, December 2020, https://www.dietaryguidelines.gov/sites/default/files/2021-03/Dietary_Guidelines_for_Americans-2020-2025.pdf.

Chapter 2

1. Charu Gupta and Ghan Prakash, "Phytonutrients as Therapeutic Agents," *Journal of Complementary & Integrative Medicine* 11, no. 3 (2014): 151–69, https://pubmed.ncbi.nlm.nih.gov/25051278/.

2. Ashley A. Thiede and Sheri Zidenberg-Cherr, "Nutrition and Health Info Sheet: Phytochemicals," Center for Nutrition in Schools, Department of Nutrition, University of California, Davis, June 2016, https://nutrition.ucdavis.edu/sites/g/files/dgvnsk426/files/content/infosheets/factsheets/fact-pro-phytochemical.pdf.

3. Ruth E. Ley et al., "Evolution of Mammals and Their Gut Microbes," *Science* 320, no. 5883 (2008): 1647–51, www.ncbi.nlm.nih.gov/pmc/articles/PMC2649005/.

4. Ghada A. Soliman, "Dietary Cholesterol and the Lack of Evidence in Cardiovascular Disease," *Nutrients* 10, no. 6 (2018): 780, www.ncbi.nlm.nih.gov/pmc/articles/PMC6024687/.

5. "Potatoes and Tomatoes Are the Most Commonly Consumed Vegetables," Economic Research Service, US Department of Agriculture, last updated December 16, 2020, https://www.ers.usda.gov/data-products/chart-gallery/gallery/chart-detail/?chartId=58340.

6. Apples and Oranges Are the Top U.S. Fruit Choices," Economic Research Service, US Department of Agriculture, last updated August 25, 2021, https://www.ers.usda.gov/data-products/chart-gallery/gallery/chart-detail/?chartId=58322.

7. Deanna M. Minich, "A Review of the Science of Colorful, Plant-Based Food and Practical Strategies for 'Eating the Rainbow,'" *Journal of Nutrition and Metabolism* (2019): 2125070, https://www.ncbi.nlm.nih.gov/pmc/articles/PMC7770496/.

8. Karen Heneman and Sheri Zidenberg-Cherr, "Publication 8381: Nutrition and Health Info Sheet: Phytochemicals," University of California, Division of Agriculture and Natural Resources, https://anrcatalog.ucanr.edu/pdf/8313.pdf.

9. Pattie Jones, "Phytonutrients: The Power of Color," University of Missouri Extension, https://health.mo.gov/living/families/wic/pdf/phytonutrientsposter.pdf.

10. D. L. Katz and S. Miller, "Can We Say What Diet Is Best for Health?" *Annual Review of Public Health* 35 (2014): 83–103, https://pubmed.ncbi.nlm.nih.gov/24641555/.

11. Marta Guasch-Ferré et al., "Nut Consumption and Risk of Cardiovascular Disease," *JACC Journals* 70, no. 20 (2017): 2519–32, www.onlinejacc.org/content/70/20/2519.full.

12. "Soy Isoflavones," National Cancer Institute, https://www.cancer.gov/publications/dictionaries/cancer-drug/def/soy-isoflavones.

13. Neela Guha et al., "Soy Isoflavones and Risk of Cancer Recurrence in a Cohort of Breast Cancer Survivors: Life After Cancer Epidemiology (LACE) Study," *Breast Cancer Research and Treatment* 118, no. 2 (2009): 395–405, https://www.ncbi.nlm.nih.gov/pmc/articles/PMC3470874/.

Chapter 3

1. Suzanne P. Murphy and Lindsay H. Allen, "Nutritional Importance of Animal Source Foods," *Journal of Nutrition* 133, no. 11 (2003): 3932S–5S, https://academic.oup.com/jn/article/133/11/3932S/4818051.

2. Marjorie J. Haskell, "The Challenge to Reach Nutritional Adequacy for Vitamin A: β-carotene Bioavailability and Conversion—Evidence in Humans," *American Journal of Clinical Nutrition* 96, no. 5 (2012): 1193S–203S, https://academic.oup.com/ajcn/article/96/5/1193S/4577160.

3. Connie M. Weaver and Robert P. Heaney, "Calcium," In: Ross C, Caballero B, Cousins RJ, Tucker KL, Ziegler TR, eds., *Modern Nutrition in Health and Disease,* 11th ed. (Baltimore, MD: Lippincott Williams & Wilkins; 2014), 133–49.

4. E. R. Monson, "Iron Nutrition and Absorption: Dietary Factors Which Impact Iron Bioavailability," *Journal of the American Dietetic Association* 88, no. 7 (1988): 786–90, https://pubmed.ncbi.nlm.nih.gov/3290310/.

5. Fady Moustarah and Shamim S. Mohiuddin, "Dietary Iron," StatPearls [Internet], last updated April 28, 2021, www.ncbi.nlm.nih.gov/books/NBK540969.

6. Nazanin Roohani, Richard Hurrell, Roya Kelishadi, and Rainer Schulin, "Zinc and Its Importance for Human Health: An Integrative Review," *Journal of Research in Medical Sciences* 18, no. 2 (2013): 144–57, www.ncbi.nlm.nih.gov/pmc/articles/PMC3724376/.

7. Janet R. Hunt, "Bioavailability of Iron, Zinc, and Other Trace Minerals from Vegetarian Diets," *American Journal of Clinical Nutrition* 78, no. 3 (2003): 633S–9S, https://academic.oup.com/ajcn/article/78/3/633S/4690005.

8. Susanne Krauss-Etschmann et al., "Effects of Fish-Oil and Folate Supplementation of Pregnant Women on Maternal and Fetal Plasma Concentrations of Docosahexaenoic Acid and Eicosapentaenoic Acid: A European Randomized Multicenter Trial," *American Journal of Clinical Nutrition* 85, no. 5 (2007): 1392–400, https://pubmed.ncbi.nlm.nih.gov/17490978/.

9. Philippe Guesnet and Jean-Marc Alessandri, "Docosahexaenoic Acid (DHA) and the Developing Central Nervous System (CNS)—Implications for Dietary Recommendations," *Biochimie* 93, no. 1 (2011): 7–12, https://pubmed.ncbi.nlm.nih.gov/20478353/.

10. Nicolas G. Bazan et al., "Docosahexaenoic Acid," ScienceDirect, www.sciencedirect.com/topics/neuroscience/docosahexaenoic-acid.

11. Emanuela Ricciotti and Garret A. FitzGerald, "Prostaglandins and Inflammation," *Arteriosclerosis, Thrombosis, and Vascular Biology* 31, no. 5 (2012): 986–1000, www.ncbi.nlm.nih.gov/pmc/articles/PMC3081099/.

12. Graham C. Burdge and Stephen A. Wootton, "Conversion of Alpha-Linolenic Acid to Eicosapentaenoic, Docosapentaenoic and Docosahexaenoic Acids in Young Women," *British Journal of Nutrition* 88, no. 4 (2002): 411–20, https://pubmed.ncbi.nlm.nih.gov/12323090/; Graham C. Burdge, Amanda E. Jones, and Stephen A. Wootton, "Eicosapentaenoic and Docosapentaenoic Acids Are the Principal Products of Alpha-Linolenic Acid Metabolism in Young Men," *British Journal of Nutrition* 88, no. 4 (2002): 355–63, https://pubmed.ncbi.nlm.nih.gov/12323085/.

13. Francois Mariotti and Christopher D. Gardner, "Dietary Protein and Amino Acids in Vegetarian Diets—A Review," *Nutrients* 11, no. 11 (2019): 2661, www.ncbi.nlm.nih.gov/pmc/articles/PMC6893534/.

14. Yingying Zhu et al., "Meat, Dairy and Plant Proteins Alter Bacterial Composition of Rat Gut Bacteria," *Scientific Reports* 5, Article Number 15220 (2015), www.nature.com/articles/srep15220.

15. David Schröter and Annika Höhn, "Role of Advance Glycation End Products in Carcinogenesis and Their Therapeutic Implications," *Current Pharmaceutical Design* 24, no. 44 (2018): 5245–51, https://pubmed.ncbi.nlm.nih.gov/30706806/.

Chapter 4

1. Center for Ecogenetics and Environmental Health, "Fast Facts about Health Risks of Pesticides in Food," January 2013, https://depts.washington.edu/ceeh/downloads/FF_Pesticides.pdf.

2. Sophie Réhault-Godbert, Nicolas Guyot, and Yves Nys, "The Golden Egg: Nutritional Value, Bioactivities, and Emerging Benefits for Human Health," *Nutrients* 11, no. 3 (2019): 684, https://www.ncbi.nlm.nih.gov/pmc/articles/PMC6470839/.

3. FoodSafety.gov, "Cold Food Storage Chart," last reviewed September 20, 2021, https://www.foodsafety.gov/food-safety-charts/cold-food-storage-charts.

4. See note 3 above.

5. Food Safety and Inspection Service, US Department of Agriculture, "Meat and Poultry Labeling Terms," last updated August 10, 2015, https://www.fsis.usda.gov/food-safety/safe-food-handling-and-preparation/food-safety-basics/meat-and-poultry-labeling-terms.

6. US Food & Drug Administration, "Mercury Levels in Commercial Fish and Shellfish (1990–2012)," last updated February 25, 2022, https://www.fda.gov/food/metals-and-your-food/mercury-levels-commercial-fish-and-shellfish-1990-2012.

7. Mashid Dehghan et al., "Association of Dairy Intake with Cardiovascular Disease and Mortality in 21 Countries from Five Continents (PURE): A Prospective Cohort Study," *The Lancet* 392, no. 10161 (2018): 2288–97, https://www.sciencedirect.com/science/article/abs/pii/S0140673618318129?via%3Dihub.

8. A. P. Simopoulos, "The Importance of the Ratio of Omega-6/Omega-3 Essential Fatty Acids," *Biomedicine and Pharmacotherapy* 56, no. 8 (2002): 365–79, https://pubmed.ncbi.nlm.nih.gov/12442909/.

nutrition info

RECIPE	PAGE	CALORIES/ SERVING	CARBO-HYDRATES (grams)	FAT (grams)	PROTEIN (grams)	NOTES
Yogurt Ranch Dressing	110	23	2	1	3	
Plant-Based Caesar Dressing	110	123	4	12	3	
Fat-Free Honey Dijon Dressing	110	74	25	0	8	
Balsamic Vinaigrette	110	86	1	9	0	
Peanut Dressing/Dip	110	72	4	6	2	
Plant-Based Avocado Green Goddess Dressing	110	95	7	8	3	
Oat Milk	112	114	18	2	4	
Any Greens Basil Pesto	114	114	1	12	2	
Quick Pico de Gallo	116	19	4	0	1	
Basic Guacamole	118	169	10	15	2	
Sweet Potato White Bean Hummus	120	99	23	4	7	
Roasted Red Pepper White Bean Hummus	120	84	21	3	7	
Avocado White Bean Hummus	120	103	20	6	7	
Roasted Garlic White Bean Hummus	120	76	19	3	7	
Plant-Based Parm	124	90	5	6	4	
Mushroom Bacon	126	186	7	16	1	
Coconut Bacon	126	143	9	7	13	
Tempeh Bacon	126	55	5	3	3	
Simple Tzatziki	128	83	4	3	9	using 2% plain Greek yogurt
No-Sugar All-Purpose Tomato Sauce	130	88	4	7	1	
50/50 Mushroom Meat Base	132	136	3	9	13	
100% Mushroom Base	132	212	9	18	7	
Chocolate Lover's Overnight Oats	138	303	48	10	9	
Apple Cinnamon Overnight Oats	138	397	55	18	9	
Banana Bread Overnight Oats	138	343	54	12	8	
Grown-Up PB&J Overnight Oats	138	435	54	21	14	
Blueberry Lemon Overnight Oats	138	283	50	7	7	
Tropical Overnight Oats	138	315	49	11	7	
Chocolate Lover's Chia Pudding	138	291	28	18	8	
Apple Cinnamon Chia Pudding	138	365	35	24	8	
Banana Bread Chia Pudding	138	329	34	20	8	
Grown-Up PB&J Chia Pudding	138	413	33	28	13	
Blueberry Lemon Chia Pudding	138	269	30	15	7	
Tropical Chia Pudding	138	301	29	19	6	
Customizable Make-Ahead Freezer Breakfast Sandwiches	140	254	24	12	14	without extra fillings
Naturally Sweetened Banana Oat Pancakes	142	256	43	6	10	
Savory Zucchini Waffle Minis	144	260	7	20	15	
Peanut Butter Cup Smoothie	146	505	66	14	34	using almond milk
Detox Green Smoothie	146	266	47	5	26	
Pumpkin Pie Smoothie	146	283	43	13	6	using almond milk
Berry Blast Smoothie	146	309	51	8	11	using nonfat yogurt and almond milk
Immunity Smoothie	146	207	46	1	9	using nonfat yogurt and almond milk
The Everyday Green Smoothie	146	343	60	7	27	using almond milk
Customizable Lower-Sugar Granola	150	223	29	10	6	using ½ c. almonds, ½ c. walnuts, 2 T. chia seeds, and 2 T. hemp seeds
Sweet Potato Toast, Savory or Sweet	152	162	37	0	4	without toppings
Very Veggie Shakshuka	154	384	37	17	21	
Basic Breakfast Burritos	156	357	42	17	13	
Blueberry Almond Blender Oat Cups	158	311	39	15	7	using almond milk
Pumpkin Spice Blender Oat Cups	158	269	36	13	5	using almond milk
Chocolate Blender Oat Cups	158	304	39	15	6	using almond milk
Zucchini Walnut Blender Oat Cups	158	329	37	19	7	using almond milk
Lemon Poppy Seed Blender Oat Cups	158	271	35	13	6	using almond milk
Raspberry Cream Cheese Blender Oat Cups	158	309	51	8	11	using almond milk
Almond Flour Bagels	162	224	23	11	9	

RECIPE	PAGE	CALORIES/ SERVING	CARBO-HYDRATES (grams)	FAT (grams)	PROTEIN (grams)	NOTES
Morning Glory Baked Oatmeal	164	338	66	7	7	using almond milk
Savory Umami Avo Toast	166	230	23	14	7	
Caprese Avo Toast	166	297	23	19	11	
Plant BLT Avo Toast	166	270	27	16	9	
Chili Mango Avo Toast	166	253	30	14	6	
Brain Booster Avo Toast	166	290	23	17	14	
Cucumber Ribbon Avo Toast	166	295	23	21	6	
Hash Brown Breakfast Casserole	170	200	26	7	11	using almond milk
Oatmeal Breakfast Cakes	172	304	38	12	11	
Mediterranean Medley Salad Jar	176	445	66	17	15	
Antioxidant Salad Jar	176	406	27	25	21	
California Cobb Salad Jar	176	392	15	33	11	
Thai Peanut Salad Jar	176	371	39	18	17	
Steakhouse Salad Jar	176	407	43	14	28	
Tempeh Taco Salad Jar	176	580	48	32	28	
Creamy Cream-Less Butternut Squash Soup	180	189	37	4	6	
Lettuce-Less Greek Salad	182	214	23	11	6	
Everyday Quinoa Salad	184	322	47	11	11	using white quinoa
Tex-Mex Chopped Salad	186	647	54	26	47	using chicken
Veggie Chili	188	260	44	5	12	
Avocado Chicken Salad	190	434	19	23	39	
Cauliflower Rice Tabbouleh	192	147	12	11	4	
Greenest Green Goddess Salad	194	247	27	16	8	
Creamy Broccoli Cauliflower Soup	196	246	37	9	10	
Kale Romaine Caesar Salad with Chickpea Croutons	198	200	17	13	6	
Romaine "Wedge" Salad	200	394	20	31	16	
Tuscan-Style Artichoke Salad	202	262	24	17	6	
Easy Taco Soup	204	480	50	13	39	
Crunchy Broccoli Cauliflower Salad	206	292	29	18	12	
Sweet Potato Fries	210	250	29	14	2	
Rosemary Parsnip Fries	210	231	41	8	3	
Smoky Jicama Fries	210	146	20	7	2	
Carrot Fries	210	154	22	8	2	
Garlic Potato Wedges	210	231	40	7	5	
Beet Fries	210	178	22	8	5	
Cowboy Caviar	214	90	11	4	4	
Lemony Blistered Shishitos	216	154	6	14	2	
Protein Pasta Chips	218	236	37	8	12	
Brownie Energy Bites	220	228	27	13	5	
Chocolate Peanut Butter Cup Energy Bites	220	247	26	15	8	
Blueberry Lemon Energy Bites	220	197	23	11	5	
Pineapple Coconut Energy Bites	220	212	26	12	4	
Garlicky Herb Roasted Cauliflower Head	224	145	9	11	4	
Rainbow Summer Rolls	226	132	26	3	2	without sauce
Balsamic Roasted Root Vegetables	228	233	32	11	4	
Spiced Chickpea Poppers	230	70	9	3	3	
"Cheezy" Chickpea Poppers	230	77	9	4	3	
Sweet Honey Chickpea Poppers	230	86	12	3	3	
Garlic Herb Chickpea Poppers	230	73	9	3	3	
BBQ Chickpea Poppers	230	81	11	3	3	
Everything Bagel Chickpea Poppers	230	80	9	3	3	
Turmeric Roasted Cauliflower	232	125	12	7	4	
Fluffy and Crispy Smashed Potatoes	234	117	18	4	3	
Everything Bagel Almond Flour Crackers	236	288	8	24	11	
Cheesy Almond Flour Crackers	236	290	6	24	13	
Roasted Vegetable Pesto Pasta	238	443	48	23	19	
Very Veggie Cauliflower Fried Rice	240	172	15	10	8	using carrots, red cabbage, and snap peas
Customizable No-Bake Granola Bars	242	246	27	12	7	using walnuts, chia seeds, and dried berries

RECIPE	PAGE	CALORIES/ SERVING	CARBO- HYDRATES (grams)	FAT (grams)	PROTEIN (grams)	NOTES
Chicken Fajitas Sheet Pan Meal	246	308	26	9	29	
Summer Shrimp Sheet Pan Meal	246	338	29	10	36	
Fall Bounty Sheet Pan Meal	246	340	34	15	24	
Tikka Sheet Pan Meal	246	398	61	11	13	
Italian Chicken Sheet Pan Meal	246	308	51	9	10	
Greek Salmon Sheet Pan Meal	246	370	44	10	26	
Portabella Bun Double Smash Burgers	252	268	6	14	29	
Simple Cauliflower Crust Pizza	254	126	7	8	7	
Drunken Veggie Noodles	256	293	17	16	20	
Spaghetti Squash Lentil Bolognese Boats	258	403	67	9	20	
Chickpea Tuna-Less Salad	260	118	15	5	4	
Loaded Cauliflower "Chip" Sheet Pan Nachos	262	330	30	19	15	
One-Skillet Greek Chicken and Veggies	264	437	52	11	34	
Turkey Avocado No-Bread Wrap	266	263	17	16	13	
Hummus and Veggie No-Bread Wrap	266	207	21	10	6	
Tempeh BLT No-Bread Wrap	266	337	22	22	14	
Easy Rotisserie Chicken Enchiladas	268	525	51	22	33	
Chipotle Burrito Bowl with Cauliflower Rice	270	434	38	12	30	
Zucchini Noodle Lasagna	272	571	19	34	46	
Burrito Loaded Sweet Potato Meal	274	545	44	23	25	
BBQ Chicken Loaded Sweet Potato Meal	274	451	44	22	18	
Chickpea Hummus Loaded Sweet Potato Meal	274	319	45	13	8	
Chickpea Carrot Burgers	278	203	25	8	8	
Baked Feta Vegetable Pasta	280	412	52	16	26	
Taco-Stuffed Zucchini Boats	282	458	40	21	32	
Deconstructed Spicy Sushi Bowl	284	419	31	23	30	using 2 T. oil
Cauliflower Cashew Ricotta–Stuffed Shells	286	465	64	19	21	
Mediterranean Lunch Box	288	417	49	20	12	
Chickpea Tuna-Less Salad Melt Lunch Box	288	387	44	17	9	
Taco Lunch Box	288	626	51	32	26	
Peanut Noodles Lunch Box	288	570	37	35	31	
Veggie Lover's Lunch Box	288	492	46	25	20	
Chicken Avocado Cups Lunch Box	288	545	33	32	35	
Pizza-Stuffed Peppers	292	393	20	23	31	using lean ground beef
Tempeh Gyros	294	335	35	16	17	
Simple Stir-Fry	296	370	46	6	34	without rice or toppings
Italian Spaghetti Squash Casserole	298	438	30	23	30	
Veggie Lover's Chickpea Flatbread	300	314	26	20	9	without feta
Lemon Tahini Buddha Bowl	302	614	62	35	18	
Caprese Cauliflower Gnocchi Skillet	304	380	65	15	24	
Baked Eggplant Parmesan Stacks	306	354	27	18	21	
Asian-Inspired Lentil Lettuce Cups	308	254	40	4	14	
Cauliflower Potato Shepherd's Pie	310	325	30	11	29	
Black Bean "Meatball" Subs	312	565	95	11	26	
Pesto Salmon Packets	314	406	13	27	32	
Better-Than-Takeout Orange Chicken Bowls	316	389	54	6	31	
Banana-Sweetened Chocolate Chip Oatmeal Cookies	320	119	16	5	3	
Any Berry Crumble Bars	322	190	10	16	4	using frozen mixed berries
Superseed Crispy Treats	324	305	27	21	5	
Peanut Butter Chocolate Candy Bites	326	142	23	6	3	
Bean Blondies	328	207	46	7	9	
3-Ingredient Strawberry Mango Sorbet	330	141	34	1	2	
Toasted Coconut and Chocolate Cluster Cookies	332	217	24	14	3	
Secret Ingredient Edible Cookie Dough	334	176	24	8	3	
4-Ingredient Fudgy Sweet Potato Brownies	336	241	23	14	5	
Single-Serve Cinnamon Apple Walnut Crisps	338	345	45	20	3	
Chocolate Chip Cookie Skillet	340	410	34	30	8	
Honey Lemon Bars	342	193	30	7	4	

allergen index

RECIPE	PAGE	MEAT FREE	FISH/ SHELLFISH FREE	DAIRY FREE	EGG FREE	NUT FREE	GLUTEN FREE	SOY FREE	SESAME FREE
Yogurt Ranch Dressing	110	x	x		x	x	x	x	x
Plant-Based Caesar Dressing	110	x	x	x	x	x		x	
Fat-Free Honey Dijon Dressing	110	x	x	x	x	x	x	x	x
Balsamic Vinaigrette	110	x	x	x	x	x	x	x	x
Peanut Dressing/Dip	110	x	x	x	x		x	x	
Plant-Based Avocado Green Goddess Dressing	110	x	x	x	x	x	x	x	x
Oat Milk	112	x	x	x	x	x	x	x	x
Any Greens Basil Pesto	114	x	x		x		x	x	
Quick Pico de Gallo	116	x	x	x	x	x	x	x	x
Basic Guacamole	118	x	x	x	x	x	x	x	x
White Bean Hummus (all flavors)	120	x	x	x	x	x	x	x	x
Plant-Based Parm	124	x	x	x	x		x	x	x
Mushroom Bacon	126	x	x	x	x				x
Coconut Bacon	126	x	x	x	x	x			x
Tempeh Bacon	126	x	x		x	x	x	x	x
Simple Tzatziki	128	x	x		x	x	x	x	x
No-Sugar All-Purpose Tomato Sauce	130	x	x	x	x	x	x	x	x
50/50 Mushroom Meat Base	132		x	x	x	x	x	x	x
100% Mushroom Base	132	x	x	x	x		x	x	x
Chocolate Lover's Overnight Oats	138	x	x		x	x	x	x	x
Apple Cinnamon Overnight Oats	138	x	x		x		x	x	x
Banana Bread Overnight Oats	138	x	x		x		x	x	x
Grown-Up PB&J Overnight Oats	138	x	x		x		x	x	x
Blueberry Lemon Overnight Oats	138	x	x		x	x	x	x	x
Tropical Overnight Oats	138	x	x		x			x	x
Chocolate Lover's Overnight Oats	138	x	x	x	x		x	x	x
Apple Cinnamon Chia Pudding	138	x	x	x	x		x	x	x
Banana Bread Chia Pudding	138	x	x	x	x		x	x	x
Grown-Up PB&J Chia Pudding	138	x	x	x	x		x	x	x
Blueberry Lemon Chia Pudding	138	x	x	x	x	x	x	x	x
Tropical Chia Pudding	138	x	x	x			x	x	x
Customizable Make-Ahead Freezer Breakfast Sandwiches	140		x			x		x	x
Naturally Sweetened Banana Oat Pancakes	142	x	x			x	x	x	
Savory Zucchini Waffle Minis	144	x	x				x	x	x
Peanut Butter Cup Smoothie	146	x	x	x	x		x	x	x
Detox Green Smoothie	146	x	x	x	x	x	x	x	x
Pumpkin Pie Smoothie	146	x	x	x	x		x	x	x
Berry Blast Smoothie	146	x	x		x	x	x	x	x
Immunity Smoothie	146	x	x		x	x	x	x	x
The Everyday Green Smoothie	146	x	x	x	x	x	x	x	x
Customizable Lower-Sugar Granola	150	x	x	x	x		x	x	x
Sweet Potato Toast, Savory or Sweet	152	x	x	x	x	x	x	x	x
Very Veggie Shakshuka	154	x	x	x		x	x	x	x
Basic Breakfast Burritos	156		x			x		x	x
Blueberry Almond Blender Oat Cups	158	x	x	x	x		x	x	x
Pumpkin Spice Blender Oat Cups	158	x	x	x	x	x	x	x	x
Chocolate Blender Oat Cups	158	x	x	x	x	x	x	x	x
Zucchini Walnut Blender Oat Cups	158	x	x	x	x		x	x	x
Lemon Poppy Seed Blender Oat Cups	158	x	x	x	x	x	x	x	x
Raspberry Cream Cheese Blender Oat Cups	158	x	x		x		x	x	x
Almond Flour Bagels	162	x	x				x	x	x
Morning Glory Baked Oatmeal	164	x	x	x	x		x	x	x
Savory Umami Avo Toast	166	x	x	x	x	x		x	

RECIPE	PAGE	MEAT FREE	FISH/SHELLFISH FREE	DAIRY FREE	EGG FREE	NUT FREE	GLUTEN FREE	SOY FREE	SESAME FREE
Caprese Avo Toast	166	X	X		X	X		X	X
Plant BLT Avo Toast	166	X	X	X	X	X			X
Chili Mango Avo Toast	166	X	X	X	X	X		X	X
Brain-Booster Avo Toast	166	X		X	X	X		X	X
Cucumber Ribbon Avo Toast	166	X	X	X	X	X			
Hash Brown Breakfast Casserole	170	X	X			X	X	X	X
Oatmeal Breakfast Cakes	172	X	X	X			X	X	X
Mediterranean Medley Salad Jar	176	X	X		X	X	X	X	X
Antioxidant Salad Jar	176		X	X	X	X	X	X	X
California Cobb Salad Jar	176		X	X	X		X	X	X
Thai Peanut Salad Jar	176	X	X	X	X			X	
Steakhouse Salad Jar	176		X		X	X			
Tempeh Taco Salad Jar	176	X	X		X	X	X		X
Creamy Cream-Less Butternut Squash Soup	180	X	X	X	X	X	X		X
Lettuce-Less Greek Salad	182	X	X		X	X	X	X	X
Everyday Quinoa Salad	184	X	X	X	X	X	X	X	X
Tex-Mex Chopped Salad	186		X		X	X		X	X
Veggie Chili	188	X	X	X	X	X	X	X	X
Avocado Chicken Salad	190		X	X	X	X	X	X	X
Cauliflower Rice Tabbouleh	192	X	X	X	X	X	X	X	X
Greenest Green Goddess Salad	194	X	X	X	X	X	X	X	X
Creamy Broccoli Cauliflower Soup	196	X	X	X	X		X	X	X
Kale Romaine Caesar Salad with Chickpea Croutons	198	X	X		X	X		X	X
Romaine "Wedge" Salad	200	X	X		X	X			X
Tuscan-Style Artichoke Salad	202	X	X	X	X	X	X	X	X
Easy Taco Soup	204		X	X	X	X	X	X	X
Crunchy Broccoli Cauliflower Salad	206		X		X	X	X	X	X
Sweet Potato Fries	210	X	X	X	X	X	X	X	X
Rosemary Parsnip Fries	210	X	X	X	X	X	X	X	X
Smoky Jicama Fries	210	X	X	X	X	X	X	X	X
Carrot Fries	210	X	X	X	X	X	X	X	X
Garlic Potato Wedges	210	X	X	X	X	X	X	X	X
Beet Fries	210	X	X		X	X	X	X	X
Cowboy Caviar	214	X	X	X	X	X	X	X	X
Lemony Blistered Shishitos	216	X	X		X	X	X	X	X
Protein Pasta Chips	218	X	X		X	X	X	X	X
Brownie Energy Bites	220	X	X	X	X			X	X
Chocolate Peanut Butter Cup Energy Bites	220	X	X	X	X			X	X
Blueberry Lemon Energy Bites	220	X	X	X	X		X		X
Pineapple Coconut Energy Bites	220	X	X	X	X		X	X	X
Garlicky Herb Roasted Cauliflower Head	224	X	X		X	X	X	X	X
Rainbow Summer Rolls	226	X	X	X	X	X	X	X	X
Balsamic Roasted Root Vegetables	228	X	X	X	X	X	X	X	X
Spiced Chickpea Poppers	230	X	X	X	X	X	X	X	X
Cheezy Chickpea Poppers	230	X	X		X	X	X	X	X
Sweet Honey Chickpea Poppers	230	X	X	X	X	X	X	X	X
Garlic Herb Chickpea Poppers	230	X	X	X	X	X	X	X	X
BBQ Chickpea Poppers	230	X	X	X	X	X	X	X	X
Everything Bagel Chickpea Poppers	230	X	X	X	X	X	X	X	
Turmeric Roasted Cauliflower	232	X	X	X	X	X	X	X	X
Fluffy and Crispy Smashed Potatoes	234	X	X	X	X	X	X	X	X
Everything Bagel Almond Flour Crackers	236	X	X	X			X	X	
Cheesy Almond Flour Crackers	236	X	X		X		X	X	X
Roasted Vegetable Pesto Pasta	238	X	X		X		X	X	X
Very Veggie Cauliflower Fried Rice	240	X	X	X		X			X
Customizable No-Bake Granola Bars	242	X	X	X	X		X	X	X
Chicken Fajitas Sheet Pan Meal	246		X	X	X	X	X	X	X

RECIPE	PAGE	MEAT FREE	FISH/SHELLFISH FREE	DAIRY FREE	EGG FREE	NUT FREE	GLUTEN FREE	SOY FREE	SESAME FREE
Summer Shrimp Sheet Pan Meal	246	X		X	X	X	X	X	X
Fall Bounty Sheet Pan Meal	246		X	X	X	X	X	X	X
Tikka Sheet Pan Meal	246	X	X	X	X	X		X	X
Italian Sheet Pan Meal	246		X	X	X	X	X	X	X
Greek Salmon Sheet Pan Meal	246	X		X	X	X	X	X	X
Portabella Bun Double Smash Burgers	252		X	X	X	X	X	X	X
Simple Cauliflower Crust Pizza	254	X	X		X		X	X	
Rainbow Veggie Noodles	256		X	X	X	X	X	X	
Spaghetti Squash Lentil Bolognese Boats	258	X	X	X	X	X	X	X	X
Chickpea Tuna-Less Salad	260	X	X	X		X	X	X	X
Loaded Cauliflower "Chip" Sheet Pan Nachos	262	X	X		X	X	X	X	X
One-Skillet Greek Chicken and Veggies	264		X	X	X	X		X	X
Turkey Avocado No-Bread Wrap	266		X	X	X	X	X	X	X
Hummus and Veggie No-Bread Wrap	266	X	X	X	X	X	X	X	X
Tempeh BLT No-Bread Wrap	266	X	X	X	X	X	X		X
Easy Rotisserie Chicken Enchiladas	268		X		X	X		X	X
Chipotle Burrito Bowl with Cauliflower Rice	270		X	X	X	X	X	X	X
Zucchini Noodle Lasagna	272		X		X	X	X	X	X
Burrito Loaded Sweet Potato Meal	274		X	X	X	X	X	X	X
BBQ Chicken Loaded Sweet Potato Meal	274		X	X		X	X	X	X
Chickpea Hummus Loaded Sweet Potato Meal	274	X	X	X	X	X	X	X	X
Chickpea Carrot Burgers	278	X	X	X	X	X	X	X	X
Baked Feta Vegetable Pasta	280	X	X		X	X	X	X	X
Taco-Stuffed Zucchini Boats	282		X		X	X	X	X	X
Deconstructed Spicy Sushi Bowl	284	X		X	X	X			X
Cauliflower Cashew Ricotta–Stuffed Shells	286	X	X					X	X
Mediterranean Lunch Box	288	X	X	X	X	X	X	X	X
Chickpea Tuna-Less Salad Melt Lunch Box	288	X	X			X	X	X	X
Taco Lunch Box	288		X	X	X	X	X	X	X
Peanut Noodles Lunch Box	288		X	X	X		X	X	X
Veggie Lover's Lunch Box	288	X	X	X			X	X	X
Chicken Avocado Cups Lunch Box	288		X	X	X		X	X	X
Pizza-Stuffed Peppers	292		X			X	X	X	X
Tempeh Gyros	294	X	X		X	X			X
Simple Stir-Fry	296		X	X	X	X			X
Italian Spaghetti Squash Casserole	298		X		X	X	X	X	X
Veggie Lover's Chickpea Flatbread	300	X	X	X	X	X	X	X	X
Lemon Tahini Buddha Bowl	302	X	X	X	X	X	X		
Caprese Cauliflower Gnocchi Skillet	304	X	X		X	X	X	X	X
Baked Eggplant Parmesan Stacks	306	X	X					X	X
Asian-Inspired Lentil Lettuce Cups	308	X	X	X	X	X			X
Cauliflower Potato Shepherd's Pie	310		X	X	X	X	X	X	X
Black Bean "Meatball" Subs	312	X	X		X	X		X	X
Pesto Salmon Packets	314	X			X		X	X	X
Better-Than-Takeout Orange Chicken Bowls	316		X	X	X	X			X
Banana-Sweetened Chocolate Chip Oatmeal Cookies	320	X	X	X	X		X	X	X
Any Berry Crumble Bars	322	X	X	X	X	X		X	X
Superseed Crispy Treats	324	X	X	X	X	X	X	X	X
Peanut Butter Chocolate Candy Bites	326	X	X	X	X		X	X	X
Bean Blondies	328	X	X	X	X		X	X	X
3-Ingredient Strawberry Mango Sorbet	330	X	X	X	X	X	X	X	X
Toasted Coconut and Chocolate Cluster Cookies	332	X	X	X	X		X	X	X
Secret Ingredient Edible Cookie Dough	334	X	X	X	X		X	X	X
4-Ingredient Fudgy Sweet Potato Brownies	336	X	X	X	X	X	X	X	X
Single-Serve Cinnamon Apple Walnut Crisps	338	X	X	X	X		X	X	X
Chocolate Chip Cookie Skillet	340	X	X	X	X		X	X	X
Honey Lemon Bars	342	X	X	X		X	X	X	X

general index